Progress in Epileptic Disorders
Volume 9
International Epilepsy Colloquium-Marburg

**The Mesial Temporal
Lobe Epilepsies**

Progress in Epileptic Disorders
Volume 9
International Epilepsy Colloquium-Marburg

The Mesial Temporal Lobe Epilepsies

Felix Rosenow
Philippe Ryvlin
Hans O. Lüders

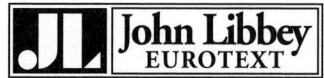

ISBN: 978-2-7420-0771-4
ISSN: 1777-4284
Vol. 9

Published by
Éditions John Libbey Eurotext
127, avenue de la République, 92120 Montrouge, France
Tél. : +33 (0)1 46 73 06 60
Website: www.jle.com

John Libbey Eurotext
42-46 High Street
Esher, Surrey
KT10 9KY
United Kingdom

© 2011, John Libbey Eurotext. All rights reserved.

Unauthorized duplication contravenes applicable laws.
It is prohibited to reproduce this work or any part of it without authorisation of the publisher or of the Centre Français d'Exploitation du Droit de Copie (CFC), 20, rue des Grands-Augustins, 75006 Paris.

Contents

Foreword IX

Workshop participants XI

Section I:
Concepts and pathophysiology of mesial temporal lobe epilepsies

The concept of mesial temporal lobe epilepsy
   Philippe Ryvlin, Philippe Kahane, Alexis Arzimanoglou 3

Ictal networks in mesial temporal lobe epilepsy
   Fabrice Bartolomei, Patrick Chauvel 11

Mesial temporal lobe epilepsy: anatomy and neuropathology
   Ingmar Blümcke 25

Genetics of mesial temporal lobe epilepsy and febrile seizures
   Jocelyn F. Bautista 37

Animal models of temporal lobe epilepsy with hippocampal sclerosis: moving beyond chemoconvulsant-induced status epilepticus
   Hemant S. Kudrimoti, Robert S. Sloviter 43

Section II:
Clinical characteristics of mesial temporal lobe epilepsies

Mesial temporal lobe epilepsy: natural history and seizure semiology
   Felix Rosenow, Soheyl Noachtar 59

Cognitive and psychiatric symptoms and their treatment in temporal lobe epilepsy: the role of the mesiotemporal structures
   Bettina Schmitz, Marco Mula, Michael Trimble 71

The clinical syndrome of mesial temporal lobe epilepsy in children
  Andras Fogarasi, Alexis Arzimanoglou 93

Mesial *versus* neocortical temporal lobe epilepsy
  Nancy Foldvary-Schaefer 109

Section III:
Clinical and experimental neurophysiology of mesial temporal lobe epilepsies

Non-invasive and invasive EEG in mesial temporal epilepsy
  Hajo M. Hamer, Philippe Kahane, Hans O. Lüders 115

Magnetoencephalograhpy findings in medial temporal lobe epilepsy
  Hideaki Shiraishi 135

The relevance of high frequency oscillations in the pathophysiology and diagnosis
of mesial temporal lobe epilepsy
  Julia Jacobs 145

Laminar electrodes in patients with temporal lobe epilepsy
  Istvan Ulbert 157

Section IV:
Imaging in mesial temporal lobe epilepsies

Structural imaging of mesial temporal lobe epilepsy
  Susanne Knake, Tim Wehner, P. Ellen Grant 165

The role of cognitive fMRI in mesial temporal lobe epilepsy
  Kirsten Labudda, Friedrich G. Woermann 175

The role of the Wada test and functional transcranial Doppler sonography
in the presurgical diagnosis of mesial temporal lobe epilepsy
  Tobias Loddenkemper, Anja Haag 189

PET and ictal SPECT in mesial temporal lobe epilepsy
  Wim Van Paesschen, Karolien Goffin, Koen Van Laere 205

Section V. Treatment of mesial temporal lobe epilepsies

Antiepileptic treatment of patients with mesial temporal lobe epilepsies
  Eugen Trinka 225

Depth electrodes (SEEG) in temporal lobe epilepsy
  Massimo Cossu, Francesco Cardinale, Laura Tassi, Francesca Gozzo, Marco Schiariti, Ivana Sartori, Laura Castana, Giorgio Lo Russo 233

Surgery for temporal lobe epilepsy: pros, cons and comparison between different procedures
  Stephan Chabardès, Shivadatta Prabhu, Taner Tanriverdi 245

Predictors of seizure outcome following resection for mesial temporal lobe epilepsy
  Alois Ebner 263

The role of automated seizure detection and prediction
  Christoph Kurth 269

Behavioural approaches: a critical review
  Bernhard J. Steinhoff 279

Foreword

In May 2008 the *First International Epilepsy Colloquium* on the mesial temporal lobe epilepsies (MTLE) was held in Marburg, Germany. It was the kick-off colloquium for a series of colloquia organized in close cooperation with colleagues from IDEE in Lyon, France (A. Arzimanoglou, P. Ryvlin and P. Kahane) and Hans Lüders from University Hospitals Cleveland, USA. This new series of Colloquia held sequentially and annually in Marburg, Lyon and Cleveland is based on the long-lasting tradition of the Bethel-Cleveland Epilepsy Symposia and likewise is focused on a specific subject of common interest to neurologists, epileptologists, neurosurgeons, neuropediatricians and neuroscientists involved in the (operative) treatment of epilepsy.

For this colloquium, we focused on mesial temporal epilepsies because this is the group of focal epilepsy syndromes (or "constellations" according to the newly proposed ILAE terminology) which is most prevalent, most frequently operated on and has therefore been at the center of interest of epileptology and neuroscience for a long time. Major progress in our understanding of MTLE has been made since the publication on MTLE-HS by Wieser and coworkers in 2004. These advances include our understanding of the neuropathological classification of MTLE, its correlation with the clinical course as well as our ability to model this disease in toxin-free animal models and to investigate and further define it through genetic, immunological studies and innovative electrophysiology methods.

We were fortunate to be able to bring together a group of outstanding international clinicians and neuroscientists involved in the study of MTLE willing to contribute to this volume of the "Progress in Epileptic Disorders" series which provides a comprehensive up to date and thought-provoking overview of a novel look at the MTLEs.

The book is organized in 5 sections covering: 1) concepts and pathophysiology; 2) clinical characteristics; 3) clinical and experimental neurophysiology; 4) structural and functional imaging findings; and 5) the treatment strategies applied to mesial temporal lobe epilepsies of variable etiology.

In the initial section, Philippe Ryvlin starts off with an in depth discussion of MTLE subsyndromes as an expression of the involvement of different networks and he proposes MTLE-plus, as a novel concept. Fabrice Bartolomei and Patrick Chauvel explain how network-properties can be characterized and quantified leading to a new understanding of and potential treatment options for MTLE. Ingmar Blümcke presents a new classification of MTLE with hippocampal sclerosis (HS) which was, in a multicenter study, correlated with clinical course and postoperative outcome. Jocelyn Bautista summarizes the available data on the genetics of MTLE-HS and febrile seizures. Finally Robert Sloviter reports on a new toxin-free rat-model of MTLE-HS induced by a specific stimulation paradigm of the perforant path.

In the second section, the natural course, different etiologies and the diagnostic relevance of ictal semiology in adults are analysed by Soheyel Noachtar, Nancy Foldvary-Schaeffer and Felix Rosenow. The semiological characteristics of MTLE seizures in children and adolescents are discussed by Andras Fogarasi and Alexis Arzimanoglou. Finally Bettina Schmitz, Marco Mula and Michael Trimble provide a detailed review on cognitive and psychiatric symptoms and related modern treatment concepts.

In the third section Hajo Hamer, Philippe Kahahne and Hans Lüders start off by providing a comprehensive review of surface and invasive EEG (including S-EEG-findings) in MTLE and Julia Jacobs provides insight into the relevance of high frequency oscillations (ripples and fast ripples) in the presurgical diagnosis of MTLE. Hideaki Shiraishi describes how MEG is used not only in the definition of the irritative zone but also of eloquent cortex. Finally Istvan Ulbert informs us about the experimental use of laminar electrodes to explore the function of the mesial temporal structures patients and animal models of MTLE.

Structural and functional imaging has undergone revolutionary changes over the last decade. In section IV, Susanne Knake, Tim Wehner and Ellen Grant summarize the state of the art including cutting egde methods of structural MRI used in MTLE. This includes the visualization of "eloquent tracts" by DTI. Kirsten Labudda and Friedrich Woermann discuss how sensitive and specific functional MRI is in deliniating irritative zone and eloquent cortical areas. The reliability and current contribution, advantages and disadvantages in lateralization of language and memory functions by the goldstandard technique Wada-test and the novel technique of functional transcranial Doppler-sonography (fTCD) are described by Anja Haag and Tobias Loddenkemper. The section is completed by Wim Van Paesschens review on the role of ictal SPECT in the presurgical diagnosis of MTLE.

The fifth and final section discusses standard as well as new treatment strategies in MTLE. Eugen Trinka discusses the available literature on syndrome related drug treatment approaches for MTLE, Giorgio LoRusso and Laura Tassi describe indications for and the techniques of SEEG-implantation in MTLE and Stephan Chabardes, Shivadatta Prabhu, and Taner Tanriverdi give a comprehensive overview of the different surgical approaches developed over the decades. Our current knowledge of predictors of postoperative seizure outcome are summarized by Alois Ebner and the methods and future role of seizure prediction/detection as well as deep brain stimulation for suppression of seizures in patients with MTLE are reviewed by Christoph Kurth. Last but not least Bernhard Steinhoff provides a critical evaluation of behavioral approaches in MTLE-treatment.

We would like to thank all the experts who invested a lot of thought and time to write detailed and thought provoking chapters covering all aspects of MTLE. We also thank the attendants at the colloquium whose active participation in the discussions during the meeting played a significant role improving the book. We also greatly appreciate the efforts of the staff of JLE who made this book a success.

Felix Rosenow Philippe Ryvlin Hans Lüders

List of Authors

Alexis Arzimanoglou, Pediatric Epileptology, University Hospitals, Lyon; Institute for children and adolescents with epilepsy IDEE, University Hospitals of Lyon, France

Fabrice Bartolomei, Inserm U751, Marseille; Aix-Marseille Medicine University, Marseille; Assistance Publique-Hôpitaux de Marseille, Timone Hospital, Department of Clinical Neurophysiology, Marseille, France

Jocelyn F. Bautista, Cleveland Clinic Lerner College of Medicine; Cleveland Clinic Epilepsy Center, Cleveland, USA

Ingmar Blümcke, Department of Neuropathology, University Hospital Erlangen, Erlangen, Germany

Francesco Cardinale, C. Munari Epilepsy Surgery Centre, Niguarda Hospital, Milan, Italy

Laura Castana, C. Munari Epilepsy Surgery Centre, Niguarda Hospital, Milan, Italy

Stephan Chabardès, Grenoble Institute of Neurosciences, Inserm U836, Joseph-Fourier University, Grenoble; Neurosurgery department, University Hospital, Grenoble, France

Massimo Cossu, C. Munari Epilepsy Surgery Centre, Niguarda Hospital, Milan, Italy

Patrick Chauvel, Inserm U751, Marseille; Aix-Marseille Medicine University, Marseille; Assistance Publique-Hôpitaux de Marseille, Timone Hospital, Department of Clinic Neurophysiology, Marseille, France

Alois Ebner, Epilepsy Clinic Mara, Epilepsy Center Bethel, Bielefeld, Germany

Nancy Foldvary-Schaefer, Cleveland Clinic, Neurological Institute, Cleveland, USA

Andras Fogarasi, Bethesda Children's Hospital, Budapest, Hungary

Karolien Goffin, Division of Nuclear Medicine, University Hospital Leuven, Leuven, Belgium

Francesca Gozzo, C. Munari Epilepsy Surgery Centre, Niguarda Hospital, Milan, Italy

P. Ellen Grant, Perinatal and Developmental Science Imaging Center, Children Hospital Boston; Harvard Medical School, Boston, USA

Anja Haag, Epilepsy Center Hessen, Department of Neurology, University Hospitals Giessen and Marburg GmbH & Philipps-University Marburg, Marburg, Germany

Hajo M. Hamer, Epilepsy Center Hessen, Department of Neurology, University Hospitals Giessen and Marburg GmbH & Philipps-University Marburg, Marburg, Germany

Julia Jacobs, Department of Neuropediatrics, University of Freiburg, Freiburg, Germany

Philippe Kahane, Department of Neurology & GIN Inserm U836-UJF-CEA, Grenoble University Hospital; CTRS-Inserm IDEE, Lyon University Hospital, France

Susanne Knake, Epilepsy Center Hessen, Department of Neurology, University Hospitals Giessen and Marburg GmbH & Philipps-University Marburg, Marburg, Germany

Hemant S. Kudrimoti, Departments of Neurology and Pharmacology, University of Arizona College of Medicine, Tucson, USA

Christoph Kurth, Epilepsiezentrum Kork, Kehl-Kork, Germany

Kirsten Labudda, Bethel Epilepsy Center, Mara Hospital, Bielefeld, Germany

Tobias Loddenkemper, Pediatric Epilepsy Center, Children's Hospital Boston, Harvard Medical School, Boston, USA

Giorgio Lo Russo, C. Munari Epilepsy Surgery Centre, Niguarda Hospital, Milan, Italy

Hans O. Lüders, Epilepsy Center, University Hospitals, Case Medical Center, Cleveland, USA

Marco Mula, Department of Neurology, Amedeo Avogadro University, Novara, Italy

Soheyl Noachtar, Epilepsy Center, Department of Neurology, University of Munich, Munich, Germany

Shivadatta Prabhu, Grenoble Institute of Neurosciences, Inserm U836, Joseph-Fourier University, Grenoble, France

Felix Rosenow, Epilepsy Center Hessen, Department of Neurology, University Hospitals Giessen and Marburg GmbH & Philipps-University Marburg, Marburg, Germany

Philippe Ryvlin, Institute for children and adolescents with epilepsy IDEE, University Hospitals of Lyon, France

Ivana Sartori, C. Munari Epilepsy Surgery Centre, Niguarda Hospital, Milan, Italy

Marco Schiariti, C. Munari Epilepsy Surgery Centre, Niguarda Hospital, Milan, Italy

Bettina Schmitz, Department of Neurology, Vivantes Humboldt-Klinikum, Berlin, Germany

Hideaki Shiraishi, Department of Pediatrics, Hokkaido University School of Medicine, Hokkaido, Japan

Robert S. Sloviter, Departments of Neurology and Pharmacology, University of Arizona College of Medicine, Tucson, USA

Bernhard J. Steinhoff, Epilepsiezentrum Kork, Kehl-Kork, Germany

Taner Tanriverdi, Department of Neurosurgery, Montreal Neurological Institute and Hospital, McGill University, Montreal, Quebec, Canada

Laura Tassi, C. Munari Epilepsy Surgery Centre, Niguarda Hospital, Milan, Italy

Michael Trimble, Institute of Neurology, Queen Square, London, United Kingdom

Eugen Trinka, Christian Doppler Klinik, Salzburg, Austria

Istvan Ulbert, Institute for Psychology, Hungarian Academy of Sciences, Budapest; Faculty of Information Technology, Pazmany Peter Catholic University, Budapest; National Institute of Neurosciences, Budapest, Hungary

Koen Van Laere, Division of Nuclear Medicine, University Hospital Leuven, Leuven, Belgium

Wim Van Paesschen, Department of Neurology, University Hospital Leuven, Leuven, Belgium

Tim Wehner, Epilepsy Center Hessen, Department of Neurology, University Hospitals Giessen and Marburg GmbH & Philipps-University Marburg, Marburg, Germany

Friedrich G. Woermann, Bethel Epilepsy Center, Mara Hospital, Bielefeld, Germany

Section I:
Concepts and pathophysiology of mesial temporal lobe epilepsies

The concept of mesial temporal lobe epilepsy

Philippe Ryvlin, Philippe Kahane, Alexis Arzimanoglou

Institute for children and adolescents with epilepsy IDEE, University Hospitals of Lyon, France

Temporal lobe epilepsy (TLE) is the most commonly reported form of refractory epilepsy and accounts for the majority of adult patients with partial seizures. Classically, mesial TLE (MTLE) refers to TLE implicating mainly the hippocampal formation, especially in the case of hippocampal sclerosis (HS). However, cases of TLE with HS have been described with other seizure onset zones or pathological findings affecting other mesial temporal structures (*e.g.* amygdala, entorhinal cortex), or the temporal pole, leading to the term "limbic epilepsy" which refers to seizures originating from temporal limbic structures (Engel, 2001; 2006). In contrast, neocortical TLE is the term used to describe temporal lateral or basal seizure onset zones, in the absence of any pathology of the mesial temporal structures.

Mesial and neocortical seizures may be distinguished clinically and electrophysiologically (O'Brien *et al.*, 1996; Foldvary *et al.*, 1997), however, there is also considerable overlap of clinical signs (Burgerman *et al.*, 1995), complicated by the fact that mesial epileptic activity may extend into the neocortex. With the advances of neuroimaging and intracerebral EEG recordings, a number of extratemporal structures were found to be frequently involved in MTLE (with HS), justifying a revision of the framework underlying this concept (Kahane & Bartolomei, 2010).

■ The origin of mesial temporal lobe epilepsy

The concept of MTLE has origins in the description of Ammon's horn sclerosis, of which the first historic report was published by Bouchet and Cazauvieilh in 1825 (Bouchet & Cazauvieilh, 1825). In this early report, hardening of the mesial temporal lobe was described in postmortem brains, as well as the hallmarks of sclerotic transformation characterised by neuronal loss within the hippocampus. Based on the studies of Bouchet and Cazauvieilh and his own, Sommer presented the first detailed histological description of Ammon's horn sclerosis, noting particular neuronal loss in an area known as Sommer's sector or CA1 (Sommer, 1880). Further detailed description by Bratz (1899) more convincingly established the role of hippocampal pathology in the pathogenesis of epilepsy.

At the same time, in the latter part of the 19th century, Hughlings Jackson, who recognised partial seizures as epileptic events, gave a clinical description of some relevant clinical findings of MTL seizures. He importantly identified the relationship between limbic-type seizures, which he referred to as "intellectual auras" or "dreamy states", and lesions described in the mesial temporal areas (Jackson, 1880; 1898). However, it was later in the middle of the 20th century that Cavanagh and Meyer brought to light a clear link between Ammon's horn sclerosis and TLE (Cavanagh & Meyer, 1956) and the characteristics of MTLE were further defined by Hill et al. (1953) and Falconer (1971). In the seminal paper of Cavanagh and Meyer (1956), the link between Ammon's horn sclerosis and TLE was pertinently suggested to be probably neither simple nor direct. An imbalance of activities generated between an atrophic hippocampus and the adjacent limbic structures (the amygdala in particular) was implicated to explain, in an indirect manner, the genesis of neuronal hyperactivity from atrophic hippocampi. This notion has since been reinvestigated from an experimental angle using hippocampus/entorhinal cortex slices by the group of Avoli and colleagues, who suggested that the ability to produce recurrent limbic seizures, as seen in patients with MTLE, is the result of changes in network interactions along with other mechanisms of synaptic plasticity (Avoli et al., 2002).

Following the early comments made by Bratz (1899), HS was controversially perceived as a consequence rather than a cause of epilepsy. This was further supported by others (Fisher et al., 1998; Berg et al., 1999). Although this point of view was not shared by all (Falconer et al., 1964), modern neuroimaging and animal models indeed indicate that early-life seizures may increase susceptibility to neuronal injury later in life.

The term "mesial temporal epilepsy" was coined by French et al. (1993), following the terms "medial temporal lobe" (Tharpe, 1979), "mesial temporal seizures" (Lieb et al., 1987) and "mesial temporal sclerosis" (Falconer & Taylor, 1968).

■ Classic clinical presentation of mesial temporal lobe epilepsy

In its typical presentation, MTLE with HS is characterized by a strong association with antecedent febrile seizures, progressive development which leads very frequently to drug-resistance, topographic distribution of interictal and ictal EEG abnormalities which tend to be focused around the anterior and basal temporal lobe regions, and neuropsychological and functional neuroimaging data which also point to MTL structures (Cendes et al., 2002). This entity is likely to produce automotor seizures, with a relative absence of tonic-clonic generalised seizures and status epilepticus. Initial loss of contact without aura is uncommon and rather suggests a mesiolateral onset of seizures (Maillard et al., 2004). Seizures often initiate with an epigastric sensation (French et al., 1993), but emotional (e.g. fear) or other psychic (e.g. déjà-vécu) auras and autonomic symptoms (flushing, palor, mydriasis, tachycardia, etc.) are also common. Some patients can have olfactory sensations (King & Ajmone-Marsan, 1977), but the question of a possible orbito-frontal involvement must be raised. Auras may occur in isolation, or progress towards a motionless stare, oroalimentary automatisms (e.g. lip smacking, chewing), less frequent verbal automatisms, and progressive clouding of consciousness. Hand automatisms are frequent and tend to be predominantly ipsilateral to the sclerotic hippocampus, due to contralateral dystonic posturing (Kotagal et al., 1989). At this stage, loss of consciousness is common, but the patient may remain responsive, even in conjunction with automatisms (Ebner et al., 1995). When present, clearly intelligible ictal or immediate postictal speech is suggestive of non-dominant hemisphere involvement (Gabr et al., 1989). Seizures typically last for one to two minutes. There is transient postictal disorientation and, with onset in the language-dominant hemisphere, there may also be some degree of postictal aphasia. Postictal nosewiping, typically performed with the hand ipsilateral to the seizure onset zone, is recognized as a frequent symptom (Leutmezer et al., 1998). Patients are most frequently amnesic of the ictal phase, however, the aura is usually remembered.

This classic ictal clinical presentation, when complete, is suggestive of MTL seizure onset, but there are no definitive characteristics which distinguish patients with HS from those with other mesiotemporal lesions or without any detectable MRI abnormalities. Yet, even typical ictal symptomatology may be due to the spread of ictal discharges from other temporal and even extratemporal areas. Conversely, although seizures may be of mesiotemporal lobe origin, they can manifest with very atypical clinical features. Overall, it is generally agreed that electroclinical features are highly variable between patients and are not specific to any form of TLE (O'Brien et al., 1996; Gil-Nagel & Risinger, 1997; Wieser et al., 2004).

■ The epileptogenic network(s) in mesial temporal lobe epilepsy

Evidence of extrahippocampal pathology in patients with MTLE was first reported in the early publication of Cavanagh and Meyer (1956). Pathological findings were then observed in various structures, including the uncus, enthorhinal cortex, amygdaloid nucleus, temporal pole and temporal neocortex (Babb & Brown, 1987; Wolf & Wiestler, 1993; Munari et al., 1994; Pasquier et al., 1996; Spanedda et al., 1997; Yilmazer-Hanke et al., 2000). Accordingly, MRI studies have demonstrated atrophy in the amygdala, entorhinal cortex, and temporal pole, but also disclosed volume reduction of the fornix, mamillothalamic tract and mamillary bodies (Moran et al., 2001; Coste et al., 2002). Likewise, FDG-PET may show extensive interictal hypometabolism, predominating over the epileptogenic mesial temporal structures and temporal pole, but also affecting the ipsilateral lateral temporal neocortex, perisylvian areas including the insula, thalamus, and at times, frontal or parietal cortex (Semah et al., 1995; Chassoux et al., 2004).

In line with these pathological, morphological and metabolic changes, intra-cerebral EEG data have shown that a hippocampal onset was reported to account for only 20-65% of seizures of patients with MTLE (Munari et al., 1994; King et al., 1997; Spanedda et al., 1997; Chabardès et al., 2005). Accordingly, animal studies have indicated that extrahippocampal structures may be particularly epileptogenic (Halonen et al., 1994; McIntyre & Kelly, 1993). Based on intracerebral electrophysiological data, Kahane and Bartolomei (2010) have recently proposed subtypes of TLE which cover both the limbic and neocortical systems, referred to as "mesial", "temporopolar", "mesiolateral", "lateral" and "temporal plus" (Figure 1). Briefly, seizures of the *mesial subtype* may start from the hippocampus, but also from the amygdala (Munari et al., 1994), both the amygdala and hippocampus (Spanedda et al., 1997), the parahippocampal gyrus (Wennberg et al., 2002) and the entorhinal cortex (Spencer & Spencer, 1994; Bartolomei et al., 2005). Clinical signs and symptoms do not necessarily derive from mesial temporal involvement (Sperling & O'Connor, 1990), and may reflect seizure spread over extra-MTL structures, such as for epigastric aura (Munari et al., 1994) which could be related to insular propagation (Isnard et al., 2000). Results of intracerebral stimulation suggest that fear aura could be more specifically related to the amygdala (Fish et al., 1993; Meletti et al., 2006), and experiential

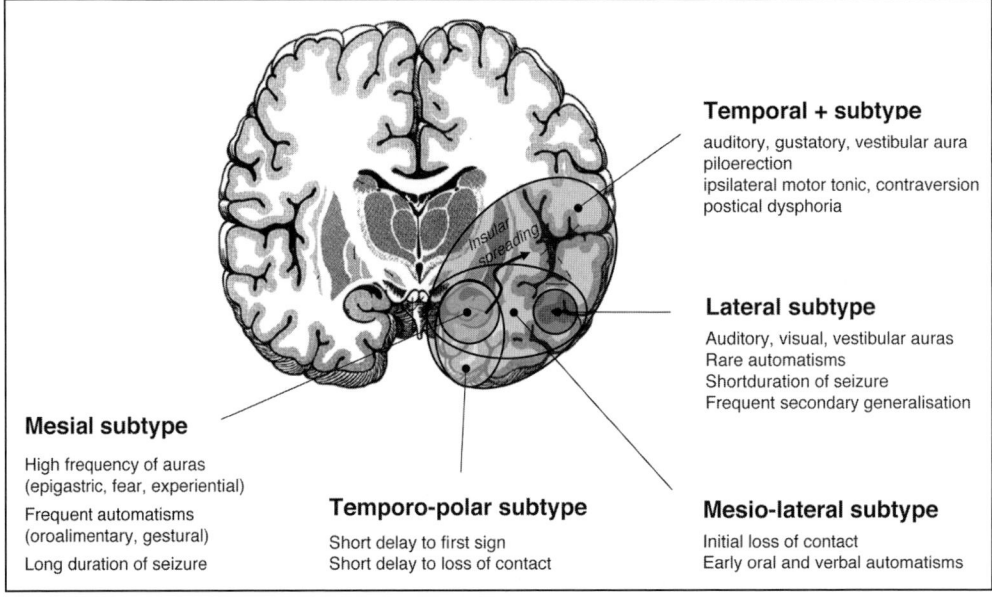

Figure 1. Classification of MTLE subtypes and their main ictal clinical features (modified from Kahane & Bartolomei, 2010).

phenomena to the involvement of the rhinal cortex (Bartolomei et al., 2004). The preferential involvement of one or more MTL structures, however, does not necessarily lead to major differences in terms of seizure symptomatology, in as much as each patient may exhibit different seizure onset zones within this complex MTL network (Spencer & Spencer, 1994; Wennberg et al., 2002). Nevertheless, patients with hippocampal onset may have predominantly epigastric auras and early oral automatisms, while those with extrahippocampal onset may have predominantly experiential auras and early motor involvement of the contralateral upper extremity without oral automatisms (Gil-Nagel & Risinger, 1997). In seizures which arise from the temporal pole alone or concurrently from MTL structures (*temporopolar subtype*), the first clinical signs and loss of awareness occur earlier than in MTL seizures, therefore suggesting that the temporal pole may play a pivotal role in seizure propagation (Chabardès et al., 2005). This subtype is possibly a variant of the *mesiolateral subtype*, in which the ictal discharge occurs simultaneously from mesial and lateral temporal lobe structures (Bartolomei et al., 1999). In fact, mesiolateral temporal lobe seizures exhibit some overlapping clinical features with temporopolar seizures, with frequent initial loss of awareness, and early oralimentary and verbal automatisms (Maillard et al., 2004). Cases of TLE with HS where seizures originate from the temporal neocortex (*lateral subtype*) are anecdotal (Arzimanoglou & Kahane, 2008). Although very rare, such cases should be suspected in the presence of auditory aura or initial loss of contact, a short duration of seizures, and frequent secondary generalisations (Maillard et al., 2004). In a more substantial number of cases, neighbouring extratemporal lobe structures, such as the orbitofrontal cortex, the insula, the frontal and parietal operculum, and the temporo-parietooccipital junction, may also be involved at onset together with temporal lobe structures, defining the *temporal plus subtype* (Ryvlin & Kahane, 2005). Clinical signs associated with this form of epilepsy include gustatory hallucinations, rotatory vertigo, auditory illusions at seizure onset, contraversive manifestations of the eyes and/or head, piloerection, ipsilateral tonic motor signs, and postictal dysphoria (Barba et al., 2007).

Overall, it appears that the epileptogenic networks which are associated with the so-called "MTLE syndrome" are rather heterogeneous, and further discussion should be addressed to establish whether this should be taken into account in order to (re)define the concept of MTLE.

■ Redefining the concept of mesial temporal lobe epilepsy

In 2004, a subcommission of the International League Against Epilepsy, chaired by Heinz-Gregor Wieser, readdressed the notion of MTLE with HS (Wieser et al., 2004). The majority of the subcommission established that MTLE with HS should be described as a syndromic entity, based on a sufficient cluster of signs and symptoms, with the suggestion that MTLE with HS is a subtype of the larger syndrome of MTLE. However, this conclusion did not reflect a consensus of the commission due to the uncertainty surrounding the progressive nature of hippocampal sclerosis, genetic predisposition and the variability of past history (febrile seizures, trauma, hypoxia, and intracranial infection). Acknowledging the existence of MTLE with HS as a syndrome has, nevertheless, been of importance since it has helped to promote early diagnostic and appropriate management for this surgically treatable condition. This concept should also be further instrumental for subsequent basic and clinical research studies. However, it is clear that the term "mesial temporal" has not been adapted to suit the above described clinical, electrophysiological and anatomo-pathological characteristics of these forms of epilepsy which should be preferentially referred to as "temporal limbic epilepsy". A better understanding of the clinical heterogeneity and variety of epileptogenic networks underlying this condition, which possibly depends on disease duration (Bartolomei et al., 2008; 2010), is required to improve the overall success rate of surgery in TLE.

References

- Avoli M, D'Antuono M, Louvel J, Köhling R, Biagini G, Pumain R, et al. Network and pharmacological mechanisms leading to epileptiform synchronization in the limbic system *in vitro*. *Prog Neurobiol* 2002; 68: 167-207.
- Arzimanoglou A, Kahane P. The ictal onset zone: general principles, pitfalls and caveats. In: Lüders HO (ed). *Textbook of Epilepsy Surgery*. London: Informa Healthcare, 2008, pp. 597-602.
- Babb TL, Brown WJ. Pathological findings in epilepsy. In: Engel J Jr (ed). *Surgical Treatment of the Epilepsies*. New York: Raven Press, 1987, pp. 511-40.
- Barba C, Barbati G, Minotti L, Hoffmann D, Kahane P. Ictal clinical and scalp-EEG findings differentiating temporal lobe epilepsies from temporal "plus" epilepsies. *Brain* 2007; 130: 1957-67.
- Bartolomei F, Wendling F, Vignal JP, Kochen S, Bellanger JJ, Badier JM, et al. Seizures of temporal lobe epilepsy: identification of subtypes by coherence analysis using stereo-electro-encephalography. *Clin Neurophysiol* 1999; 110: 1741-54.
- Bartolomei F, Barbeau E, Gavaret M, Guye M, McGonigal A, Régis J, Chauvel P. Cortical stimulation study of the role of rhinal cortex in *déjà vu* and reminiscence of memories. *Neurology* 2004; 63: 858-64.

- Bartolomei F, Khalil M, Wendling F, Sontheimer A, Régis J, Ranjeva JP, et al. Entorhinal cortex involvement in human mesial temporal lobe epilepsy: an electrophysiologic and volumetric study. Epilepsia 2005; 46: 677-87.
- Bartolomei F, Chauvel P, Wendling F. Epileptogenicity of brain structures in human temporal lobe epilepsy: a quantified study from intracerebral EEG. Brain 2008; 131: 1818-30.
- Bartolomei F, Cosandier-Rimele D, McGonigal A, Aubert S, Régis J, Gavaret M, et al. From mesial temporal lobe to temporoperisylvian seizures: A quantified study of temporal lobe seizure networks. Epilepsia 2010; 51: 2147-58.
- Berg AT, Shinnar S, Levy SR, et al. Childhood-onset epilepsy with and without preceding febrile seizures. Neurology 1999; 53: 1742-8.
- Bouchet C, Cazauvieilh JB. De l'épilepsie considérée dans ses rapports avec l'aliénation mentale. Arch Gen Med 1825; 9: 510-42.
- Bratz E. Ammonshornbefunde bei Epileptischen. Arch Psychiat Nervenkr 1899; 31: 820-35.
- Cavanagh JB, Meyer A. Aetiological aspects of Ammon's horn sclerosis associated with temporal lobe epilepsy. Br Med J 1956; 2: 1403-7.
- Cendes F, Kahane P, Brodie M, Andermann F. The mesiotemporal lobe epilepsy syndrome. In: Roger J, Bureau M, Dravet C, Genton P, Tassinari CA, Wolf P (eds). Epileptic Syndromes in Infancy, Childhood and Adolescence, 3rd edition. London: John Libbey & Co Ltd, 2002, pp. 513-530.
- Chabardès S, Kahane P, Minotti L, Tassi L, Grand S, Hoffmann D, Benabid AL. The temporopolar cortex plays a pivotal role in temporal lobe seizures. Brain 2005; 128: 1818-31.
- Chassoux F, Semah F, Bouilleret V, Landre E, Devaux B, Turak B, et al. Metabolic changes and electroclinical patterns in mesiotemporal lobe epilepsy: a correlative study. Brain 2004; 127: 164-74.
- Coste S, Ryvlin P, Hermier M, Ostrowsky K, Adeleine P, Froment JC, Mauguière F. Temporopolar changes in temporal lobe epilepsy: a quantitative MRI-based study. Neurology 2002; 59: 855-61.
- Ebner A, Dinner DS, Noachtar S, Lüders H. Automatisms with preserved responsiveness: a lateralizing sign in psychomotor seizures. Neurology 1995; 45: 61-4.
- Engel J Jr. A proposed diagnostic scheme for people with epileptic seizures and with epilepsy: report of the ILAE Task Force on Classification and Terminology. Epilepsia 2001; 42: 796-803.
- Engel J Jr. Report of the ILAE Classification Core Group. Epilepsia 2006; 47: 1558-68.
- Falconer MA. Genetic and related aetiological factors in temporal lobe epilepsy. Epilepsia 1971; 12: 13-31.
- Falconer MA, Serafetinides EA, Corsellis JAN. Etiology and pathogenesis of temporal lobe epilepsy. Arch Neurol 1964; 10: 233-48.
- Falconer M A, Taylor DC. Surgical treatment of drug-resistant epilepsy due to mesial temporal sclerosis. Archives of Neurology (Chic) 1968; 19: 353-61.
- Fish DR, Gloor P, Quesney FL, Olivier A. Clinical responses to electrical brain stimulation of the temporal and frontal lobes in patients with epilepsy. Pathophysiological implications. Brain 1993; 116: 397-414.
- Fisher PD, Sperber EF, Moshé SL. Hippocampal sclerosis revisited. Brain Dev 1998; 20: 563-73.
- Foldvary N, Lee N, Thwaites G, Mascha E, Hammel J, Kim H, Friedman AH, Radtke RA. Clinical and electrographic manifestations of lesional neocortical temporal lobe epilepsy. Neurology 1997; 49: 757-63.
- French JA, Williamson PD, Thadani VM, Darcey TM, Mattson RH, Spencer SS, Spencer DD. Characteristics of medial temporal lobe epilepsy: I. Results of history and physical examination. Ann Neurol 1993; 34: 774-80.
- Gabr M, Lüders H, Dinner D, Morris H, Wyllie E. Speech manifestations in lateralization of temporal lobe seizures. Ann Neurol 1989; 25: 82-7.

- Gil-Nagel A, Risinger MW. Ictal semiology in hippocampal *versus* extrahippocampal temporal lobe epilepsy. *Brain* 1997; 120: 183-92.
- Halonen T, Tortorella A, Zrebeet H, *et al*. Posterior piriform and perirhinal cortex relay seizures evoked from the area tempestas: role of excitatory and inhibitory amino acid receptors. *Brain Res* 1994; 652: 145-8.
- Hill D, Falconer MA, Pampiglione G, Liddell DW. Discussion on the surgery of temporal lobe epilepsy. *Proc R Soc Med* 1953; 46: 965-76.
- Isnard J, Guénot M, Ostrowsky K, Sindou M, Mauguière F. The role of the insular cortex in temporal lobe epilepsy. *Ann Neurol* 2000; 48: 614-23.
- Kahane P, Bartolomei F. Temporal lobe epilepsy and hippocampal sclerosis: lessons from depth EEG recordings. *Epilepsia* 2010; 51 (Suppl 1): 59-62.
- King DW, Ajmone-Marsan C. Clinical features and ictal patterns in epileptic patients with EEG temporal lobe foci. *Ann Neurol* 1977; 2: 138-47.
- King D, Spencer SS, McCarthy G, Spencer DD. Surface and depth EEG findings in patients with hippocampal atrophy. *Neurology* 1997; 48: 1363-7.
- Kotagal P, Lüders HO, Morris HH, Dinner DS, Wyllie E, Godoy J, Rothner AD. Dystonic posturing in complex partial seizures of temporal lobe onset: a new lateralizing sign. *Neurology* 1989; 39: 196-201.
- Leutmezer F, Serles W, Lehrner J, *et al*. Postictal nose wiping: a lateralizing sign in temporal lobe complex partial seizures. *Neurology* 1998; 51: 1175-7.
- Lieb JP, Hoque K, Skomer CE, Song XW. Inter-hemispheric propagation of human mesial temporal lobe seizures: a coherence/phase analysis. *Electroencephalogr Clin Neurophysiol* 1987; 67: 101-19.
- Maillard L, Vignal JP, Gavaret M, Guye M, Biraben A, McGonigal A, Chauvel P, Bartolomei F. Semiologic and electrophysiologic correlations in temporal lobe seizure subtypes. *Epilepsia* 2004; 45: 1590-9.
- McIntyre DC, Kelly ME. Are differences in dorsal hippocampal kindling related to amygdala-piriform area excitability? *Epilepsy Res* 1993; 14: 49-61.
- Meletti S, Tassi L, Mai R, Fini N, Tassinari CA, Russo GL. Emotions induced by intracerebral electrical stimulation of the temporal lobe. *Epilepsia* 2006; 47 (Suppl 5): 47-51.
- Moran NF, Lemieux L, Kitchen ND, Fish DR, Shorvon SD. Extrahippocampal temporal lobe atrophy in temporal lobe epilepsy and mesial temporal sclerosis. *Brain* 2001; 124: 167-75.
- Munari C, Tassi L, Kahane P, Francione S, Di Leo M, Quarato PP. Analysis of clinical symptomatology during stereo-EEG recorded mesiotemporal seizures. In: Wolf P (ed). *Epileptic Seizures and Syndromes*. London: John Libbey, 1994, pp. 335-357.
- O'Brien TJ, Kilpatrick C, Murrie V, Vogrin S, Morris K, Cook MJ. Temporal lobe epilepsy caused by mesial temporal sclerosis and temporal neocortical lesions. A clinical and electroencephalographic study of 46 pathologically proven cases. *Brain* 1996; 119: 2133-41.
- Pasquier B, Bost F, Peoc'h M, Barnoud R. Données neuropathologiques dans l'épilepsie partielle pharmaco-résistante. Étude d'une série de 195 observations. *Ann Pathol* 1996; 16: 174-81.
- Ryvlin P, Kahane P. The hidden causes of surgery-resistant temporal lobe epilepsy: extratemporal or temporal plus? *Curr Opin Neurol* 2005; 18: 125-7.
- Semah F, Baulac M, Hasboun D, Frouin V, Mangin JF, Papageorgiou S, *et al*. Is interictal temporal hypometabolism related to mesial temporal sclerosis? A positron emission tomography/magnetic resonance imaging confrontation. *Epilepsia* 1995; 36: 447-56.
- Sommer W. Erkrankung des Ammonshorns als aetiologisches Moment der Epilepsie. *Arch Psychiat Nervenkr* 1880; 10: 631-75.
- Spanedda F, Cendes F, Gotman J. Relations between EEG seizure morphology, interhemispheric spread, and mesial temporal atrophy in bitemporal epilepsy. *Epilepsia* 1997; 38: 1300-14.

- Spencer SS, Spencer DD. Entorhinal-hippocampal interactions in medial temporal lobe epilepsy. *Epilepsia* 1994; 35: 721-7.
- Sperling MR, O'Connor MJ. Auras and subclinical seizures: characteristics and prognostic significance. *Ann Neurol* 1990; 28: 320-8.
- Tharp BR. Transient global amnesia: manifestation of medial temporal lobe epilepsy. *Clin Electroencephalogr* 1979; 10: 54-6.
- Wennberg R, Arruda F, Quesney LF, Olivier A. Preeminence of extrahippocampal structures in the generation of mesial temporal seizures: evidence from human depth electrode recordings. *Epilepsia* 2002; 43: 716-26.
- Wieser HG, et al. ILAE Commission on Neurosurgery of Epilepsy. ILAE Commission Report. Mesial temporal lobe epilepsy with hippocampal sclerosis. *Epilepsia* 2004; 45: 695-714.
- Wolf HK, Wiestler OD. Surgical pathology of chronic epileptic seizure disorders. *Brain Pathol* 1993; 3: 371-80.
- Yilmazer-Hanke DM, Wolf HK, Schramm J, et al. Subregional pathology of the amygdala complex and entorhinal region in surgical specimens from patients with pharmacoresistant temporal lobe epilepsy. *J Neuropathol Exp Neurol* 2000; 59: 907-20.

Ictal networks in mesial temporal lobe epilepsy

Fabrice Bartolomei, Patrick Chauvel

Inserm U751, Marseille, France; Aix-Marseille Medicine University, Marseille, France; Assistance Publique-Hôpitaux de Marseille, Timone Hospital, Department of Clinical Neurophysiology, Marseille, France

Mesial temporal lobe seizures (MTLS) are the most common form of partial epileptic seizures originating in the temporal lobe (Williamson et al., 1998). They are frequently resistant to antiepileptic drug treatments. Depth-EEG recordings performed with intracerebral electrodes during presurgical evaluation have demonstrated that MTLS are generated within the mesial part of the temporal lobe (Bancaud, 1981; Engel et al., 1989; Spencer et al., 1992). However, the precise functional anatomical organization of the epileptogenic zone (EZ) and the region from where seizures start are still matters of debate (Bartolomei et al., 2001b; Bertram et al., 1998).

According to the "focal" model, a single pathological region is responsible for the generation of seizures. Accordingly, in the past, most studies have focused on the role of hippocampal alterations in temporal lobe epilepsies (TLEs) and some of these studies also established a link between the presence of hippocampal atrophy and the area of seizure onset (King et al., 1997).

In contrast, the "network" model holds that seizures result from a more extensive alteration of limbic networks within the temporal lobe (Bartolomei et al., 2001b; Bertram et al., 1998). Recent studies have lent strength to this last model. Besides the classic finding of hippocampal atrophy, neuroradiological studies have demonstrated a statistical reduction in the volume of other limbic regions, particularly the entorhinal cortex in patients with TLEs (Bernasconi et al., 1999; Bernasconi et al., 2000; Briellmann et al., 2004; Jutila et al., 2001), corroborating previous neuropathological data (Du et al., 1995). More direct arguments are based on experimental studies showing that the substrate of seizure onset in TLEs more frequently simultaneously involves several limbic regions rather than a unique site (Bertram et al., 1998). In addition, it has been shown that other mesial temporal lobe structures may play a key role in seizure genesis, such as the entorhinal cortex (Bartolomei et al., 2005; Spencer & Spencer, 1994) or the limbic part of the temporal pole (Chabardès et al., 1999).

This brief review deals with the emerging concept that seizures in mesial temporal lobe epilepsy (MTLE) are probably more appropriately described as a consequence of diseased mesial temporal lobe networks, rather than a focal process. As a result, these seizures constitute a good example of so-called "epileptogenic networks", a concept that may be applicable to other types of partial seizures (Bartolomei et al., 2008).

Intracerebral recordings are the only way to directly study the electrical behaviour of the different temporal lobe structures. Progress made in stereotactic approaches have led to the possibility of recording all the brain structures which are potentially involved in the production of ictal discharge in TLE. In particular, stereoelectroencephalography (SEEG) allows recording of intracerebral EEG via orthogonal electrodes, giving access to both lateral (neocortical) and medial (limbic) temporal structures, as well as extratemporal cortices. Using several electrodes, it is now possible to sample the different mesial and neocortical structures and thus study their "collective" behaviour during seizures (*Figure 1*), alleviating the sampling problem inherent to intracerebral recordings.

In the present chapter, we summarise some work performed by our group, focusing on studies using quantification of SEEG signals in mesial temporal lobe seizures.

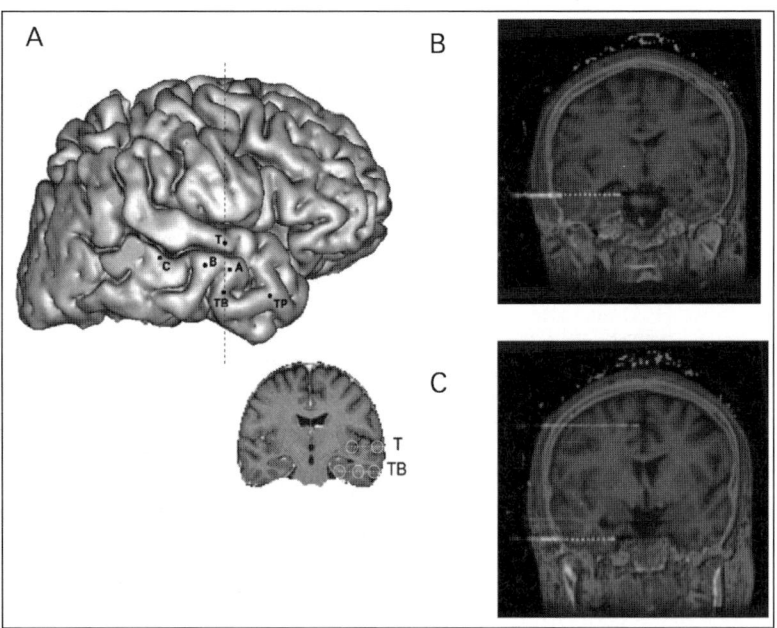

Figure 1. A. Example of depth electrode implantation for stereoelectroencephalographic (SEEG) exploration in temporal lobe epilepsy. Lateral view of depth electrodes superimposed on a 3D reconstruction of the neocortical surface of the brain. In this case, brain structures were explored with six intracerebral multiple contact electrodes denoted by the letters A, B, C, Tp, Tb and T. Internal contacts of electrodes Tp, A, B, and C recorded four mesial structures (the internal part of the temporal pole, the amygdala, the anterior hippocampus, and the posterior hippocampus, respectively). The external contacts recorded four lateral structures (the external part of the temporal pole, the anterior, the middle, and the posterior part of middle temporal gyrus, respectively). Internal and external electrode T contacts were used to explore two main structures (the insula and the superior temporal gyrus, respectively). Internal contacts of electrode Tb reached the entorhinal cortex. The reconstruction of the trajectory of the electrodes Tb and B, superimposed on the coronal MRI view, is also shown. **B.** Superimposition of electrode B traces on MRI; internal contacts are within the hippocampus. **C.** Superimposition of electrode TB on MRI; internal contacts are within the entorhinal cortex.

Electrophysiology of pure mesial temporal lobe seizures

Seizure genesis according to SEEG/intracerebral recordings

The brain regions where seizures initiate are classically defined as the epileptogenic zone (EZ) (Bancaud et al., 1965). In MTLE, the EZ consists of different structures of the medial part of the temporal lobe.

Based on hippocampal recordings, the transition between the interictal period and ictal rapid discharges (RDs) has been shown to schematically take the form of two classic patterns (Engel et al., 1989; Spencer et al., 1992; Velasco et al., 2000). In the first pattern ("type 1"), the transition from interictal to ictal activity is characterized by the emergence of a low-frequency high-amplitude rhythmic spiking followed by an RD (*Figure 2A*). In the second pattern ("type 2"), the seizure onset is characterized by the emergence of an RD without prior spiking (*Figure 2A*). Pattern 1 has been shown to be more restricted to the hippocampus than pattern 2, which tends to be more "regional". The mean duration of the RD has been found to be 8.9±3.2 seconds with frequencies ranging from 12 to 35 Hz (Bartolomei et al., 2004) (*Figure 2B*).

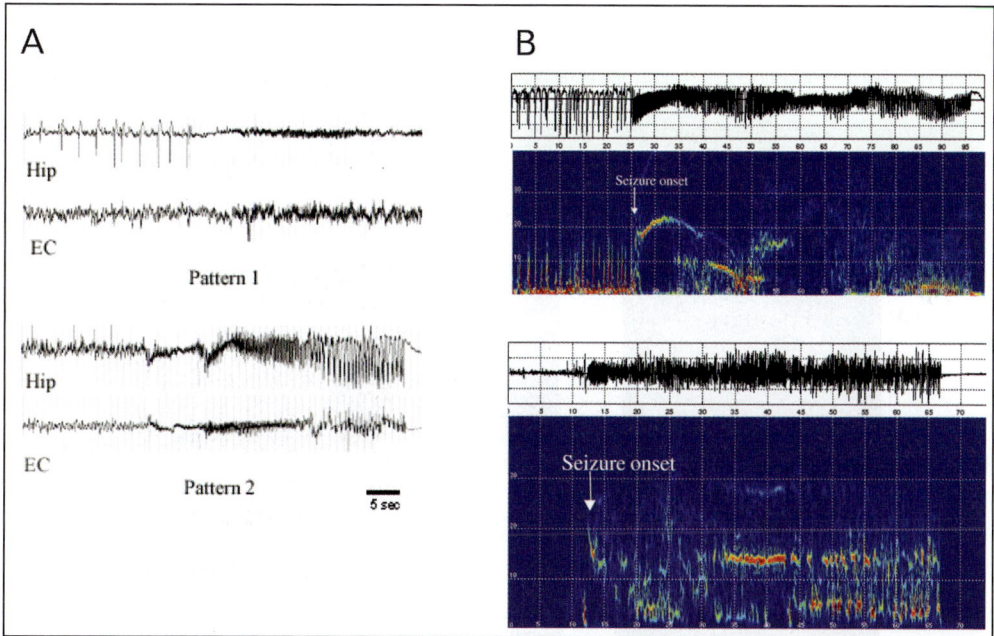

Figure 2. A. Patterns of ictal onset in mesial temporal seizures. Type 1: pre-ictal spiking followed by rapid discharge; type 2: rapid discharge without pre-ictal spiking. **B.** Time-frequency representation shows rapid discharges with frequency ranging from 15 to 25. Hip: hippocampus; EC: entorhinal cortex.

An important feature is the extension of the discharges through the mesial temporal lobe. Indeed, it is normal for distinct structures of the mesial part of the temporal lobe to be conjointly involved at the beginning of seizures. This point is illustrated in *Figures 3* and *4* in which seizures start by RDs over several mesial structures. In addition, in pure mesial seizures the neocortical part of the temporal lobe is only secondarily affected by the ictal discharge, a major criterion for the distinction between pure mesial seizures and other types of TLEs.

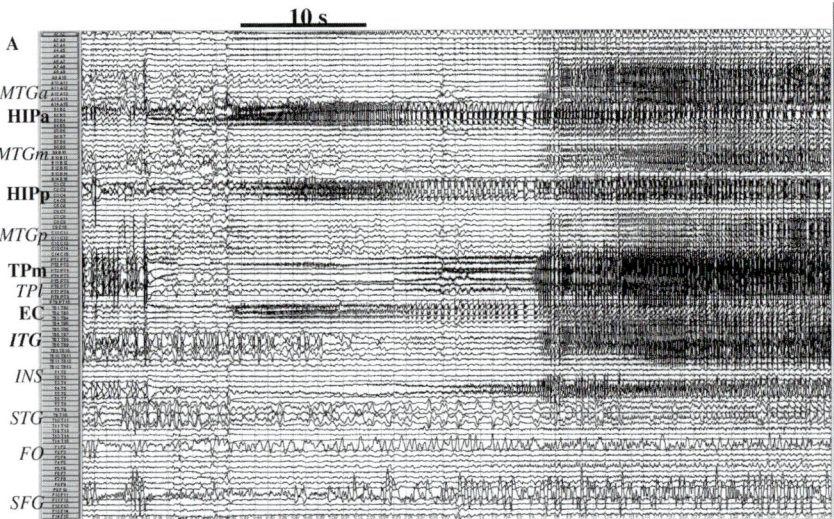

Figure 3. Example of a mesial temporal lobe seizure (type 2 pattern).
The seizure onset is marked by the emergence of rapid discharge affecting the medial structures: amygdala (A), entorhinal cortex (EC), anterior hippocampus (HIPa), posterior hippocampus (HIPp) and internal part of the temporal pole (TPi). Other structures are affected later; the middle temporal gyrus (MTG), insular cortex (INS), superior temporal gyrus (STG) and frontal regions (orbitofrontal [FO] and superior frontal gyrus [SFG]). Each line represents the recording between two adjacent contacts. The involvement of several structures is indicated, including neocortical regions during seizure propagation, approximately 30 seconds after the onset. Bold: mesial structures; italics: lateral structures.

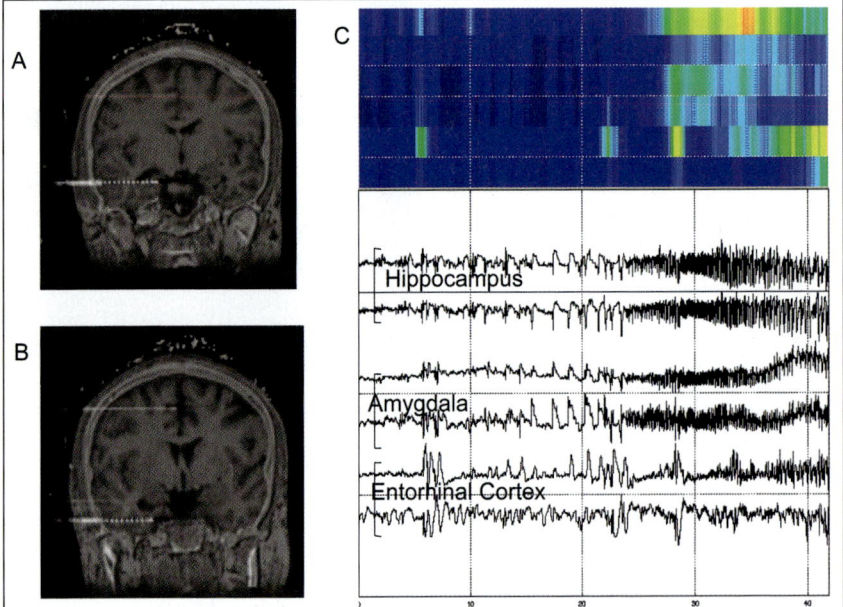

Figure 4. Another example of a seizure starting with pre-ictal spiking (pattern 1).
Three mesial structures are represented disclosing pre-ictal changes followed by rapid discharge. The upper part of the figure shows a map of beta/gamma activity showing the onset of rapid discharge in the three structures.

Quantification of SEEG signal interdependencies: an analysis of network dynamics

As indicated above, the seizure onset characterized by the RD often involves distant and functionally distinct brain sites almost simultaneously. Thus, it could be hypothesized that a "synchronizing phenomenon" gives rise to the simultaneous start of fast oscillations. This hypothesis prompted us to study the spatio-temporal dynamics of these phenomena by measuring the interdependencies between generated signals.

Epileptic phenomena have been known for a long time to be associated with dramatic changes in brain synchrony mechanisms (Brazier, 1972) and subsequent studies have shown that seizures in humans are associated with abnormal synchronization of distant structures (Bartolomei et al., 1999; Gotman, 1996; Le Van Quyen et al., 1998). This synchronization can be quantified by measuring the interdependencies between signals recorded in different brain regions involved in the EZ. Numerous methods have been proposed over the past decades, often categorized according to their ability to assess the linear (such as coherence or linear regression analysis) or non-linear (mutual information, non-linear regression analysis and similarity between state-space trajectories reconstructed from observed signals) properties of the relationship (Ansari-Asl et al., 2006). Using these methods, it is therefore possible to study functional associations between several brain regions which may or may not be involved at seizure onset. The use of non-linear approaches is probably best suited as it does not require assumptions on the nature of the relationship (Bartolomei et al., 2001a). In this context, the so called non-linear regression analysis was introduced by Pijn et al. (Pijn & Lopes Da Silva, 1993) in the middle of the '90s. This provides a parameter, referred to as the non-linear correlation coefficient h^2, with values of between 0 and 1. Low values of he denote the independence of two signals X and Y under analysis. On the other hand, high values of h^2 indicate that the second signal Y may be explained by a transformation (possibly non-linear) of the first signal X (*i.e.* both signals are dependent). In addition, this method offers the possibility of studying the direction of the coupling between neuronal populations which is an important parameter to determine the "leader region" responsible for the "driving" input in the system. In addition to the estimation of h^2, a second parameter has been proposed (Bartolomei et al., 2001a) which provides information about the "causal relationship" of the association. This parameter, referred to as the direction index D, takes into account both the estimated time delay between signals X and Y (latency) and the asymmetry property of the non-linear correlation coefficient h^2 (values of the he coefficient are different according to whether computation is performed from X to Y or from Y to X). Values of parameter D range from -1.0 (X is driven by Y) to 1.0 (Y is driven by X). These methods have been mainly applied in the last five years for the study of temporal lobe seizures (TLS) (Bartolomei et al., 1999; 2001a; 2004; 2005; Wendling et al., 2001). Results of signal quantification demonstrate that the regions involved in the EZ establish preferential functional links during a seizure and militate in favour of the existence of a network organization of the EZ. In addition, the study of the statistical relationship between SEEG signals at seizure onset has allowed us to identify four subtypes of TLE according to the interactions between mesial (amygdala-hippocampus-entorhinal cortex) and neocortical structures: mesial, mesial-lateral, lateral-mesial and lateral (Bartolomei et al., 1999; 2001a).

MTLS are the most frequent type of TLS; a typical example investigated using non-linear correlation is shown in *Figure 5*. In this group, functional coupling between several regions belonging to the mesial structures is observed. Absence of coupling between mesial and neocortical structures at seizure onset is also a characteristic feature of these seizures.

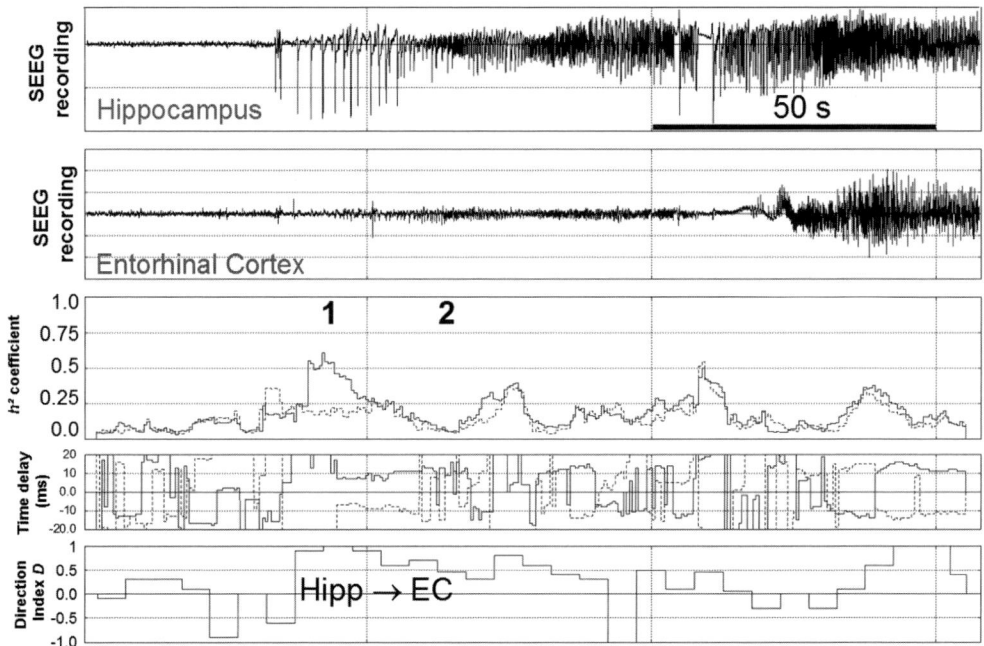

Figure 5. A study of functional coupling between the entorhinal cortex and hippocampus in a patient with mesial temporal lobe seizures. An increase in synchrony (1) during the phase of pre-ictal spiking is observed, as measured by the coefficient h^2 between the two structures. The direction index D indicates that the activity in the hippocampus (Hipp) "leads" that recorded in the entorhinal cortex (EC). Note that the rapid discharge is associated with a decrease in correlation (2).

A more general phenomenon is that the coupling between mesial temporal structures at seizure onset is maximal before the emergence of the low-voltage RD and tends to decrease thereafter and then increase once again later during the course of the seizure. This phenomenon is illustrated in *Figure 5*. This "pre-ictal" synchronization has been particularly quantified in a group with MTLE, by studying the interactions between entorhinal cortex, hippocampus and amygdala (Bartolomei et al., 2004).

Relative to the pattern of ictal onset, we identified that seizures starting with a fast discharge seemed to be predominantly under the control of the entorhinal cortex (pattern 2), while seizures starting with "pre-ictal" periodic spiking were probably more likely to be triggered by the hippocampus (pattern 1) (Bartolomei et al., 2004; 2005). Finally, the pattern of synchronization/desynchronization between regions forming the EZ appears to be a characteristic property of the EZ which may be observed in many different forms of partial seizures (Schindler et al., 2007). Synchronization before the emergence of RD was found to predominantly involve low frequencies (Ponten et al., 2007).

The EZ may be thus considered as a set of hyperexcitable structures which transiently "couple" their activity and generate RDs. It is remarkable that even in the interictal state, the structures belonging to the EZ are probably characterized by an increase of synchronization (Bettus et al., 2008; Schevon et al., 2007), in part, linked to the interictal spikes (Bettus et al., 2008). This state of hypersynchronicity probably "primes" the system for ictal genesis. The mechanisms of seizure generation are, however, unknown. According to simulation studies, ictal genesis in the mesial temporal lobe has been proposed to depend on the gradual decrease of dendritic inhibition with preserved somatic inhibition of the principal cells (Wendling et al., 2002; 2005).

Later, in the course of the seizure, synchronization occurs between distant structures which do not belong to the EZ and may involve neocortical interactions (Bartolomei et al., 2002), as well as interactions between neocortex and subcortical structures, such as the thalamus (Guye et al., 2006). It is noteworthy that most of the clinical symptoms of TLE seizures are related to the extent of the discharge outside the zone of seizure onset. In particular, loss of consciousness has been reported to occur when seizures involve the thalamus and neocortical associative cortices (Arthuis et al., 2008; Guye et al., 2006) (Figure 6).

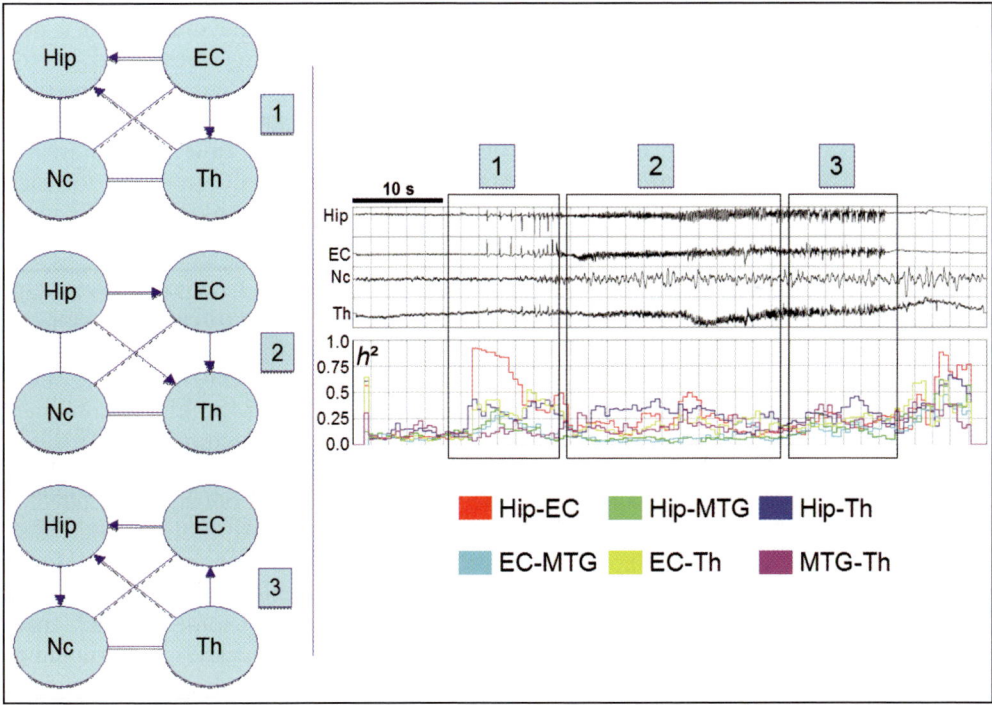

Figure 6. Example of a seizure with early synchrony between the thalamus and temporal lobe structures in a case of MTLE (with normal MRI). Non-linear correlation was studied between the temporal lobe structures (Hip: hippocampus; EC: entorhinal cortex; NC: temporal neocortex) and the midline thalamus (TH). A large increase in correlation (determined by the coefficient h^2) between temporal lobe and thalamus is observed as soon as the seizure starts (1).

Quantification of the "epileptogenic zone" using the "epileptogenicity index" method in mesial temporal lobe epilepsies

For clinicians facing the problem of definition of the EZ based on analysis of intracerebral EEG signals, two parameters are generally considered in order to qualitatively determine the degree of "epileptogenicity" of a given structure and its subsequent contribution to the EZ. The first parameter is the capability of a given structure to generate RDs typically in the beta and/or the gamma range of frequency, as measured by classic Fourrier transform analysis (Alarcon et al., 1995; Allen et al., 1992; Wendling et al., 2003). RDs have long been recognized to be one of the most characteristic patterns of the EZ in focal epilepsy (Bancaud et al., 1965). The second parameter is the delay of involvement of the structure with respect to the onset of the seizure. Indeed, it is generally accepted that the earlier the appearance of an RD in a given brain area, the more epileptogenic this area. Therefore, both the spectral content and the delay of appearance of the fast ictal activity appear as crucial parameters for determining the EZ. However, until recently, no attempt to quantify the combination of these two phenomena (appearance of high-frequency oscillations and latency with respect to seizure onset time) has been made. We have proposed a new approach to quantify the "epileptogenicity" of recorded brain structures based on the analysis of intracerebral EEG signals (Bartolomei et al., 2008). This approach is based on an "epileptogenicity index" (EI), which combines both spectral and temporal parameters, related to the propensity of a brain area to generate RDs and the time for this area to become involved in the seizure process, respectively. After normalization and for each quantified structure, the EI values may vary between 0 (no epileptogenicity) and 1 (maximal epileptogenicity) (for further explanation, refer to *Figure 7*).

In this study, the epileptogenicity index was determined in mesial (including hippocampus, entorhinal cortex, temporal pole and amygdala) and lateral structures of the temporal lobe in patients with MTLE. Two types of MTLE were included; one with hippocampal sclerosis and the other with normal MRI (the so-called "paradoxical MTLE" [Cohen-Gadol et al., 2005]). As indicated in *Figure 8*, the highest values of the EI were obtained in the mesial structures but were not restricted to a single mesial structure (*i.e.* a "focus"), but rather corresponded to a set of mesial structures, mostly in the anterior part of the temporal region. This result is in line with the view that extended networks are affected in MTLEs. Even if MTLE is considered to be a relatively homogeneous entity, individual results clearly show variable epileptogenicity profiles from one patient to another. However, taken as a whole, results indicated that the two most epileptogenic structures in MTLE are the anterior hippocampus and the entorhinal cortex. For some patients (three in this group) high values were disclosed in the amygdala. Future studies are required to better determine if subgroups of MTLE may be distinguished according to the distinct epileptogenicity of mesial structures.

Another interesting result of this study is the evidence of a correlation between the extension of the epileptogenic zone and the duration of epilepsy. It has long been proposed that epileptogenesis is an active process that could develop over years. Some studies have reported a significant relationship between the duration of epilepsy and the degree of mesial temporal atrophy (Bernasconi et al., 2005; Liu et al., 2005). We found that the extent of the EZ, characterized by the number of structures disclosing high EI values, was strongly correlated with the duration of epilepsy. This finding may be interpreted as the gradually increasing propensity of epileptogenic networks to generate RDs. This interpretation also relates to the so called process of "secondary epileptogenesis". In the long term,

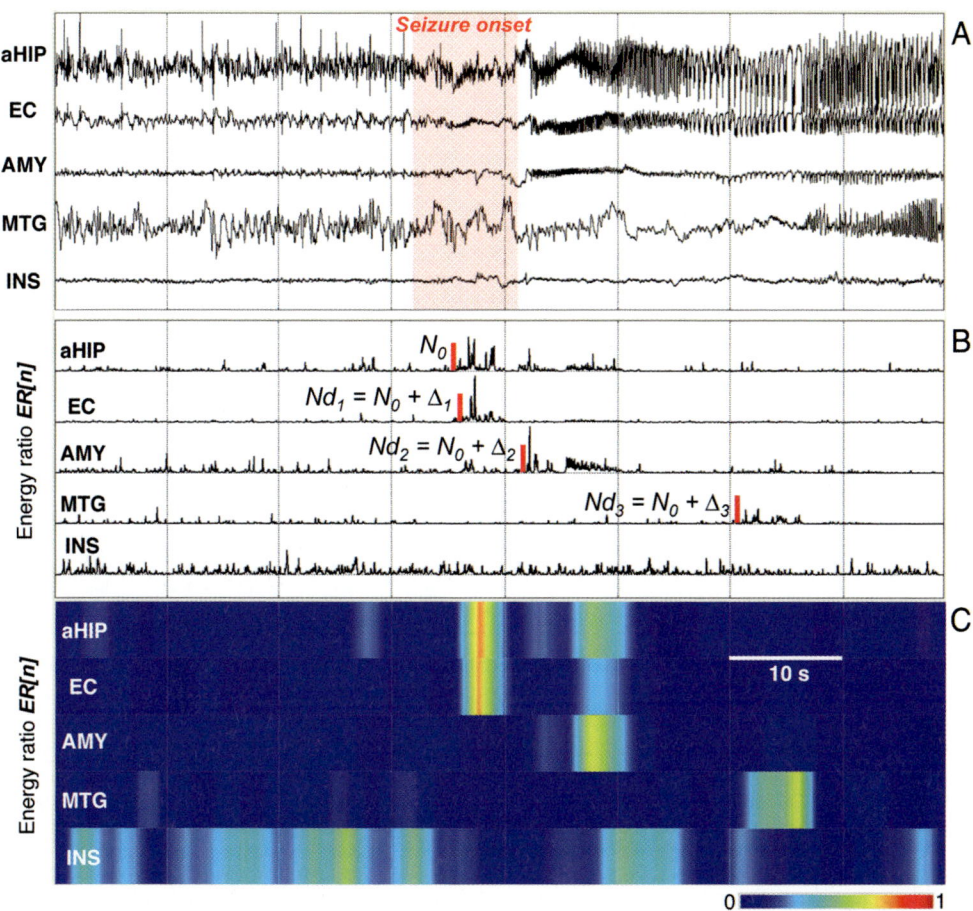

Figure 7. Determination of the epileptogenicity index (EI).
A. Example of an intracerebral EEG recording (limited to 5 channels). **B.** The Page-Hinkley algorithm provides a detection time Ndi (in red) for each brain structure involved in the generation of a rapid discharge. The first detection time is arbitrarily defined as the reference time N0 (aHIP in this case). For each EEG signal recorded from a given brain structure (EC, AMY, etc.), the EI is then defined as the energy ratio ER[n] (ratio of the energy in gamma and beta sub-bands divided by the energy in theta and alpha bands) divided by the delay δi of involvement of the considered structure with respect to time N0 (time interval following detection). The signal energy ratio (ER) is determined, between high (β[12.4-24 Hz] and γ[24-90 Hz]) and low (θ[3.4-7.4 Hz] and α[7.4-12.4 Hz]) frequency bands of the EEG from the signal spectral density $\Gamma(w)$ (squared modulus of its Fourier transform). **C.** Colour-coded map showing the evolution of the energy ratio with time (same information as in **B**. From top to bottom, this representation displays the early involvement of the anterior hippocampus (aHIP) and the entorhinal cortex (EC), as well as the delayed rapid discharge in the amygdala (AMY) and subsequently in the middle temporal gyrus (MTG). Note that the algorithm does not detect any rapid discharge in the insula (INS). (Adapted with permission from Bartolomei et al., 2008).

these changes lead to epileptic discharges in the other structures and provoke an extension of epileptogenic networks (Morrell, 1989; Sutula, 2001; Wilder, 2001). Our findings add strong arguments for the existence of such mechanisms in human epilepsy and support the results of Janszky et al. (2005) that early surgery is more effective in patients with drug-resistant MTLE.

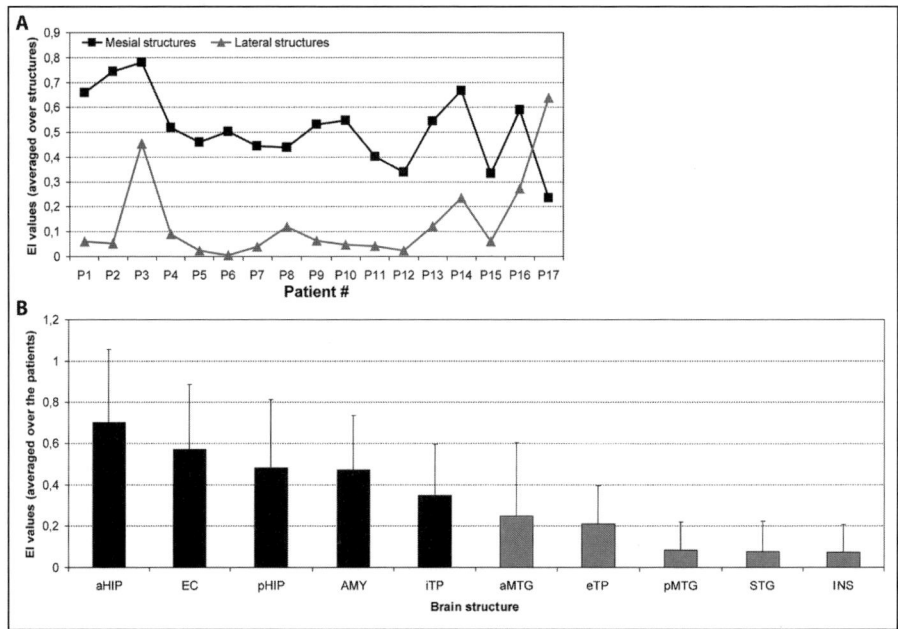

Figure 8. Values of the epileptogenicity index (EI) determined from mesial and lateral structures of the temporal lobe in 17 patients with MTLE.
A. EI values were averaged from the 17 patients. Mean EI values were significantly higher in mesial (EI averaged from the mesial structures) than lateral structures (EI averaged from the lateral structures). The values of averaged EI from the 17 patients is presented graphically for mesial structures (M) and lateral structures (L). Most of the EI values are greater than 0.3 for mesial structures and less than 0.3 for lateral cortices. **B.** Mean and standard deviation of IE values obtained from the different explored brain regions averaged over the 17 patients for each structure. Black columns: mesial structures; grey columns: lateral structures; aHIP: anterior hippocampus; EC: entorhinal cortex; pHIP: posterior hippocampus; AMY: amygdala; iTP: internal temporal pole; aMTG: anterior middle temporal gyrus; eTP: external temporal pole; pMTG: posterior part of the middle temporal gyrus; STG: superior temporal gyrus; INS: insular cortex. (Adapted with permission from Bartolomei et al., 2008).

■ The distinction between mesial seizures and other forms of temporal lobe epilepsy seizures

Pure mesial seizures are not the only anatomo-functional subtype of TLE seizures, even if the current literature generally tends to underestimate the other forms of TLE seizures. TLE is classically recognized to include two types of EZ; the mesial temporal lobe subtype (the EZ is localized in the temporal mesial lobe) or the lateral subtype (the EZ is localized within the neocortex) (Commission, 1989). These two forms may be distinguished according to the aetiology or the ictal electroclinical semiology. This dichotomous classification has, however, been challenged by studies using lateral/orthogonal depth electrodes (SEEG) showing that other forms of TLE may exist (Bancaud et al., 1965; Bartolomei et al., 1999; Wieser, 1983). It has been shown that a great number of TLEs are in fact characterized by a more complex EZ including both mesial (M) and lateral (L) cortices (mesio-lateral subtypes) (Bartolomei et al., 1999; 2001a). Mesio-lateral (ML) subtypes are more frequently associated with lesional temporal lobe epilepsies (Maillard et al., 2004; Usui et al., 2008).

In these situations, the seizure onset takes place in both mesial and neocortical compartments of the temporal lobe. An example of ML seizures is shown in *Figure 9*. In these seizures, a rapid "tonic" discharge is observed over the temporal neocortex at the onset of the seizure (Bartolomei, et al., 1999). Quantitative analysis has shown an initial increase in non-linear correlation coefficient or coherence between neocortex and mesial structures (Bartolomei et al., 1999; 2001a). This subtype is rarely associated with hippocampal sclerosis (Maillard et al., 2004).

Recently, complex epileptogenic networks, including temporal lobe structures and adjacent extratemporal cortices (ET), have been referred to as "temporal plus" seizures (T+S) (Barba et al., 2007). T+S may be suspected when clinical features are suggestive of extra-temporal involvement (such as gustatory hallucinations) with important EEG abnormalities. The extension of the EZ outside the limit of the surgical procedure is thought to be a major determinant of epilepsy surgery failure particularly when focal or conservative surgery has been proposed in a given patient.

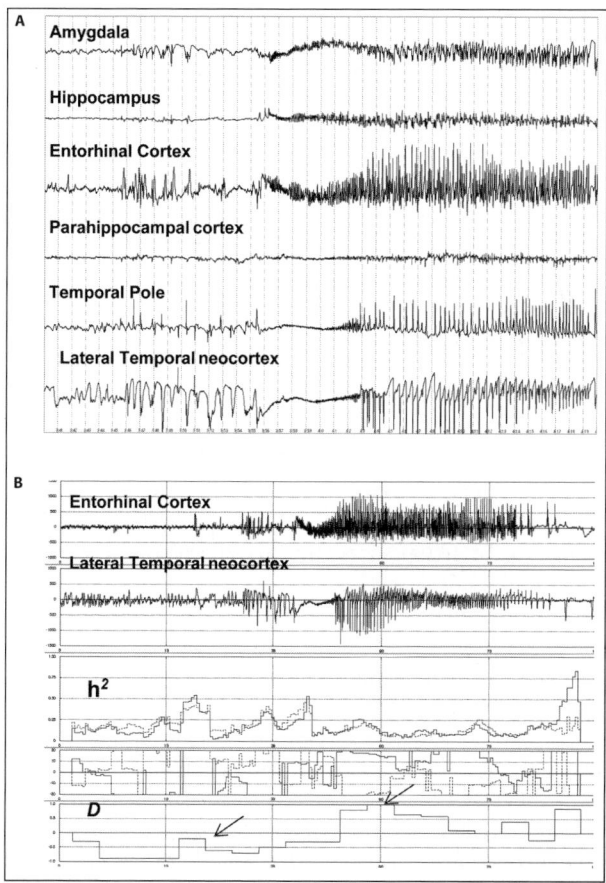

Figure 9. A. Ictal discharges involving both the temporal neocortex and the mesial temporal structures (a latero-mesial seizure) in a patient with a latero-basal lesion (tumour) of the temporal lobe. **B.** Non-linear correlation analysis of the coupling between the lateral temporal cortex and the entorhinal cortex. The h^2 coefficient increases at the beginning of the seizure during the phase of spiking, before decreasing. The direction index D indicates that during the synchronization phase, the lateral neocortex is the "leading" structure.

References

- Alarcon G, Binnie CD, Elwes RD, Polkey CE. Power spectrum and intracranial EEG patterns at seizure onset in partial epilepsy. *Electroencephalogr Clin Neurophysiol* 1995; 94: 326-37.
- Allen PJ, Fish DR, Smith SJ. Very high-frequency rhythmic activity during SEEG suppression in frontal lobe epilepsy. *Electroencephalogr Clin Neurophysiol* 1992; 82: 155-9.
- Ansari-Asl K, Senhadji L, Bellanger JJ, Wendling F. Quantitative evaluation of linear and non-linear methods characterizing interdependencies between brain signals. *Phys Rev E Stat Nonlin Soft Matter Phys* 2006; 74: 031916.
- Arthuis M, Valton L, Régis J, Chauvel P, Wendling F, Naccache L, et al. Impaired consciousness during temporal lobe seizures is related to increased long-distance cortical-subcortical synchronization. *Brain* 2009; 132: 2091-101.
- Bancaud J. Epileptic attacks of temporal lobe origin in man. *Jap J EEG EMG* 1981 (Suppl): 61-71.
- Bancaud J, Talairach J, Bonis A, Schaub C, Szikla G, Morel P, et al. La stéréoélectroencéphalographie dans l'épilepsie: informations neurophysiopathologiques apportées par l'investigation fonctionnelle stereotaxique. Paris: Masson, 1965.
- Barba C, Barbati G, Minotti L, Hoffmann D, Kahane P. Ictal clinical and scalp-EEG findings differentiating temporal lobe epilepsies from temporal "plus" epilepsies. *Brain* 2007; 130: 1957-67.
- Bartolomei F, Chauvel P, Wendling F. Epileptogenicity of brain structures in human temporal lobe epilepsy: a quantified study from intracerebral EEG. *Brain* 2008.
- Bartolomei F, Khalil M, Wendling F, Sontheimer A, Regis J, Ranjeva JP, et al. Entorhinal cortex involvement in human mesial temporal lobe epilepsy: an electrophysiologic and volumetric study. *Epilepsia* 2005; 46: 677-87.
- Bartolomei F, Wendling F, Bellanger J, Regis J, Chauvel P. Neural networks involved in temporal lobe seizures: a nonlinear regression analysis of SEEG signals interdependencies. *Clin Neurophysiol* 2001a; 112: 1746-60.
- Bartolomei F, Wendling F, Bellanger JJ, Regis J, Chauvel P. Neural networks involving the medial temporal structures in temporal lobe epilepsy. *Clin Neurophysiol* 2001b; 112: 1746-60.
- Bartolomei F, Wendling F, Regis J, Gavaret M, Guye M, Chauvel P. Pre-ictal synchronicity in limbic networks of mesial temporal lobe epilepsy. *Epilepsy Res* 2004; 61: 89-104.
- Bartolomei F, Wendling F, Vignal J, Kochen S, Bellanger J, Badier J, et al. Seizures of temporal lobe epilepsy: identification of subtypes by coherence analysis using stereo-electro-encephalography. *Clin Neurophysiol* 1999; 110: 1741-54.
- Bartolomei F, Wendling F, Vignal JP, Chauvel P, Liegeois-Chauvel C. Neural networks underlying epileptic humming. *Epilepsia* 2002; 43: 1001-12.
- Bernasconi N, Bernasconi A, Andermann F. Entorhinal cortex in temporal lobe epilepsy. *Neurology* 1999; 52: 1870-6.
- Bernasconi N, Bernasconi A, Caramanos Z, Andermann F, Dubeau F, Arnold DL. Morphometric MRI analysis of the parahippocampal region in temporal lobe epilepsy. *Ann N Y Acad Sci* 2000; 911: 495-500.
- Bernasconi N, Natsume J, Bernasconi A. Progression in temporal lobe epilepsy: differential atrophy in mesial temporal structures. *Neurology* 2005; 65: 223-8.
- Bertram EH, Zhang DX, Mangan P, Fountain N, Rempe D. Functional anatomy of limbic epilepsy: a proposal for central synchronization of a diffusely hyperexcitable network. *Epilepsy Res* 1998; 32: 194-205.
- Bettus G, Wendling F, Guye M, Valton L, Regis J, Chauvel P, et al. Enhanced EEG functional connectivity in mesial temporal lobe epilepsy. *Epilepsy Res* 2008; 81: 58-68.

- Brazier MAB. Spread of seizure discharges in epilepsy: anatomical and electrophysiological consideration. *Exp Neurol* 1972; 36: 263-72.
- Briellmann RS, Jackson GD, Pell GS, Mitchell LA, Abbott DF. Structural abnormalities remote from the seizure focus: a study using T2 relaxometry at 3 T. *Neurology* 2004; 63: 2303-8.
- Chabardès S, Kahane P, Hoffman D, Munari C, Benabid AL. Role of the temporo-polar region in the genesis of temporal lobe seizures. *Epilepsia* 1999; 40 (Suppl 7): 78.
- Cohen-Gadol AA, Bradley CC, Williamson A, Kim JH, Westerveld M, Duckrow RB, et al. Normal magnetic resonance imaging and medial temporal lobe epilepsy: the clinical syndrome of paradoxical temporal lobe epilepsy. *J Neurosurg* 2005; 102: 902-9.
- Commission. Commission on classification and terminology of the International League Against Epilepsy: Proposal for revised classification of epilepsies and epileptic syndromes. *Epilepsia* 1989; 30: 389-99.
- Du F, Eid T, Lothman EW, Kohler C, Schwarcz R. Preferential neuronal loss in layer III of the medial entorhinal cortex in rat models of temporal lobe epilepsy. *J Neurosci* 1995; 15: 6301-13.
- Engel J, Jr., Babb TL, Crandall PH. Surgical treatment of epilepsy: opportunities for research into basic mechanisms of human brain function. *Acta Neurochir (Wien)* 1989; 46 (Suppl): 3-8.
- Gotman J, Levtova, V. Amygdala-hippocampus relationships in temporal lobe seizures: a phase coherence study. *Epilepsy Res* 1996; 25: 51-7.
- Guye M, Regis J, Tamura M, Wendling F, McGonigal A, Chauvel P, et al. The role of cortico-thalamic coupling in human temporal lobe epilepsy. *Brain* 2006; 129: 1917-28.
- Janszky J, Janszky I, Schulz R, Hoppe M, Behne F, Pannek HW, et al. Temporal lobe epilepsy with hippocampal sclerosis: predictors for long-term surgical outcome. *Brain* 2005; 128: 395-404.
- Jutila L, Ylinen A, Partanen K, Alafuzoff I, Mervaala E, Partanen J, et al. MR volumetry of the entorhinal, perirhinal, and temporopolar cortices in drug-refractory temporal lobe epilepsy. *AJNR Am J Neuroradiol* 2001; 22: 1490-501.
- King D, Bronen RA, Spencer DD, Spencer SS. Topographic distribution of seizure onset and hippocampal atrophy: relationship between MRI and depth EEG. *Electroencephalogr Clin Neurophysiol* 1997; 103: 692-7.
- Le Van Quyen M, Adam C, Baulac M, Martinerie J, Varela F. Nonlinear interdependencies of EEG signals in human intracranially recorded temporal lobe seizures. *Brain Res* 1998; 792: 24-40.
- Liu RS, Lemieux L, Bell GS, Sisodiya SM, Bartlett PA, Shorvon SD, et al. Cerebral damage in epilepsy: a population-based longitudinal quantitative MRI study. *Epilepsia* 2005; 46: 1482-94.
- Maillard L, Vignal JP, Gavaret M, Guye M, Biraben A, McGonigal A, et al. Semiologic and electrophysiologic correlations in temporal lobe seizure subtypes. *Epilepsia* 2004; 45: 1590-9.
- Morrell F. Varieties of human secondary epileptogenesis. *J Clin Neurophysiol* 1989; 6: 227-75.
- Pijn J, Lopes Da Silva F. Propagation of electrical activity: nonlinear associations and time delays between EEG signals. In: Zschocke and Speckmann, eds. *Basic Mechanisms of the EEG*. Boston: Birkauser, 1993.
- Ponten S, Bartolomei F, Stam C. Small-world networks and epilepsy: Graph theoretical analysis of intracerebrally recorded mesial temporal lobe seizures. *Clin Neurophysiol* 2007; 118: 918-27.
- Schevon CA, Cappell J, Emerson R, Isler J, Grieve P, Goodman R, et al. Cortical abnormalities in epilepsy revealed by local EEG synchrony. *Neuroimage* 2007; 35: 140-8.
- Schindler K, Leung H, Elger CE, Lehnertz K. Assessing seizure dynamics by analysing the correlation structure of multichannel intracranial EEG. *Brain* 2007; 130: 65-77.
- Spencer S, Guimaraes P, Katz A, Kim J, Spencer D. Morphological patterns of seizures recorded intracranially. *Epilepsia* 1992; 33: 537-45.
- Spencer S, Spencer D. Entorhinal-hippocampal interactions in medial temporal lobe epilepsy. *Epilepsia* 1994; 35: 721-7.

- Sutula TP. Secondary epileptogenesis, kindling, and intractable epilepsy: a reappraisal from the perspective of neural plasticity. *Int Rev Neurobiol* 2001; 45: 355-86.
- Usui N, Mihara T, Baba K, Matsuda K, Tottori T, Umeoka S, et al. Intracranial EEG findings in patients with lesional lateral temporal lobe epilepsy. *Epilepsy Res* 2008; 78: 82-91.
- Velasco A, Wilson C, Babb T, Engel J. Functional and anatomic correlates of two frequently observed temporal lobe seizure-onset patterns. *Neural Plasticity* 2000; 7: 49-63.
- Wendling F, Bartolomei F, Bellanger J, Chauvel P. Interpretation of interdependencies in epileptic signals using a macroscopic physiological model of EEG. *Clin Neurophysiol* 2001; 112: 1201-18.
- Wendling F, Bartolomei F, Bellanger JJ, Bourien J, Chauvel P. Epileptic fast intracerebral EEG activity: evidence for spatial decorrelation at seizure onset. *Brain* 2003; 126: 1449-59.
- Wendling F, Bartolomei F, Bellanger JJ, Chauvel P. Epileptic fast activity can be explained by a model of impaired GABAergic dendritic inhibition. *Eur J Neurosci* 2002; 15: 1499-508.
- Wendling F, Hernandez A, Bellanger JJ, Chauvel P, Bartolomei F. Interictal to ictal transition in human temporal lobe epilepsy: insights from a computational model of intracerebral EEG. *J Clin Neurophysiol* 2005; 22: 343-56.
- Wieser H. *Electroclinical features of the psychomotor seizures*. London: Butterworths, 1983.
- Wilder BJ. The mirror focus and secondary epileptogenesis. *Int Rev Neurobiol* 2001; 45: 435-46.
- Williamson P, Engel P, Munari C. Anatomic classification of localization-related epilepsies. In: Engel J, Pedley T (eds). *Epilepsy: a comprehensive textbook*. New Yok: Lippincott-Raven, 1998.

Mesial temporal lobe epilepsy: anatomy and neuropathology

Ingmar Blümcke

Department of Neuropathology, University Hospital Erlangen, Germany

The temporal lobe is amongst the anatomical brain regions most susceptible to seizures in mammals. One of the central structures is the hippocampus, localized at the mesial part, bordering the inferior horn of the lateral ventricle. An intriguing observation is the selective vulnerability of hippocampal subregions when tissue specimens obtained from patients with chronic drug-resistant epilepsies are analysed. Based on astroglial "scarring" of the affected brain tissue, the term Ammon's horn sclerosis was coined as early as 1880. Nowadays, the classification of specific histopathological patterns is increasingly recognized and helpful for the prediction of postsurgical seizure control in individual patients. The most frequent pattern of mesial temporal sclerosis (MTS, also known as hippocampal sclerosis and Ammon's horn sclerosis) involves neuronal loss in all hippocampal segments (MTS type 1a and 1b) and is associated with favourable seizure relief after surgical resection. However, atypical patterns, with cell loss restricted either to the CA1 region (MTS type 2) or CA4 segment (MTS type 3), should also be recognized by histopathological inspection. These patients experience their first seizures at a significantly later time point and have less favourable seizure relief after surgery. The majority of MTS patients also present with alterations within the dentate gyrus (DG), an anatomically distinct region but functionally tightly connected to the hippocampal formation. There is increasing knowledge that granule cell loss in the dentate gyrus is associated with cognitive dysfunction. Thus, systematic neuropathological investigations are helpful to further explore epileptogenic pathomechanisms, as well as compromised memory function, in patients with mesial temporal lobe epilepsies.

■ Microscopic anatomy of the human hippocampus

The anatomical description of the human hippocampus has a long and varied history led by Julius Caesar Arantius in 1587, a pupil of the famous Italian anatomist Andreas Vesalius (Lewis, 1923). Arantius compared the anatomical elevations within the inferior horn of the lateral ventricles with that of a seahorse *(hippocampus)*, with the animal's head pointing either to the third ventricle or the anterior part of the temporal lobe. Confusion was further promoted by de Garengeot in 1742, who compared the mesial view of the hippocampus with the Ammon's horn adopted from the Egyptian god Ammun Kneph (Lewis, 1923; Walther, 2002). The pyramidal cell layer of the various hippocampal subregions is now microscopically recognized as the Cornu Ammonis (the CA areas) and, indeed, also resembles a ram's horn *(Figure 1)*. The anatomical classification of hippocampal subfields is no less contradictory with many classification systems available, in some cases due to differences between rodent and human hippocampi. The classification introduced by Lorente de Nó in 1933 (Lorente de Nó, 1933) is predominantly used and comprises four designated hippocampal sectors, namely CA1 to CA4. The transition areas between CA1 and the subiculum or between the CA3 and CA4 regions remain, however, difficult to clarify using routine staining techniques.

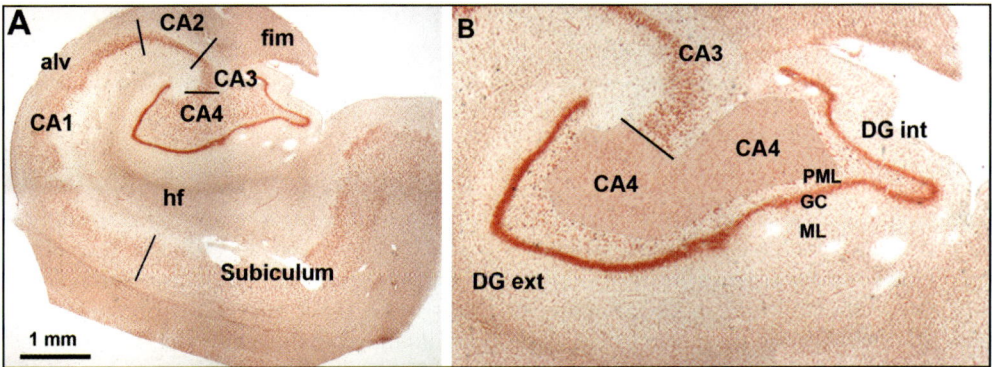

Figure 1. Microscopic anatomy of the human hippocampus.
A. Coronar section through the mid-body of the human hippocampus. Pigment-Nissl-staining of a 40 µm vibratome section. Borders between pyramidal cell layers are not always sharp nor easy to define at low magnification. This applies in particular to transition areas between CA1 and subiculum or CA3 – CA4. **B.** Higher magnification of the Dentate Gyrus (from *Figure 1A*). The three-layered Dentate Gyrus is composed of a molecular layer (ML), granule cell layer (GC) and polymorphic layer (PML). In addition, two blades can be developmentally distinguished (Altman & Bayer 1990), *i.e.*, the external (DGext) vs. internal limb (DGint). The term "Hilus" should be restricted to the rodent hippocampus, and is not defined by Lorente de No (1933). The same applies for the term "Endfolium", which is not a proper anatomical terminology for this region.
Hf: hippocampal fissure; fim: fimbria; alv; alveus. Scale bar: 1 mm.

■ Clinico-pathological findings in mesial temporal sclerosis

Histopathological studies in patients with pharmacoresistant temporal lobe epilepsies have identified MTS as a major histopathological finding (Blümcke *et al.*, 2002; Thom *et al.*, 2005b). In a large series of 3,311 patients suffering from TLE, MTS was identified in 48%. Within our entire cohort of 4,512 epilepsy patients undergoing surgical resection for various aetiologies, MTS was recognized in 35.2%, with 5% presenting as dual pathology, *i.e.* in combination with focal cortical dysplasia (FCD), tumours or scars (see below). Although the pathogenesis of MTS remains to be identified, clinical histories follow a characteristic pattern in most patients. In one cohort, approximately 50% of patients were reported to suffer from an "initial precipitating injury" before the age of four years and complex febrile seizures were the most frequently noted events (Blümcke *et al.*, 2002). Birth trauma, head injury or meningitis are other early childhood lesions observed in TLE patients. The mean age at onset of spontaneous complex partial seizures is reported to be 11.5 years (Blümcke, 2009). Molecular or functional analysis can usually not be obtained at this early and clinically silent period, and the diagnosis of MTS is verified after a long, frustrating period of antiepileptic medication. The mean age at the time of surgery is 34.6 years with a history of epileptic seizures over 23.3 years. As in most other series reported so far, both genders are equally affected and a familial history of TLE is very rare, indicating that hereditary factors do not play a major role in MTS-associated TLE.

MTS is characterized at the histopathological level by segmental pyramidal cell loss in CA1 (Sommer's sector), CA3 and CA4, whereas CA2 pyramidal and DG granule cells are more "resistant" to seizures (Sommer, 1880). Notwithstanding, several interneuronal cell populations are also affected, *i.e.* neuropeptide Y, somatostatin-immunoreactive interneurons and/or mossy cells in the CA4 sector (Blümcke et al., 2000; de Lanerolle et al., 2003). Neuronal cell loss is invariably associated with reactive astrogliosis, resulting in stiffening of the tissue, and gives rise to the traditional term of "Ammon's horn sclerosis" (Sommer, 1880). What determines the mechanisms of selective neuronal vulnerability between these morphologically similar neuronal cell populations is an intriguing question, however, this topic is a matter of ongoing studies and will not be further discussed here. Abnormal neuronal circuitries (aberrant mossy fibre sprouting) (Sutula et al., 1989) and molecular rearrangement/plasticity of ion channel and neurotransmitter receptor expression (Becker et al., 2002; Bernard et al., 2004) are some of the many major pathomechanisms described.

Clinical studies assume mesial temporal lobe epilepsies to be a heterogeneous entity with different aetiologies and clinical histories (Janszky et al., 2005; Mathern et al., 1995a; Wieser, 2004). Hence, neuropathological investigations have described different patterns of neuronal cell loss within hippocampal subfields and adjacent temporal lobe structures (de Lanerolle et al., 2003; Mathern et al., 1995b; Wyler et al., 1992). An intriguing aspect, therefore, is the identification of determining factors of hippocampal pathology patterns. A reliable neuropathological classification system will be helpful to separate distinct pathological subgroups and to better predict postsurgical seizure control. A first systematic attempt was published in 1992 by Wyler (Wyler et al., 1992), referring to percentages of neuronal cell loss within identified hippocampal subfields CA1-CA4. The Wyler score is well established in the neuropathological work-up of MTS and threshold values are defined as either 10% (Wyler score 1 = mild MTS) or 50% neuronal loss. Classification includes five grades (W0: normal, W1: mild, W2: moderate, W3: classic hippocampal sclerosis and W4: severe hippocampal sclerosis). Cell loss restricted to CA4 is described as "Endfolium sclerosis" by Wyler et al. and subsumed into W2. In previous investigations, certain difficulties evolved using the Wyler score to identify mild hippocampal sclerosis on the basis of 10% neuronal cell loss within CA1 and CA3/CA4. Our own analysis identified 10% neuronal loss within the first standard deviation of age-matched control individuals. An extension and revision of the Wyler score was subsequently published by Proper (Proper et al., 2001; Wyler et al., 1992) to include mossy fibre sprouting. Mossy fibre sprouting as well as reactive gliosis are frequently associated with long-term mesial temporal lobe epilepsy, and both were confirmed in a variety of different animal models (Blümcke et al., 1999; Borges et al., 2003; Mathern et al., 1995b; Nadler, 2003; Parent et al., 1997; Proper et al., 2000). However, any histopathological classification system should be intentionally based on general histopathological techniques and staining protocols applicable to any pathology laboratory worldwide (Wieser, 2004).

A novel clinico-pathological classification system for hippocampal cell loss has been proposed for patients suffering from mesial temporal lobe epilepsies (Blümcke et al., 2007). In this, five distinct patterns were proposed (*Figure 2*), based on association with specific clinical histories and probability for postsurgical seizure control (Blümcke et al., 2007; Stefan et al., 2009).

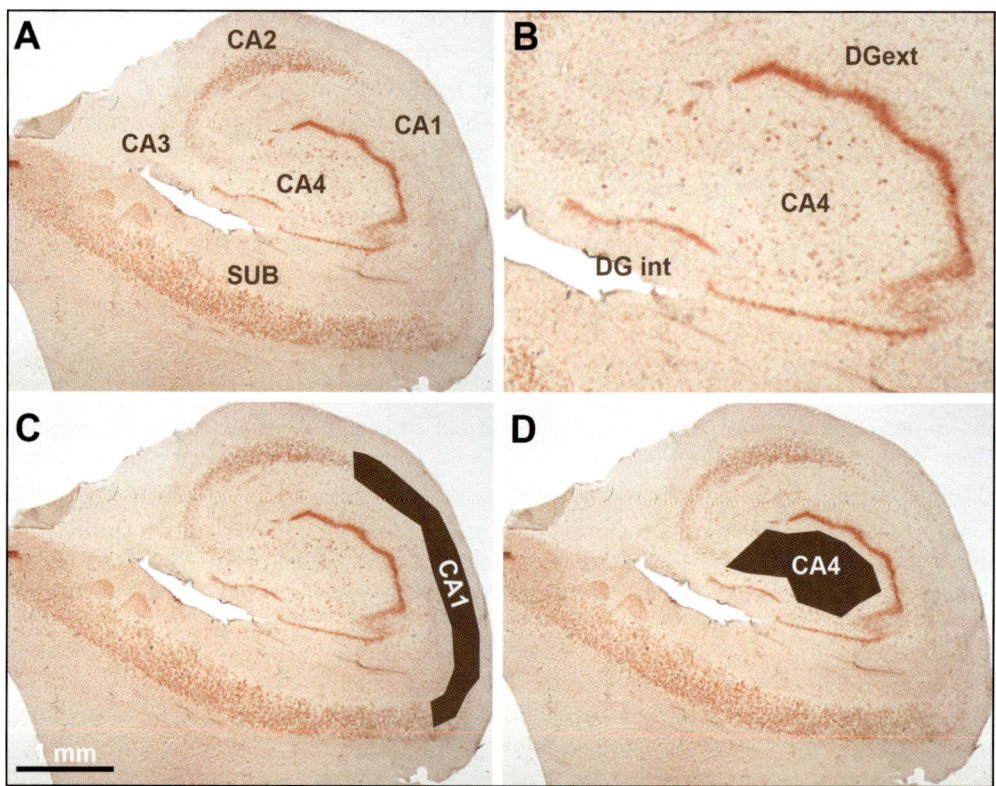

Figure 2. New mesial temporal sclerosis classification system.
A. Microscopic examination of surgical hippocampus specimens revealed distinct neuropathological subgroups (Blumcke et al., 2007). Classical patterns of hippocampal sclerosis encounter major cell loss in all pyramidal cell layers with the exception of CA2 (MTS Type 1a). Severe MTS (MTS Type 1b; not shown) involves also CA2. **B.** Granule cell loss is often variable. In the presented example (higher magnification from *Figure 1A*), granule cell loss is pronounced in the internal (DGint) compared to the external limb (DGext). This finding is frequently associated with impaired memory in the affected patient (Pauli et al., 2006). **C.** Atypical MTS patterns need to be histopathologically distinguished. MTS Type 2 refers to pronounced cell loss only in the CA1 sector (shaded region). **D.** MTS Type 3 refers to pronounced cell loss in the CA4 sector (shaded region; similar to the description of "endfolium sclerosis" [Margerison & Corsellis, 1966]). These patients experienced their first seizures at a significant later time point and have less favorable seizure relief after surgery.

■ Mesial temporal sclerosis variants in patients with mesial temporal lobe epilepsy

No mesial temporal sclerosis

Despite electrophysiological evidence for mesial temporal lobe generation of seizures, microscopic features of neuronal cell loss were reported to be absent in approximately 20% of mesial temporal lobe epilepsy (MTLE) patients (Blümcke et al., 2007). Moreover, cell density measurements were not significantly different from age-matched autopsy controls (a 10% difference in either more or less neuronal cell density was obtained, relative to controls, based on standard deviation). We designated this group "No mesial temporal sclerosis" (no MTS). This observation has been frequently reported in neuropathological surveys of similar MTS series (Blümcke et al., 2002; Thom et al., 2005b). The epileptogenic pathomechanisms of hippocampal seizure generation remain to be further determined, but are suggested to be similar to kindling in TLE animal models.

Mesial temporal sclerosis type 1a and 1b (classic and severe hippocampal sclerosis)

The largest group of MTS cases presents with a classic (MTS type 1a) or severe pattern (MTS type 1b) of segmental neuronal cell loss affecting CA1-CA4. There are, however, considerable similarities between MTS type 1a and 1b which may be distinguished based on the degree of CA3 and CA2 pyramidal cell loss; MTS type 1a is associated with moderate CA2 cell loss and MTS type 1b with severe CA2 cell loss. This distinction is reasonably similar to Wyler scores W3 and W4 (Wyler et al., 1992). Correlation with clinical data points to an early age of preceding events (< 3 years) which is an important predictor of classic and severe hippocampal pathology patterns.

Atypical mesial temporal sclerosis type 2 (CA1-sclerosis) and type 3 (CA4-sclerosis)

Two atypical variants are characterized either by severe neuronal loss restricted to sector CA1 (MTS type 2) or CA4 (MTS type 3). In MTS type 2, preceding events are documented at a later age (mean of six years), whereas in MTS type 3 and normal appearing hippocampus (no MTS) the first event appears beyond the ages of 13 and 16 years, respectively.

This novel MTS classification system allows some prediction of postsurgical outcome (Blümcke et al., 2007; Stefan et al., 2009). The most favourable outcome was achieved in patients presenting with MTS type 1a and MTS type 1b (> 83% seizure freedom), whereas only half of patients with atypical MTS patterns (type 2 and type 3) became seizure-free. However, this classification system will need further confirmation in independent patient cohorts to assess inter-observer reliability.

■ Mesial temporal lobe epilepsy: associated pathology of the dentate gyrus

The population of DG granule cells is pathologically affected in the vast majority of MTS patients. Lesional patterns in this anatomically distinct compartment range from granule cell dispersion in almost 50% of patients (Blümcke et al., 2002) to severe cell loss in patients with MTS type 1a and 1b (*Figure 3*). Neuropathological criteria for granule cell alterations have not been firmly established (Wieser, 2004). Increased granule cell lamination above 10 layers, with smaller perikarya and larger intercellular gaps, is proposed to be pathognomonic. Ectopic cluster and bilamination within the molecular layer can also be identified, although to a lesser extent. Since granule cell pathology is not internationally standardized, clinico-pathological studies have yielded complementary as well as controversial results (El Bahh et al., 1999; Harding & Thom, 2001; Houser, 1990; Houser et al., 1992; Mathern et al., 1997; Sagar & Oxbury, 1987; Thom et al., 2005a).

We recently proposed a clinico-pathological classification of DG pathology based on the examination of 96 surgically resected hippocampal specimens (Blümcke et al., 2009). Three different histopathological patterns were described: 1) normal granule cell layer (no granule

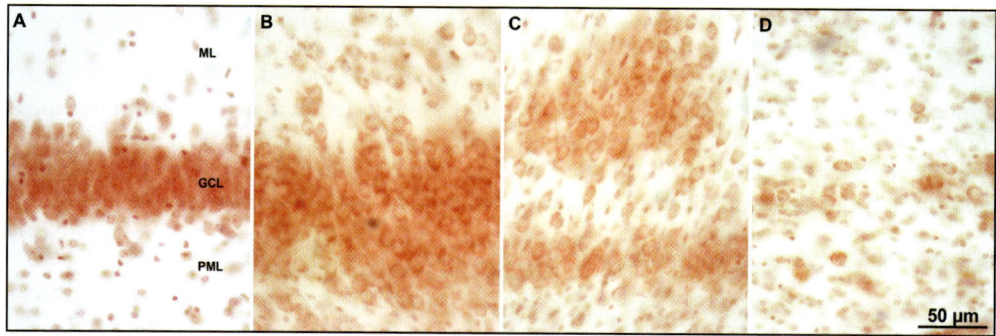

Figure 3. Granule cell pathology in mesial temporal sclerosis.
Different patterns of granule cell pathologies can be observed in surgical MTS specimens. **A.** Normal, densely packed granule cell layer of the dentate gyrus (ML – molecular layer; GCL – granule cell layer; PML – pleomorphic cell layer). **B.** A frequent finding comprises granule cell dispersion with a broader thickness of GCL and increased gaps between individual neurons (GCP Type II). Compared to controls, borders to adjacent layers are always less distinguishable in GC pathologies. **C.** A cluster of ectopic granule cells is displaced into the molecular layer (GCP Type II). **D.** Granule cell loss is, however, evident in many TLE patients (GCP Type I). Scale bar in D: 50 µm (applies also to A, B and C).

cell pathology, no-GCP); 2) substantial granule cell loss (GCP type 1); and 3) architectural abnormalities including one or more of the following features: granule cell dispersion, ectopic neurons or clusters of neurons displaced into the molecular layer, or bi-lamination (GCP type 2). Cell loss was always encountered for the latter group. There was a significant association between DG pathology patterns and older patient age at epilepsy surgery and longer epilepsy duration. No correlation was observed between GCP patterns and MTS scores (*i.e.* extent of pyramidal cell loss in adjacent hippocampal segments) or with postsurgical seizure relief (Blümcke et al., 2009).

The significant association between the loss of dentate granule cells and memory impairment remains an intriguing observation (Blümcke et al., 2009; Pauli et al., 2006; Stefan et al., 2009). This further highlights the importance of granule cells within hippocampal circuitries and the fact that the anatomical integrity of the human dentate gyrus correlates with the capacity to acquire new memory. Interestingly, professional training of spatial memory may increase hippocampal volumes (Maguire et al. 2000; Stefan et al. 2009). Also, functional imaging has indicated the involvement of the hippocampal subregions including the dentate gyrus in the formation of new memory (Zeineh et al., 2003), although structural resolution remains too unrefined to precisely differentiate between anatomical subregions. Ample evidence obtained from animal studies, however, demonstrates that the recruitment of new neurons into the dentate gyrus granule cell layer is necessary for learning (Coras et al., 2010; Gould et al., 1999; Jessberger et al., 2009; Schmidt-Hieber et al., 2004; Shors et al., 2001).

Studies addressing the molecular pathomechanism of granule cell dispersion (GCD) point to a compromised reelin signalling pathway. An inverse correlation was described between the degree of GCD and reelin mRNA expression in epilepsy patients with hippocampal sclerosis (Haas et al., 2002). While the compact layer organization may be associated with abundant reelin mRNA expression, TLE patients with pronounced GCD showed significantly reduced reelin mRNA levels, as well as increased promoter methylation of the reelin gene (Kobow et al., 2009). Reelin is synthesized and secreted by Cajal-Retzius cells, which are amongst the earliest neurons to be generated (Del Rio et al., 1997). Biochemical and functional studies using either organotypic slice cultures or knock-out mice have confirmed the relevance of reelin signalling in the formation of a densely packed granule cell layer (Haas & Frotscher, 2009; Muller et al., 2009; Zhao et al., 2004).

■ Dual pathology

In a proportion of patients with MTS, more widespread areas of epileptiform activity involving both mesial and lateral temporal lobe regions have been characterized using depth electrode recordings and intraoperative electrocorticography (Fauser & Schulze-Bonhage, 2006; Fauser et al., 2004; Tassi et al., 2002). Based on neuroimaging and neuropathological studies, it is well established that MTS can occur in combination with a second temporal lobe epileptogenic pathology such as cortical dyslamination (Tassi et al., 2002; Thom et al., 2009), ectopic white matter neurons or low grade glio-neuronal tumours (Blümcke et al., 2002; Bruton, 1988; Kuzniecky et al., 1997; Levesque et al., 1991; Li et al., 1999; Palmini et al., 2004; Raymond et al., 1994; Tassi et al., 2002). There are also occasional reports of distinct hippocampal malformations occurring with MTS (Baulac et al., 1998) and structural hippocampal abnormalities on MRI which appear to precede MTS (Fernandez et al., 1998; Grunewald et al., 2001). In the German Neuropathological Database for Epilepsy Surgery[1], dual pathologies were identified in approximately 5% of cases. In the presence of "dual pathology" (i.e. MTS type 3), less severe hippocampal neuronal loss may be evidenced. In these cases, "kindling" of the hippocampus by the adjacent temporal lobe lesion may play a role. There is some evidence for progressive hippocampal atrophy in patients with longer duration of seizures (Fuerst et al., 2001; Kalviainen et al., 1998; Tasch et al., 1999). It has been shown, however, that surgical removal of both lesions results in favourable postoperative seizure control for dual pathologies (Li et al., 1999; Marusic et al., 2007), indicating that each component contributes to the genesis of seizures. The coincidence of dual temporal lobe pathologies also raises the important question of a common predisposing malformative process for both lesions.

A major complication is the poor inter-rater concordance for the definition of dual pathology in epilepsy patients. The term "dual pathology" should be restricted to the combination of MTS with another principal lesion within the ipsilateral temporal lobe, i.e. MTS and tumours or MTS and vascular lesions. White matter neuronal ectopy and cortical dyslamination of the temporal lobe may not inevitably fit this assumption and, therefore, require careful attention (Blümcke et al., 2011). The same holds true for the frequent association between epilepsy-associated tumours and cortical dysplasias, which may arise from the same pathogenic mechanisms. It remains to be clarified, however, whether dual pathologies associate with distinct pathogenic aetiologies.

---

1. The Neuropathological Reference Center for Epilepsy Surgery is a consortium of colleagues from the following German epilepsy centers: *Berlin*: H.J. Meencke, N.T. Lehmann; *Bielefeld*: V. Hans, A. Ebner, H.W. Pannek, F. Woermann; *Bonn*: A. Becker, P. Niehusmann, C. Elger, C. G. Bien, C. Helmstaedter, J. Schramm, H. Clusmann, H. Urbach; *Erlangen*: I. Blümcke, R. Coras, H. Stefan, B. Kasper, E. Pauli, M. Buchfelder, D. Weigel; *Freiburg/Kehl-Kork*: B. Steinhoff, A. Schulze-Bonhage, S. Fauser, J. Zentner, C. Scheiwe; *Greifswald*: S. Vogelesang. *Marburg*: F. Rosenow, H. Hamer, S. Knake; *Munich*: S. Noachtar. *Radeberg*: K. Grohme, T. Mayer; *Stuttgart*: P. Winkler; *Tübingen*: H. Lerche; *Ulm*: Y. Weber; *Vogtareuth*: H. Holthausen, P.A. Winkler, T. Pieper.

■ A pathogenic model for mesial temporal sclerosis: associated temporal lobe epilepsy

Available data suggest that MTS is an early disorder which compromises normal development of mesial temporal lobe organization and hippocampal formation (Blümcke, 2009; Blümcke et al., 2002). Whether a genetic/epigenetic component plays a role, i.e. affecting neurodevelopmental signalling pathways such as the reelin cascade, can not yet be excluded (Kobow et al., 2009). However, increased neurogenesis and/or persistence of Cajal-Retzius cells in TLE patients with MTS points towards a prolonged and abnormal maturation period (Siebzehnrubl & Blümcke, 2008) and may be regarded as predisposition/susceptibility factor(s) for seizures and neuronal cell loss. This hypothesis is supported by the notion that long-term epilepsies *per se* do not inevitably damage the hippocampus, as repetitively shown in cohorts of TLE patients with poorly controlled seizures (Thom et al., 2005b).

During a latency period, which usually extends into the "teenager period", a number of structural and molecular reorganization mechanisms can be assumed. This model is difficult to address in human surgical tissue specimens obtained at a late stage of the disease. However, there is ample evidence from animal models of limbic epilepsy indicating a number of activity-dependent reorganization events preceding the onset of spontaneous seizure activity. In particular, neurotransmitter receptor complexes dramatically change their molecular composition in a region-specific manner. Such modulatory changes can functionally reduce seizure threshold levels in the hippocampus (Becker et al., 2003; Brooks-Kayal et al., 1998; Shumate et al., 1998).

Following the onset of spontaneous seizure activity within the hippocampal formation and mesial temporal lobe structures during adolescence, secondary changes associated with excitotoxic cell damage may lead to the full-blown pattern of MTS (Blümcke et al., 2002). This model does not rule out that segmental neuronal cell loss may already occur during an earlier period. We do, however, propose that limbic seizure activity alone cannot induce MTS without preceding anatomical and functional alterations in the hippocampus/dentate gyrus network. This assumption is supported by our studies in lesion-associated TLE, in which patients suffer from low grade tumours, malformations or vascular lesions. In these patients, the hippocampus does not unequivocally reveal neuropathological changes although seizure semiology and clinical history can be very similar to MTS-associated TLE patients (Blümcke et al., 2002).

Adult onset MTLE with histopathologically proven hippocampal sclerosis has been described following limbic encephalitis (Bien et al., 2007; Kroll-Seger et al., 2009). Further clarification is required to establish whether such distinct clinical MTLE histories readily adhere to the aforementioned concept. It is tempting to speculate, however, that hippocampal cell loss patterns reveal significant differences in late-onset MTLE corresponding to "atypical MTS variants" (Bien, personal communication). In conclusion, systematic neuropathological evaluation is a helpful tool to characterize distinct pathogenic patterns and better understand focal onset, drug-resistant chronic epilepsies.

Acknowledgements

I am grateful to Dr. Roland Coras for his critical comments and proof reading of the manuscript. This work is supported by the European Community (LSH-CT-2006-037315 EPICURE).

References

- Altman J, Bayer SA. Mosaic organization of the hippocampal neuroepithelium and the multiple germinal sources of dentate granule cells. *J Comp Neurol* 1990; 301: 325-42.
- Baulac M, De Grissac N, Hasboun D, et al. Hippocampal developmental changes in patients with partial epilepsy: magnetic resonance imaging and clinical aspects. *Ann Neurol* 1998; 44: 223-33.
- Becker AJ, Chen J, Zien A, et al. Correlated stage- and subfield-associated hippocampal gene expression patterns in experimental and human temporal lobe epilepsy. *Eur J Neurosci* 2003; 18: 2792-802.
- Becker AJ, Urbach H, Scheffler B, et al. Focal cortical dysplasia of Taylor's balloon cell type: mutational analysis of the TSC1 gene indicates a pathogenic relationship to tuberous sclerosis. *Ann Neurol* 2002; 52: 29-37.
- Bernard C, Anderson A, Becker A, Poolos NP, Beck H, Johnston D. Acquired dendritic channelopathy in temporal lobe epilepsy. *Science* 2004; 305: 532-5.
- Bien CG, Urbach H, Schramm J, et al. Limbic encephalitis as a precipitating event in adult-onset temporal lobe epilepsy. *Neurology* 2007; 69: 1236-44.
- Blümcke I. Neuropathology of focal epilepsies: a critical review. *Epilepsy Behav* 2009; 15: 34-9.
- Blümcke I, Kistner I, Clusmann H, et al. Towards a clinico-pathological classification of granule cell dispersion in human mesial temporal lobe epilepsies. *Acta Neuropathol* 2009; 117: 535-44.
- Blümcke I, Pauli E, Clusmann H, et al. A new clinico-pathological classification system for mesial temporal sclerosis. *Acta Neuropathol* 2007; 113: 235-44.
- Blümcke I, Suter B, Behle K, et al. Loss of hilar mossy cells in Ammon's horn sclerosis. *Epilepsia* 2000; 41: S174-S80.
- Blümcke I, Thom M, Aronica E, et al. The clinico-pathological spectrum of focal cortical dysplasias: a consensus classification proposed by an ad hoc Task Force of the ILAE Diagnostics Methods Commission. *Epilepsia* 2011; 52: 158-74.
- Blümcke I, Thom M, Wiestler OD. Ammon's horn sclerosis: a maldevelopmental disorder associated with temporal lobe epilepsy. *Brain Pathol* 2002; 12: 199-211.
- Blümcke I, Zuschratter W, Schewe JC, et al. Cellular pathology of hilar neurons in Ammon's horn sclerosis. *J Comp Neurol* 1999; 414: 437-53.
- Borges K, Gearing M, McDermott DL, et al. Neuronal and glial pathological changes during epileptogenesis in the mouse pilocarpine model. *Exp Neurol* 2003; 182: 21-34.
- Brooks-Kayal AR, Shumate MD, Jin H, Rikhter TY, Coulter DA. Selective changes in single cell GABA(A) receptor subunit expression and function in temporal lobe epilepsy. *Nat Med* 1998; 4: 1166-72.
- Bruton CJ. The neuropathology of temporal lobe epilepsy. In: Russel G, Marley E, Williams P, eds. *Maudsley monographs*. London: Oxford University Press, 1988: 1-158.
- Coras R, Siebzehnrubl FA, Pauli E, et al. Low proliferation and differentiation capacities of adult hippocampal stem cells correlate with memory dysfunctions in humans. *Brain* 2010; 133: 3359-72.
- de Lanerolle NC, Kim JH, Williamson A, et al. A retrospective analysis of hippocampal pathology in human temporal lobe epilepsy: evidence for distinctive patient subcategories. *Epilepsia* 2003; 44: 677-87.
- Del Rio JA, Heimrich B, Borrell V, et al. A role for Cajal-Retzius cells and reelin in the development of hippocampal connections. *Nature* 1997; 385: 70-4.
- El Bahh B, Lespinet V, Lurton D, Coussemacq M, Le Gal La Salle G, Rougier A. Correlations between granule cell dispersion, mossy fiber sprouting, and hippocampal cell loss in temporal lobe epilepsy. *Epilepsia* 1999; 40: 1393-401.

- Fauser S, Schulze-Bonhage A. Epileptogenicity of cortical dysplasia in temporal lobe dual pathology: an electrophysiological study with invasive recordings. *Brain* 2006; 129: 82-95.
- Fauser S, Schulze-Bonhage A, Honegger J, et al. Focal cortical dysplasias: surgical outcome in 67 patients in relation to histological subtypes and dual pathology. *Brain* 2004; 127: 2406-18.
- Fernandez G, Effenberger O, Vinz B, et al. Hippocampal malformation as a cause of familial febrile convulsions and subsequent hippocampal sclerosis. *Neurology* 1998; 50: 909-17.
- Fuerst D, Shah J, Kupsky WJ, et al. Volumetric MRI, pathological, and neuropsychological progression in hippocampal sclerosis. *Neurology* 2001; 57: 184-8.
- Gould E, Beylin A, Tanapat P, Reeves A, Shors TJ. Learning enhances adult neurogenesis in the hippocampal formation. *Nat Neurosci* 1999; 2: 260-5.
- Grunewald RA, Farrow T, Vaughan P, Rittey CD, Mundy J. A magnetic resonance study of complicated early childhood convulsion. *J Neurol Neurosurg Psychiatry* 2001; 71: 638-42.
- Haas CA, Dudeck O, Kirsch M, et al. Role for reelin in the development of granule cell dispersion in temporal lobe epilepsy. *J Neurosci* 2002; 22: 5797-802.
- Haas CA, Frotscher M. Reelin deficiency causes granule cell dispersion in epilepsy. *Exp Brain Res* 2009.
- Harding B, Thom M. Bilateral hippocampal granule cell dispersion: autopsy study of 3 infants. *Neuropathol Appl Neurobiol* 2001; 27: 245-51.
- Houser CR. Granule cell dispersion in the dentate gyrus of humans with temporal lobe epilepsy. *Brain Res* 1990; 535: 195-204.
- Houser CR, Swartz BE, Walsh GO, Delgado-Escueta AV. Granule cell disorganization in the dentate gyrus: possible alterations of neuronal migration in human temporal lobe epilepsy. *Epilepsy Res Suppl* 1992; 9: 41-8.
- Janszky J, Janszky I, Schulz R, et al. Temporal lobe epilepsy with hippocampal sclerosis: predictors for long-term surgical outcome. *Brain* 2005; 128: 395-404.
- Jessberger S, Clark RE, Broadbent NJ, et al. Dentate gyrus-specific knockdown of adult neurogenesis impairs spatial and object recognition memory in adult rats. *Learn Mem* 2009; 16: 147-54.
- Kalviainen R, Salmenpera T, Partanen K, Vainio P, Riekkinen P, Pitkanen A. Recurrent seizures may cause hippocampal damage in temporal lobe epilepsy. *Neurology* 1998; 50: 1377-82.
- Kobow K, Jeske I, Hildebrandt M, et al. Increased reelin promoter methylation is associated with granule cell dispersion in human temporal lobe epilepsy. *J Neuropathol Exp Neurol* 2009; 68: 356-64.
- Kroll-Seger J, Bien CG, Huppertz HJ. Non-paraneoplastic limbic encephalitis associated with antibodies to potassium channels leading to bilateral hippocampal sclerosis in a pre-pubertal girl. *Epileptic Disord* 2009; 11: 54-9.
- Kuzniecky R, Hetherington H, Pan J, et al. Proton spectroscopic imaging at 4.1 tesla in patients with malformations of cortical development and epilepsy. *Neurology* 1997; 48: 1018-24.
- Levesque MF, Nakasato N, Vinters HV, Babb TL. Surgical treatment of limbic epilepsy associated with extrahippocampal lesions: the problem of dual pathology. *J Neurosurg* 1991; 75: 364-70.
- Lewis FT. The significance of the term hippocampus. *J Comp Neurol* 1923; 35: 213-30.
- Li LM, Cendes F, Andermann F, et al. Surgical outcome in patients with epilepsy and dual pathology. *Brain* 1999; 122: 799-805.
- Lorente de Nó R. Studies on the structure of the cerebral cortex. I. The area entorhinalis. *J Psychol Neurol (Lpz)* 1933; 45: 381-438.
- Maguire EA, Gadian DG, Johnsrude IS, et al. Navigation-related structural change in the hippocampi of taxi drivers. *Proc Natl Acad Sci USA* 2000; 97: 4398-403.
- Margerison JH, Corsellis JA. Epilepsy and the temporal lobes. A clinical, electroencephalographic and neuropathological study of the brain in epilepsy, with particular reference to the temporal lobes. *Brain* 1966; 89: 499-530.

- Marusic P, Tomasek M, Krsek P, et al. Clinical characteristics in patients with hippocampal sclerosis with or without cortical dysplasia. *Epileptic Disord* 2007; 9 (Suppl 1): S75-82.
- Mathern GW, Babb TL, Vickrey BG, Melendez M, Pretorius JK. The clinical-pathogenic mechanisms of hippocampal neuron loss and surgical outcomes in temporal lobe epilepsy. *Brain* 1995; 118: 105-18.
- Mathern GW, Kuhlman PA, Mendoza D, Pretorius JK. Human fascia dentata anatomy and hippocampal neuron densities differ depending on the epileptic syndrome and age at first seizure. *J Neuropathol Exp Neurol* 1997; 56: 199-212.
- Mathern GW, Pretorius JK, Babb TL. Quantified patterns of mossy fiber sprouting and neuron densities in hippocampal and lesional seizures. *J Neurosurg* 1995b; 82: 211-9.
- Muller MC, Osswald M, Tinnes S, et al. Exogenous reelin prevents granule cell dispersion in experimental epilepsy. *Exp Neurol* 2009; 216: 390-7.
- Nadler JV. The recurrent mossy fiber pathway of the epileptic brain. *Neurochem Res* 2003; 28: 1649-58.
- Palmini A, Najm I, Avanzini G, et al. Terminology and classification of the cortical dysplasias. *Neurology* 2004; 62: S2-8.
- Parent JM, Yu TW, Leibowitz RT, Geschwind DH, Sloviter RS, Lowenstein DH. Dentate granule cell neurogenesis is increased by seizures and contributes to aberrant network reorganization in the adult rat hippocampus. *J Neurosci* 1997; 17: 3727-38.
- Pauli E, Hildebrandt M, Romstock J, Stefan H, Blümcke I. Deficient memory acquisition in temporal lobe epilepsy is predicted by hippocampal granule cell loss. *Neurology* 2006; 67: 1383-9.
- Proper EA, Jansen GH, van Veelen CW, van Rijen PC, Gispen WH, de Graan PN. A grading system for hippocampal sclerosis based on the degree of hippocampal mossy fiber sprouting. *Acta Neuropathol (Berl)* 2001; 101: 405-9.
- Proper EA, Oestreicher AB, Jansen GH, et al. Immunohistochemical characterization of mossy fibre sprouting in the hippocampus of patients with pharmaco-resistant temporal lobe epilepsy. *Brain* 2000; 123: 19-30.
- Raymond AA, Fish DR, Stevens JM, Cook MJ, Sisodiya SM, Shorvon SD. Association of hippocampal sclerosis with cortical dysgenesis in patients with epilepsy. *Neurology* 1994; 44: 1841-5.
- Sagar HJ, Oxbury JM. Hippocampal neuron loss in temporal lobe epilepsy: correlation with early childhood convulsions. *Ann Neurol* 1987; 22: 334-40.
- Schmidt-Hieber C, Jonas P, Bischofberger J. Enhanced synaptic plasticity in newly generated granule cells of the adult hippocampus. *Nature* 2004; 429: 184-7.
- Shors TJ, Miesegaes G, Beylin A, Zhao M, Rydel T, Gould E. Neurogenesis in the adult is involved in the formation of trace memories. *Nature* 2001; 410: 372-6.
- Shumate MD, Lin DD, Gibbs JWr, Holloway KL, Coulter DA. GABA(A) receptor function in epileptic human dentate granule cells: comparison to epileptic and control rat. *Epilepsy Res* 1998; 32: 114-28.
- Siebzehnrubl F, Blümcke I. Neurogenesis in the human hippocampus and its relevance to temporal lobe epilepsies. *Epilepsia* 2008; 49 55-65.
- Sommer W. Die erkrankung des ammonshorns als aetiologisches moment der epilepsie. *Arch Psychiat Nervenkr* 1880; 308: 631-75.
- Stefan H, Hildebrandt M, Kerling F, et al. Clinical prediction of postoperative seizure control: structural, functional findings and disease histories. *J Neurol Neurosurg Psychiatry* 2009; 80: 196-200.
- Sutula TP, Cascino G, Cavazos J, Parada I, Ramirez L. Mossy fiber synaptic reorganization in the epileptic human temporal lobe. *Ann Neurol* 1989; 26: 321-30.
- Tasch E, Cendes F, Li LM, Dubeau F, Andermann F, Arnold DL. Neuroimaging evidence of progressive neuronal loss and dysfunction in temporal lobe epilepsy. *Ann Neurol* 1999; 45: 568-76.

- Tassi L, Colombo N, Garbelli R, et al. Focal cortical dysplasia: neuropathological subtypes, EEG, neuroimaging and surgical outcome. *Brain* 2002; 125: 1719-32.
- Thom M, Eriksson S, Martinian L, et al. Temporal lobe sclerosis associated with hippocampal sclerosis in temporal lobe epilepsy: neuropathological features. *J Neuropathol Exp Neurol* 2009; 68: 928-38.
- Thom M, Martinian L, Williams G, Stoeber K, Sisodiya SM. Cell proliferation and granule cell dispersion in human hippocampal sclerosis. *J Neuropathol Exp Neurol* 2005a; 64: 194-201.
- Thom M, Zhou J, Martinian L, Sisodiya S. Quantitative post-mortem study of the hippocampus in chronic epilepsy: seizures do not inevitably cause neuronal loss. *Brain* 2005b; 128: 1344-57.
- Walther C. Hippocampal terminology: concepts, misconceptions, origins. *Endeavour* 2002; 26: 41-4.
- Wieser HG. ILAE Commission Report. Mesial temporal lobe epilepsy with hippocampal sclerosis. *Epilepsia* 2004; 45: 695-714.
- Wyler AR, Dohan FC, Schweitzer JB, Berry AD. A grading system for mesial temporal pathology (hippocampal sclerosis) from anterior temporal lobectomy. *J Epilepsy* 1992; 5: 220-5.
- Zeineh MM, Engel SA, Thompson PM, Bookheimer SY. Dynamics of the hippocampus during encoding and retrieval of face-name pairs. *Science* 2003; 299: 577-80.
- Zhao S, Chai X, Forster E, Frotscher M. Reelin is a positional signal for the lamination of dentate granule cells. *Development* 2004; 131: 5117-25.

Genetics of mesial temporal lobe epilepsy and febrile seizures

Jocelyn F. Bautista

Cleveland Clinic Lerner College of Medicine; Cleveland Clinic Epilepsy Center, USA

Mesial temporal lobe epilepsy (MTLE) has traditionally been considered a purely acquired disorder, however, there have been a number of familial temporal lobe epilepsy syndromes described in recent years. Such syndromes have provided insight into the phenotypic spectrum of MTLE. This chapter will review the familial mesial temporal lobe epilepsy (FMTLE) syndromes, the genetics of sporadic MTLE, and the genetics of febrile seizures.

■ Familial mesial temporal lobe epilepsy

Clinical features

FMTLE was first described in a study of 38 affected individuals from 13 unrelated families (Berkovic *et al.*, 1996). Affected individuals had a mean age of epilepsy onset of 24 years, and no history of febrile seizures or other risk factors. Epilepsy was relatively mild in these individuals, with seizures either in remission or well controlled by medication. Some individuals had only *déjà-vu* aura. For those who underwent MRI, there was no evidence of hippocampal sclerosis. Pedigree analysis suggested autosomal dominant inheritance with incomplete penetrance. This initial description of FMTLE painted a picture quite distinct from the refractory sporadic MTLE commonly seen in epilepsy surgery centres.

Since this initial report, several other families have been identified, and it has become clear that not all FMTLE is benign. In a study of 36 affected individuals from 11 families (Cendes *et al.*, 1998), 41% had pharmacoresistant epilepsy, and 22% had a history of febrile seizures. Four affected individuals had hippocampal atrophy on MRI and three underwent epilepsy surgery; surgical pathology confirmed hippocampal sclerosis. In a related study of MRI in asymptomatic family members, hippocampal atrophy was observed in 34% with associated abnormal T2 signal in 27% (Kobayashi *et al.*, 2002).

Clearly, there is a great deal of intra- and interfamilial variability in FMTLE. Kobayashi *et al.* classified families into those with: benign MTLE in which all affected family members have seizures either in remission or well controlled by antiepileptic medication (41% of their population), severe MTLE in which all affected family members have pharmacoresistant MTLE (5% of their population), and both benign and severe MTLE (54% of their population) (Kobayashi et al., 2001).

If we compare individuals with refractory/pharmacoresistant FMTLE to those with refractory/pharmacoresistant sporadic, or non-familial MTLE, are there any differences, particularly with regards to surgical outcome or surgical pathology? One concern is that individuals with a familial or genetic epilepsy syndrome are at higher risk of more diffuse brain abnormalities which could negatively impact prognosis following epilepsy surgery. In a study of 20 patients with FMTLE who underwent surgery (six with selective amygdalohippocampectomy and 14 with anterior temporal lobectomy with resection of mesial structures) 17 (85%) were found to be in Engel class I (free of disabling seizures) following surgery (Kobayashi et al., 2003). In another study comparing 20 individuals with FMTLE and 39 with sporadic MTLE, 15/20 (75%) of the familial cases, compared to 36/39 (92%) of the sporadic cases, were classified as Engel class I following epilepsy surgery with mean follow-up of 4.3 years (Andrade-Valenca et al., 2008). This difference did not reach statistical significance, however, the study may not have been sufficiently powered to detect a difference of this size. This study also compared surgical pathological results and found no clear differences in hippocampal cell density but did find greater mossy fibre sprouting in sporadic, compared to familial, cases. The exact significance of these pathological findings is not entirely clear and it remains to be seen whether there is a true difference in outcome following epilepsy surgery in familial *vs.* sporadic MTLE patients.

Genetics of familial mesial temporal lobe epilepsy

To date, a handful of loci have been identified in families with MTLE. Linkage to 12q22 was identified in one five-generation family with 22 affected members (10 with febrile seizures and TLE, 11 with TLE, and one with febrile seizures alone) (Claes et al., 2004). Spontaneous remission was seen in 11 patients while three patients developed pharmacoresistant epilepsy. Hippocampal sclerosis was not observed on MRI. A genome scan was performed and linkage to 12q22 was identified; the disease haplotype was observed in all 22 affected and in four asymptomatic individuals, suggesting incomplete penetrance.

Evidence for digenic inheritance was observed in one three-generation French family with nine affected individuals (Baulac et al., 2001). All nine affected individuals had simple febrile seizures before five years of age; eight developed subsequent epilepsy, seven had focal epilepsy and one had generalised tonic-clonic seizures without clear focality. Outcome was "good" in seven patients (antiepileptic medication was withdrawn by 24 years of age) and one had pharmacoresistant epilepsy. A genome scan was performed and linkage was identified to 18qter and 1q25 with haplotype analysis suggesting digenic inheritance.

In a third family with 11 affected individuals over three generations, linkage was observed to 4q13 (Hedera et al., 2007). Affected individuals had no history of febrile seizures and all had a benign course. Two candidate genes were excluded: *SLC4*, which encodes for a sodium bicarbonate cotransporter and is important for tissue excitability, and *CCN1* which encodes for cyclin 1 and plays a role in cell migration. A number of other families with MTLE have been described, but specific genetic defects have yet to be identified for FMTLE.

Genetics of sporadic mesial temporal lobe epilepsy

There have been a number of association studies implicating various polymorphisms in non-familial or sporadic MTLE, but for the most part, the evidence has been inconclusive and findings have been difficult to replicate. Associations with sporadic TLE have been reported with several genes including the IL-1beta gene, *PRNP* (cellular prion protein gene), *PDYN* (prodynorphin gene), and *GABBR1*, but follow-up studies are conflicting (Cavalleri et al., 2005). Discordant reports are common in case-control association studies of susceptibility alleles and may be due to differences in study design, case definition, and population ethnicity and genetic background. In addition, multiple testing, ascertainment bias, and small sample sizes lacking statistical power often play a role.

The association between MTLE and febrile seizures is a consistent finding. In some retrospective surgical series, 60-80% of TLE patients have a history of febrile seizures. Given that not all children with fever develop febrile seizures, and that, furthermore, not all children with complex febrile seizures go on to develop epilepsy, there appears to be a role for genetic susceptibility in the risk for febrile seizures as well as subsequent epilepsy. The exact relationship between febrile seizures and MTLE is complex and a matter of debate, however, the association has led some to wonder whether FMTLE is simply a reflection of an underlying susceptibility to febrile seizures.

Genetics of febrile seizures

We know from twin studies, family studies, and segregation analysis that febrile seizures have a genetic component. While a small proportion of febrile seizures are due to monogenic or simple inheritance, the vast majority are likely to exhibit complex genetic inheritance, due to multiple genes and multiple environmental factors.

There are several loci (FEB1-10) associated with familial febrile seizures. Two loci (FEB3 and FEB4) were shown to be associated with specific genetic defects. The FEB4 locus was identified in one large Japanese family and subsequently confirmed in 39 nuclear families (Nakayama et al., 2000). Of 48 families with familial febrile seizures, mutations were identified in the *MASS1* (monogenic audiogenic seizure susceptibility) gene at the FEB4 locus in one family with febrile and afebrile seizures (Nakayama et al., 2002). A mutation in the *SCN1A* gene at the FEB3 locus was later identified in another family with 12 individuals with afebrile seizures, of whom three developed subsequent MTLE (Mantegazza et al., 2005). Mutations in *SCN1A* are also seen in generalised epilepsy with febrile seizures plus (GEFS+). The GEFS+ phenotype is quite broad, but the "classic" phenotype consists of febrile seizures persisting beyond six years of age. Individuals subsequently develop afebrile seizures, typically dialeptic (absence) or generalised tonic-clonic seizures. While afebrile seizures are typically generalised, focal epilepsy syndromes have also been described in individuals with GEFS+. One report described a proband with pharmacoresistant MTLE, preceded by prolonged febrile seizures beyond six years of age, with evidence of hippocampal sclerosis based on MRI (Abou-Khalil et al., 2001). Of the total 27 affected family members, 19 also had febrile seizures (11 with generalised epilepsy, seven with focal, and one undetermined). All affected individuals, regardless of their epilepsy syndrome, had the same *SCN1A* mutation.

It is not clear how fever causes seizures, but there is some evidence to suggest that temperature-dependent changes in GABA receptors may play a role. In a study of the *GABRG2* mutations seen in GEFS+ individuals, Kang et al. expressed mutant *GABRG2* sequences of subunits and measured the surface expression of mutant channels (Kang et al., 2006). They found that increases in temperature produced decreased surface expression of GABA receptors. The implication is that fever causes a reduction in inhibitory GABA function in the brain, leading to network excitability.

■ Conclusions

There are multiple possible genetic mechanisms at play in the development of febrile seizures and/or MTLE, from single major genes in the familial forms to the combination of multiple genetic and non-genetic factors in the sporadic forms (Figure 1), however, we are still in the early stages of identifying and understanding these factors. FMTLE is a heterogeneous disorder with intra and inter-familial variability. While a significant portion of individuals with FMTLE appear to have a relatively mild epilepsy, those individuals with pharmacoresistant FMTLE are difficult to distinguish from those with pharmacoresistant sporadic MTLE. Surgical outcome appears to be similar, thus a familial form of MTLE is not a contraindication for surgery. The relationship between MTLE and febrile seizures in humans is complex and not well understood, but there are clearly genetic factors which underlie both febrile seizures and MTLE.

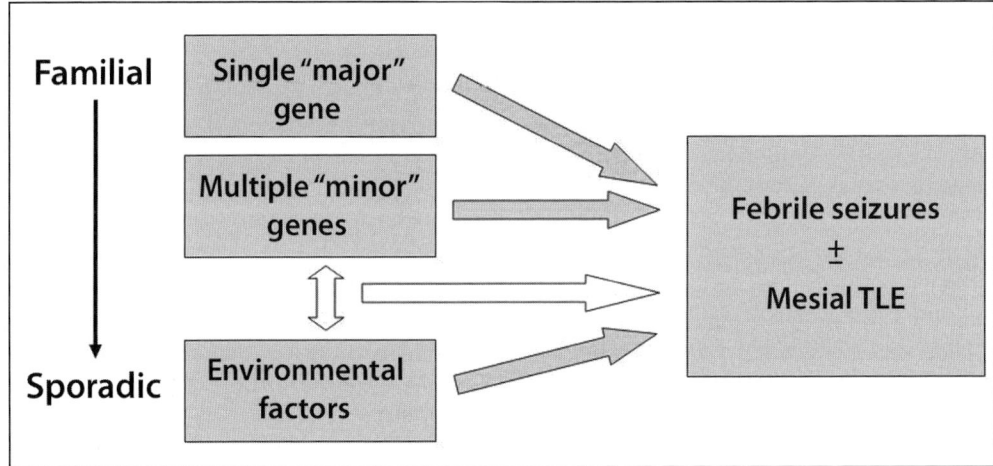

Figure 1. Genetics of mesial temporal lobe epilepsy (TLE) and febrile seizures.

While a great deal of progress has been made in the genetics of epilepsy, we still have a long way to go. Further work in this field is expected to lead to improved methods of diagnosis and treatment, the ability to predict response and ultimately prevent epilepsy in those at risk.

References

- Abou-Khalil B, Ge Q, Desai R, Ryther R, Bazyk A, Bailey R, et al. Partial and generalized epilepsy with febrile seizures plus and a novel SCN1A mutation. Neurology 2001; 57: 2265-72.
- Andrade-Valença LP, Valença MM, Velasco TR, Carlotti CG Jr, Assirati JA, Galvis-Alonso OY, et al. Mesial temporal lobe epilepsy: clinical and neuropathologic findings of familial and sporadic forms. Epilepsia 2008; 49: 1046-54.

- Baulac S, Picard F, Herman A, Feingold J, Genin E, Hirsch E, et al. Evidence for digenic inheritance in a family with both febrile convulsions and temporal lobe epilepsy implicating chromosomes 18qter and 1q25-q31. *Ann Neurol* 2001; 49: 786-92.
- Berkovic SF, McIntosh A, Howell RA, Mitchell A, Sheffield LJ, Hopper JL. Familial temporal lobe epilepsy: a common disorder identified in twins. *Ann Neurol* 1996; 40: 227-35.
- Cavalleri GL, Lynch JM, Depondt C, Burley MW, Wood NW, Sisodiya SM, Goldstein DB. Failure to replicate previously reported genetic associations with sporadic temporal lobe epilepsy: where to from here? *Brain* 2005; 128: 1832-40.
- Cendes F, Lopes-Cendes I, Andermann E, Andermann F. Familial temporal lobe epilepsy: a clinically heterogeneous syndrome. *Neurology* 1998; 50: 554-7.
- Claes L, Audenaert D, Deprez L, Van Paesschen W, Depondt C, Goossens D, et al. Novel locus on chromosome 12q22-q23.3 responsible for familial temporal lobe epilepsy associated with febrile seizures. *J Med Genet* 2004; 41: 710-4.
- Hedera P, Blair MA, Andermann E, Andermann F, D'Agostino D, Taylor KA, et al. Familial mesial temporal lobe epilepsy maps to chromosome 4q13.2-q21.3. *Neurology* 2007; 68: 2107-12.
- Kang JQ, Shen W, Macdonald RL. Why does fever trigger febrile seizures? GABAA receptor gamma2 subunit mutations associated with idiopathic generalized epilepsies have temperature-dependent trafficking deficiencies. *J Neurosci* 2006; 26: 2590-7.
- Kobayashi E, Lopes-Cendes I, Guerreiro CA, Sousa SC, Guerreiro MM, Cendes F. Seizure outcome and hippocampal atrophy in familial mesial temporal lobe epilepsy. *Neurology* 2001; 56: 166-72.
- Kobayashi E, Li LM, Lopes-Cendes I, Cendes F. Magnetic resonance imaging evidence of hippocampal sclerosis in asymptomatic, first-degree relatives of patients with familial mesial temporal lobe epilepsy. *Arch Neurol* 2002; 59: 1891-4.
- Kobayashi E, D'Agostino MD, Lopes-Cendes I, Andermann E, Dubeau F, Guerreiro CA, et al. Outcome of surgical treatment in familial mesial temporal lobe epilepsy. *Epilepsia* 2003; 44: 1080-4.
- Mantegazza M, Gambardella A, Rusconi R, Schiavon E, Annesi F, Cassulini RR, et al. Identification of an Na(v)1.1 sodium channel (SCN1A) loss-of-function mutation associated with familial simple febrile seizures. *Proc Nat Acad Sci* 2005; 102: 18177-82.
- Nakayama J, Hamano K, Iwasaki N, Nakahara S, Horigome Y, Saitoh H, et al. Significant evidence for linkage of febrile seizures to chromosome 5q14-q15. *Hum Mol Genet* 2000; 9: 87-91.
- Nakayama J, Fu YH, Clark AM, Nakahara S, Hamano K, Iwasaki N, et al. A nonsense mutation of the MASS1 gene in a family with febrile and afebrile seizures. *Ann Neurol* 2002; 52: 654-7.

Animal models of temporal lobe epilepsy with hippocampal sclerosis: moving beyond chemoconvulsant-induced status epilepticus

Hemant S. Kudrimoti, Robert S. Sloviter

Departments of Neurology and Pharmacology, University of Arizona College of Medicine, Tucson, USA

Understanding the aetiologies and mechanisms of any human neurological disorder requires animal models that have at least some of the features and mechanisms of that disorder. Although an obvious truism, it is also correct to say that, for practical reasons, we use the models that we have always used, others have used, are easy to use, and know how to use. Animals subjected to chemoconvulsant-induced status epilepticus (SE) have long been suggested to be models of human mesial temporal lobe epilepsy (MTLE) with hippocampal sclerosis (Pisa et al., 1980; Nadler, 1981; Ben-Ari, 1985), and this has been the dominant view for years (Leite et al., 2002; Stables et al., 2003). However, the results of several decades of research on possible epileptogenic mechanisms have raised the question of whether animals subjected to prolonged, chemoconvulsant-induced SE resemble human patients with MTLE and hippocampal sclerosis. It seems obvious, in retrospect, that prolonged convulsive SE in animals is an excellent model for prolonged convulsive SE in humans, which may cause extensive brain damage, cognitive impairment, and spontaneous seizures as part of a larger syndrome of severe brain damage (Fujikawa et al., 2000; Mikaeloff et al., 2006). The question we raise here is whether prolonged convulsive SE in animals produces an animal model that resembles the much more subtle condition of human MTLE with hippocampal sclerosis.

The primary appeal of chemoconvulsant-treated animals is that they can be easily produced simply by injecting a chemoconvulsant agent into a normal rodent, and virtually all of the animals that develop convulsive SE, and do not die, have widespread brain damage and are chronically epileptic (Cavalheiro et al., 1991). However, the assumption that all surviving animals become spontaneously epileptic because they have specifically undergone "hippocampal epileptogenesis" has led to the secondary assumption that any hippocampal abnormalities that can be detected following convulsive SE can be linked to epileptogenic mechanisms, even though these animals have not been shown to exhibit hippocampal-onset seizures (Harvey & Sloviter, 2005). The assumption that the hippocampus of epileptic animals is reliably "epileptic" has had profound consequences for the interpretation of experimental results because it has been assumed that the occurrence of spontaneous motor seizures in extensively brain-damaged animals is a reliable indication that a process of hippocampal epileptogenesis has occurred (Harvey & Sloviter, 2005). It is particularly strange that this assumption has become so well-established given that the initial thorough pathological study of kainate-treated rats clearly stated that the hippocampus was among the least affected structures following systemic injection of kainate (Schwob et al., 1980). In this chapter, we focus on the features of human MTLE, and the issue of whether animals subjected to prolonged convulsive SE exhibit any of the defining features of human MTLE.

Which features of human mesial temporal lobe epilepsy need to be modelled?

MTLE, the most common epilepsy syndrome, is seen in a majority of patients with partial-onset epilepsy (Semah et al., 1998; Engel, 2001). Patients with relatively innocuous MTLE symptoms (e.g. gustatory or olfactory auras) or secondary generalised seizures have only subtle functional neurological deficits interictally (e.g. short-term memory complaints), often present no clear history of risk factors for epilepsy (e.g., family history, head injuries, encephalitis, or febrile seizures), usually have normal routine neurological examinations, and often have normal MRI scans of the brain. Indeed, only a small percentage of newly-diagnosed MTLE patients have visually detectable hippocampal sclerosis (Berg et al., 2000; Salmenperä et al., 2005), let alone widespread brain damage. Although the syndrome of MTLE with hippocampal sclerosis may constitute approximately 44% of refractory MTLE cases (Semah et al., 1998) and between 50 and 70% of surgical MTLE cases (Cavanagh & Meyer, 1956; Bruton, 1988), hippocampal atrophy was noted on initial MRI in only 8% of partial-onset epilepsy cases, and serial MRIs scheduled after 1-5 years of treatment showed that only 13% of patients developed hippocampal volume decreases during this period (Salmenperä et al., 2005). These and earlier observations (Van Paesschen et al., 1997; Liu et al., 2002; Lehericy et al., 1997) suggest that the true prevalence of MRI-detectable hippocampal sclerosis in the overall MTLE patient population is approximately 10%. The large patient subpopulation lacking detectable hippocampal atrophy presumably includes patients with: 1) minimal or no detectable hippocampal neuron loss, and; 2) those with relatively selective neuron loss in the dentate hilus (endfolium sclerosis), which alone does not cause significant hippocampal shrinkage detectable by routine MRI. Epilepsy in a brain that does not exhibit severe hippocampal atrophy or any other obvious brain abnormality may be relatively amenable to drug treatment, and the presence of classic hippocampal sclerosis is a sign of the most refractory form of temporal lobe epilepsy. This is suspected, but not known with certainty (Cardoso et al., 2006). Because patients with MTLE and classic hippocampal sclerosis may report an antecedent episode of febrile seizures (Sagar & Oxbury, 1987; Kuks et al., 1993; Maher & McLachlan, 1995), head injury with loss of consciousness or amnesia (Falconer et al., 1964; Williamson et al., 1993; Marks et al., 1995) or meningoencephalitis (French et al., 1993), an initial brain injury is a suspected cause of both hippocampal sclerosis and hippocampal epileptogenesis.

MTLE with hippocampal sclerosis is only rarely associated with a history of generalised SE (Bruton, 1988; French et al., 1993). Afebrile convulsive SE usually does not lead to hippocampal sclerosis (Scott et al., 2002), and has significant associated morbidity and mortality as a result of widespread brain damage and refractory seizures, the sources of which are not clearly identifiable (Cavanagh & Meyer, 1956; Teitelbaum et al., 1990; DeLorenzo et al., 1996, Lowenstein & Alldredge, 1998; Fujikawa et al., 2000). Patients who survive prolonged SE can develop diffuse cortical atrophy and significant neurological deficits including severe cognitive impairment, in addition to intractable epilepsy (Jambaqué et al., 2006; Mikaeloff et al., 2006; Bauer et al., 2006; Korngut et al., 2007; Chevret et al., 2008). Conversely, most patients with MTLE and hippocampal sclerosis, have relatively innocuous risk factors, do not have functional neurological deficits according to history or routine neurological examination (French et al., 1993), and do not have evidence of extensive brain injury on routine brain MRI scans, even if scans demonstrate hippocampal sclerosis (Van Paesschen et al., 1997). MTLE patients have relatively subtle cognitive impairment, but often have medically refractory seizures of temporal lobe origin (Engel, 2001; Spencer, 2002a). Thus, unlike the syndrome of severe brain damage, cognitive impairment, and recurrent seizures that can result from a prolonged episode of convulsive SE (e.g., Mikaeloff et al., 2006), MTLE is characterized by unprovoked seizures that develop following relatively subtle brain damage in otherwise relatively normal patients (French et al., 1993; Engel, 1996).

■ The possible significance of classic hippocampal sclerosis

Hippocampal sclerosis refers to a specific pattern of selective hippocampal neuron loss and survival that has been recognized as a distinct pathological entity since the early 19th century (Bouchet & Cazauvieilh, 1825), and was subsequently described histologically (Sommer, 1880; Bratz, 1899). However, a detailed clinico-pathological post-mortem analysis of chronically hospitalised epilepsy patients was not made until the study of Margerison and Corsellis (1966). Their autopsy study of the entire brain of 55 patients revealed that: 1) a minority of patient brains exhibited classic hippocampal sclerosis (extensive hilar and pyramidal layer neuron loss with partial or predominant survival of dentate granule cells and CA2 pyramidal cells [the "resistant zone"]); 2) the only common pathology present in all epileptic patients with any detectable hippocampal pathology was neuron loss in the hilus of the dentate gyrus (endfolium sclerosis); and 3) some patients exhibited no obvious hippocampal neuron loss (Margerison & Corsellis, 1966). Importantly, Margerison and Corsellis emphasised that most patients did not exhibit widespread or severe brain damage, and noted that temporal lobe epilepsy was associated with multifocal, but limited, brain damage (Margerison & Corsellis, 1966). Thus, unlike animals subjected to prolonged convulsive SE (Harvey & Sloviter, 2005), MTLE patients with classic hippocampal sclerosis do not have evidence of extensive extrahippocampal or extratemporal brain injury on routine brain MRI scans, rarely have a history of convulsive status epilepticus (Bruton, 1988; Van Paesschen et al., 1997), and often have medically refractory seizures of temporal lobe origin (Engel 2001; French et al., 1993; Jackson et al., 2004; de Lanerolle et al., 2005).

Although classic hippocampal sclerosis occurs in a small minority of all MTLE patients (Blümcke et al., 2007), it is of special significance since a sclerotic and atrophied hippocampus is often the only obvious pathology in medically-intractable patients, and its presence is an indicator of a good surgical outcome (Semah et al., 1998; Wiebe et al., 2001). Because patients with MTLE and classic hippocampal sclerosis may report an antecedent episode of febrile seizures, infection, or head trauma (French et al., 1993), an initial brain injury is a suspected cause of both hippocampal sclerosis and hippocampal epileptogenesis (Mathern et al., 1994). However, the vast majority of children who experience febrile seizures do not subsequently develop epilepsy (Annegers et al., 1987; Berg & Shinnar, 1997; Berg et al., 1999) and some patients with MTLE and hippocampal sclerosis do not report any clinical risk factors, suggesting that other factors may be involved. A recent series of case reports has described hippocampal oedema following prolonged focal febrile seizures that subsequently resulted in hippocampal atrophy (Van Landingham et al., 1998, Perez et al., 2000; Grünewald et al., 2001; Scott et al., 2002; 2003; 2006; Sokol et al., 2003, Farrow et al., 2006; Natsume et al., 2007, Provenzale et al., 2008). These reports suggest the possibility of a pre-existing hippocampal abnormality (Fernández et al., 1998) provoking focal febrile status epilepticus in children, resulting in MTLE with classic hippocampal sclerosis later (Kälviäinen et al., 1998). On the other hand, brief febrile seizures and subsequent afebrile epilepsy may be two unconnected effects of a pre-existing abnormality (Annegers et al., 1987; Auer et al., 2008) that manifests itself at early age as febrile seizures, and later as recurrent, unprovoked, afebrile seizures. Brief febrile seizures may be innocuous in most children, however, if particularly prolonged (Maher & McLachlan, 1995) or of a certain frequency or intensity (Sloviter et al., 2007), the prolonged excitation at an early age (Marks et al., 1992) produces classic hippocampal sclerosis immediately, followed by the refractory form of MTLE. Alternatively, brief febrile seizures may damage only the most vulnerable neurons (Sloviter, 1994a) or cause other subtle effects (Dubé et al., 2006), and the extensive loss of hippocampal neurons that characterises classic hippocampal sclerosis may be the progressive result of many years of recurrent afebrile seizures (Briellmann et al., 2002; Pitkänen & Sutula, 2002; Fuerst et al., 2003: Gorter et al., 2003). Whether classic hippocampal sclerosis is caused by a single initial insult in a minority of patients or by years of spontaneous seizures following an initial injury, is still unclear. In either scenario, other factors need to be taken into account, including the possible roles of inflammation and elevated temperature in the aetiology of epileptic pathology (Vezzani et al., 2008).

The possible causal or synergistic relationship between brain insults, the presence of hippocampal sclerosis in the absence of widespread brain injury, and the development of epilepsy raises many questions about the roles of injury and cell death in epileptogenesis, as well as the relative importance of cell loss and the secondary processes that cell loss may trigger (Tauck & Nadler, 1985; Sloviter, 1992). Although its aetiology and its exact pathophysiological significance are incompletely understood, hippocampal atrophy has long been considered to be a sign of a seizure focus in refractory patients because depth electrode recordings demonstrate hypersynchronous electrical activity associated with auras originating from this region, and surgical removal of the hippocampus and adjacent medial temporal structures generally reduces seizure frequency (Wiebe et al., 2001). Assuming that the atrophic hippocampus is a source of seizures, which surviving hippocampal neurons become the source of the seizures? Does the initial loss of vulnerable hippocampal neurons cause an immediate network defect that results in hippocampal hyperexcitability, or does initial neuron loss have little direct role other than as a trigger of a delayed secondary epileptogenic process? Since the atrophic hippocampus and its closely related structures are the apparent source of many of the spontaneous seizures that define the disorder (Spencer, 1998; 2002a; Jackson et al., 2004), surviving dentate granule cells and subicular neurons are among the most commonly suspected sources (Sloviter, 1987; 1994b; Cohen et al., 2002). Although the injured hippocampus is believed to be a critical epileptogenic component, growing evidence points to additional temporal lobe sources of seizure onset (Margerison and Corsellis, 1966; Du et al., 1993; Spencer, 1998, 2002a; Salmenperä et al., 2000; Schwarcz et al., 2000; Bertram et al., 2001; Wennberg et al., 2002; Bernasconi et al., 2003; see also Bartolomei in this book).

If extrahippocampal temporal lobe structures are frequent sources of seizures (Spencer, 1998; 2002a), is the severely atrophic hippocampus really crucial for clinical seizures to occur, or is it little more than the remaining visual evidence of past involvement, before the most extensive cell loss occurred? The answers to these questions involve many variables that include the relationships between pre-existing defects, brief febrile seizures, prolonged febrile seizures, head injuries, temporal lobe pathology, the latent period between injury and epilepsy, the putative mechanisms that mediate epileptogenesis including neuronal loss and reorganization, and the network, cellular, and molecular changes that result from neuronal injury (Sloviter, 1991; 1992; 1994a; 1994b). None of these questions are readily answered by studying human patients because patients are highly heterogeneous, historical information is incomplete, different patients have different pathologies and clinical characteristics, and few experimental manipulations or analyses are possible in human patients. Thus, human data are valuable, not because they provide definitive answers to compelling questions, but because they generate testable hypotheses based on clinico-pathological correlations.

The difficulty inherent in studying patients in order to understand the epileptogenic process gives experimental animal models unparalleled heuristic value. A principal issue considered here is whether any of the existing convulsive SE-based animal models resemble MTLE with hippocampal sclerosis, and more importantly, whether an abnormality in one brain structure of an epileptic rat, when the structure(s) responsible for the seizures is unknown, can be causally related to the epileptogenic mechanism. The implications of using prolonged convulsive SE to produce epileptic animals go beyond whether the lesions produced in animals closely resemble the pathologies seen in human surgical pathology specimens. Clearly, the often small proportion of rats that survive the initial episode of convulsive SE go on to have epilepsy, but do these seizures arise from mesial temporal lobe structures, or even involve the hippocampus? Is the brain injury relatively limited, as seen in humans, or is there evidence of widespread brain damage, not typically present in patients with MTLE? Mindful of the defining features of the human neurological condition that we are trying to reproduce in animals, we consider below some of the assumptions that underlie current conceptions about the nature and duration of the epileptogenic process, and we address the properties and possible deficiencies of some of the animal models most commonly used to identify likely mechanisms underlying refractory MTLE with classic hippocampal sclerosis.

■ Main assumptions about animal models of temporal lobe epilepsy

Current conceptions of hippocampal epileptogenesis in animal models have been significantly influenced, historically and experimentally, by three factors: 1) the assertion that prolonged convulsive status epilepticus in animals produces pathology, including hippocampal sclerosis, that resembles the pathology of human MTLE (Nadler, 1981; Ben-Ari, 1985); 2) the assumption that following prolonged convulsive status epilepticus, animals reliably exhibit a seizure-free, "pre-epileptic" latent period before spontaneous seizures begin (Leite et al., 2002; Stables et al., 2003); and 3) animals subjected to prolonged convulsive status epilepticus have specifically undergone a process of hippocampal epileptogenesis, which underlies the widespread assumption that the hippocampus is the source of the spontaneous seizures that develop in these animals (Tauck & Nadler, 1985; Wuarin & Dudek, 1996).

Convulsive status epilepticus-induced brain damage

Although the features of human refractory MTLE typically include extensive hippocampal atrophy and limited extrahippocampal damage (Margerison & Corsellis, 1966), animals subjected to prolonged convulsive status epilepticus exhibit the reverse pattern of pathology, i.e. extensive extrahippocampal damage, but limited hippocampal pathology (Schwob et al., 1980; Turski et al., 1983; Chen & Buckmaster, 2005; Harvey & Sloviter, 2005; Niessen et al., 2005). Convulsive SE in rats produces widespread injury to extrahippocampal structures (Schwob et al., 1980; Brandt et al., 2003; Chen & Buckmaster, 2005; Harvey & Sloviter, 2005), confounding determination of the role of hippocampal injury in epileptogenesis. Moreover, the human pattern of hippocampal pathology is not replicated in these animal models (Sloviter et al., 2007), and the hippocampus may not be a source of seizure onset in these models (Harvey & Sloviter, 2005). Convulsive SE, induced by systemically administered chemoconvulsants, is associated with a high rate of mortality (Glien et al., 2001; Goffin et al., 2007), which means a biased population is comprised of only the animals available, i.e. those that survive, presumably because their seizures are less severe. The death of the "best" animals may explain why surviving animals have variable and often minimal hippocampal damage (Schwob et al., 1980), i.e. hippocampal involvement may exacerbate seizure spread and lethality, leaving animals that had less seizure-related hippocampal involvement. Chemoconvulsants initiate seizure activity in multiple sites by unknown mechanisms, result in highly variable patterns of excitotoxic brain damage, and often involve severe vascular changes that cause ischaemic injury (Sloviter, 2005; Fabene et al., 2007). Since most animals subjected to SE-induced injury exhibit spontaneous seizures within days of injury (Raol et al., 2006; Goffin et al., 2007; Jung et al., 2007; Bumanglag & Sloviter, 2008), the observation that some animals exhibit a delay before the first generalised motor seizure is detected (Cavalheiro et al., 1982; Hamani & Mello, 2002; Gorter et al., 2001; Mazarati et al., 2002; van Vliet et al., 2004; D'Ambrosio et al., 2005; El-Hassar et al., 2007) may reflect differences in the extent or location of damage, rather than the development of a delayed secondary process that must mature before epilepsy develops. There appears, therefore, to be little justification for the widespread notion that the brains of rats that survive kainate or pilocarpine-induced convulsive status epilepticus, resemble the limited pathology and the pattern of hippocampal injury present in the brains of MTLE patients.

The latent period

Few issues have had a greater impact on how we think about the epileptogenic process than the concept of the latent period. Determination of the interval between a brain injury and the onset of clinical epilepsy led to the idea of the latent period, as the time it takes for a slowly progressing epileptogenic process to "ripen" (Earle et al., 1953). The notion that the initial post-SE absence of clinical seizures reflects a quiescent "pre-epileptic" state after injury, and that the duration of this state accurately reflects the duration of a slowly developing process of hippocampal epileptogenesis, has logically led to the search for molecular, cellular, and network changes that are initially absent, but subsequently develop gradually during the period before spontaneous epileptic seizures begin

(Chang & Lowenstein, 2003). The concept of the latent period, as the time required for a distinct secondary process to mature, involves several significant conceptual problems. First, a significant proportion of patients with MTLE and hippocampal sclerosis do not have any obvious history of brain injury from which a latent period might be calculated. Second, latent periods are calculated as the time between a presumed injury and the emergence of clinical epilepsy. However, many injuries that can be remembered by a patient under questioning may have had no causal role in the development of the epilepsy. Third, injury-induced epileptogenesis may result in an abnormal, epileptic brain long before the first clinical seizure is verified by a physician. Fourth, it is not at all clear whether the duration of the latent period is an accurate reflection of the duration of the epileptogenic process. If so, it is difficult to conceive of a molecular or structural process that may take 30 years to mature, and is, furthermore, impractical to study. Latent periods can be very short or very long, possibly depending on the severity or nature of the insult (French et al., 1993; Mathern et al., 1994; Lhatoo et al., 2001; Mikaeloff et al., 2006), and it is doubtful that different latent periods reflect uniquely different processes that mature at different rates.

It is difficult to overemphasize the conceptual importance of the latent period to the design and interpretation of many of the experimental epilepsy studies conducted during the past 25 years. The notion that rats subjected to kainate or pilocarpine-induced convulsive SE exhibit a seizure-free (pre-epileptic) "latent period" before spontaneous seizures occur was the primary justification for suggesting that delayed secondary processes, such as synaptic reorganization or neurogenesis, are likely epileptogenic mechanisms (Tauck & Nadler, 1985; Parent et al., 1997; Chang & Lowenstein, 2003). Clearly, if rats are epileptic in the first days after SE (either subclinically or clinically), when neurons are actively degenerating, there would be no time for delayed secondary processes to be involved in the causation of the spontaneous seizures, and epileptogenesis would then be coincident with the initial injury, rather than a delayed secondary process (Mazarati et al., 2002; Bumanglag & Sloviter, 2008; Mouri et al., 2008).

We attribute the enduring notion of a seizure-free, "pre-epileptic" period of several weeks duration after convulsive SE in rats (Leite et al., 2002; Stables et al., 2003) to the way in which the discovery of spontaneous seizures in kainate-treated rats was first reported, and how it has been reinforced by non-continuous behavioural monitoring methods. In the first description of spontaneous seizures after SE, of which we are aware, Pisa and colleagues (1980) reported that spontaneous seizures were observed 35-77 days post-SE. However, these authors only started their behavioural observations on day 35 post-SE, presumably because they were addressing the issue of whether, and not when, spontaneous seizures developed. The notion of the post-SE latent period being an extended period when epileptogenesis slowly develops has been repeatedly reinforced by studies using non-continuous monitoring methods (Cavalheiro et al., 1982; Nissinen et al., 2000; Glien et al., 2001; Brandt et al., 2003). However, recent studies of rats monitored continuously after chemoconvulsant-induced SE have reported that spontaneous seizures begin less than one week post-SE (Raol et al., 2006; Goffin et al., 2007). Importantly, a recent study which involved continuous monitoring only on days three and six post-SE reported that pilocarpine-treated rats were spontaneously epileptic during the first week after convulsive SE which lasted for only one hour (Jung et al., 2007). The development of spontaneous hippocampal-onset seizures after chemoconvulsant and perforant pathway stimulation-induced SE during the early neurodegenerative phase (Bumanglag & Sloviter, 2008) would seem to preclude even hypothetical involvement of delayed secondary changes in these animal models.

The hippocampus as the presumed source of spontaneous seizures in chemoconvulsant-treated animals

Despite widespread brain damage and a lack of information regarding which brain regions might be the source of the spontaneous seizures that develop following convulsive SE, the hippocampus has nonetheless been assumed to have undergone "epileptogenesis," and to be the source of the spontaneous seizures that develop in these rats. More specifically, the suggestion that granule cell axon sprouting, or other secondary changes in granule cells, are epileptogenic (Tauck & Nadler, 1985) depends entirely on the assumption that the granule cells of the dentate gyrus are the source of the seizures that develop in rats after widespread brain injury. It is difficult to understand why epileptic chemoconvulsant-treated rats, with widespread brain damage and frequent spontaneous seizures of unknown origin, have been so widely assumed to have "epileptic" hippocampi in general, and "epileptic" granule cells in particular, since this has never been demonstrated *in vivo*. Several studies have reported cellular abnormalities in hippocampal slices taken from chronically epileptic rats, and causally related these abnormalities to the epileptogenic process (Tauck & Nadler, 1985; Wuarin & Dudek, 1996), despite a lack of evidence that the hippocampus was in any way involved in generating the spontaneous seizures that defined these often severely brain-damaged animals as "epileptic." On the contrary, studies of neuropathology following systemic kainate or pilocarpine-induced SE have shown that convulsive SE produces widespread and variable brain damage depending on which brain pathways are activated during SE, and that extrahippocampal brain regions are more severely damaged than the hippocampus (Schwob et al., 1980; Turski et al., 1983; André et al., 2007). Furthermore, *in vivo* studies have shown that granule cells in chronically epileptic kainate or pilocarpine-treated rats appear hyperinhibited, rather than hyperexcitable (Sloviter, 1992; Buckmaster & Dudek, 1997; Harvey & Sloviter, 2005; Sloviter et al., 2006). Also, depth recordings from the granule cell layers in awake, epileptic pilocarpine-treated rats during spontaneous seizures have shown that the hippocampus appears to be minimally involved during spontaneous seizures (Harvey & Sloviter, 2005). Thus, there appears to be little experimental justification for assuming that the hippocampus of chemoconvulsant-treated rats has undergone an epileptogenic process simply because the rats exhibit spontaneous behavioural seizures of unknown origin.

■ Conclusions and new directions

Based on the extensive body of information now available on electrical stimulation, and chemoconvulsant-based animal models, the following conclusions serve as a rationale for developing animal models that more closely resemble a human neurological disorder. For the purpose of assessing whether any model replicates classic hippocampal sclerosis, it is important to consider that most MTLE patients have limited, highly localized pathologies, rather than severe and widespread brain damage, and that they exhibit spontaneous seizures of temporal lobe, and often hippocampal, origin (Spencer, 2002b). Given these features of the human neurological condition, an animal model of injury-initiated hippocampal epileptogenesis should ideally and reproducibly involve endfolium or classic hippocampal sclerosis, limited extrahippocampal brain damage, and verified spontaneous hippocampal-onset seizures.

A latent period between injury and clinical epilepsy, although perhaps not a requirement, is nonetheless important as a therapeutic "window" for the development of anti-epileptogenic strategies (White, 2002). Regardless, the duration of the latent period needs to be determined accurately by continuous recording (Goffin *et al.*, 2007) rather than by intermittent observation, which results in an inherently inaccurate overestimate of the length of the latent period because the first behavioural seizures, and all subclinical seizures, are likely to be overlooked. Unlike chemoconvulsants, electrical stimulation of the perforant pathway initiates seizure activity in one focal location by a known mechanism, forces the hippocampus to discharge throughout the duration of stimulation and produces a highly reproducible pattern of hippocampal injury, as well as confirmed hippocampal-onset epileptic seizures (Sloviter *et al.*, 2007; Bumanglag & Sloviter, 2008). By varying stimulus intensity, frequency, and duration, perforant path stimulation produces spontaneously epileptic animals that exhibit endfolium sclerosis or classic hippocampal sclerosis, limited extratemporal damage, minimal mortality, and no non-responders (Sloviter *et al.*, 2007; Bumanglag & Sloviter, 2008). Despite the greater technical effort needed for chronic electrode implantation, the use of newly developed *in vivo* models, in which the temporal lobe is selectively activated throughout the period of stimulation, and that reliably exhibit hippocampal sclerosis and hippocampal-onset seizures (Sloviter *et al.*, 2007; Bumanglag & Sloviter, 2008), should make mechanistic studies of epileptogenesis, neuroprotection, and antiepileptogenesis more feasible and easier to interpret than is currently possible.

Supported by grants NS50181 and NS18201 from the National Institute of Neurological Disorders and Stroke.

References

- André V, Dubé C, François J, Leroy C, Rigoulot MA, Roch C, Namer IJ, Nehlig A. Pathogenesis and pharmacology of epilepsy in the lithium-pilocarpine model. *Epilepsia* 2007; 48 (Suppl 5): 41-7.
- Annegers JF, Hauser WA, Shirts SB, Kurland LT. Factors prognostic of unprovoked seizures after febrile convulsions. *N Engl J Med* 1987; 316: 493-8.
- Auer T, Barsi P, Bone B, Angyalosi A, Aradi M, Szalay C, *et al.* History of simple febrile seizures is associated with hippocampal abnormalities in adults. *Epilepsia* 2008; 49: 1562-9.
- Bauer G, Gotwald T, Dobesberger J, Embacher N, Felber S, Bauer R, *et al.* Transient and permanent magnetic resonance imaging abnormalities after complex partial status epilepticus. *Epilepsy Behav* 2006; 8: 666-71.
- Ben-Ari Y. Limbic seizure and brain damage produced by kainic acid: mechanisms and relevance to human temporal lobe epilepsy. *Neuroscience* 1985; 14: 375-403.
- Berg AT, Shinnar S. Do seizures beget seizures? An assessment of the clinical evidence in humans. *J Clin Neurophysiol* 1997; 14: 102-10.
- Berg AT, Shinnar S, Levy SR, Testa FM. Childhood-onset epilepsy with and without preceding febrile seizures. *Neurology* 1999; 53: 1742-8.
- Berg AT, Testa FM, Levy SR, Shinnar S. Neuroimaging in children with newly diagnosed epilepsy: a community-based study. *Pediatrics* 2000; 106: 527-32.
- Bernasconi N, Bernasconi A, Caramanos Z, Antel SB, Andermann F, Arnold DL. Mesial temporal damage in temporal lobe epilepsy: a volumetric MRI study of the hippocampus, amygdala and parahippocampal region. *Brain* 2003; 126: 462-9.
- Bertram EH, Mangan PS, Zhang D, Scott CA, Williamson JM. The midline thalamus: alterations and a potential role in limbic epilepsy. *Epilepsia* 2001; 42: 967-78.
- Blümcke I, Zuschratter W, Schewe JC, Suter B, Lie AA, Riederer BM, *et al.* 1999. Cellular pathology of hilar neurons in Ammon's horn sclerosis. *J Comp Neurol* 1999; 414: 437-53.

- Bouchet M, Cazauvieilh M. De l'épilepsie considérée dans ses rapports avec l'aliénation mentale. Recherche sur la nature et le siège de ces deux maladies. *Arch Gen Med* 1825; 9: 510-42.
- Brandt C, Glien M, Potschka H, Volk H, Loscher W. Epileptogenesis and neuropathology after different types of status epilepticus induced by prolonged electrical stimulation of the basolateral amygdala in rats. *Epilepsy Res* 2003; 55: 83-103.
- Bratz E. Ammonshornbefunde der Epileptischen. *Arch Psychiat Nervenkr* 1899; 31: 820-36.
- Briellmann RS, Berkovic SF, Syngeniotis A, King MA, Jackson GD. Seizure-associated hippocampal volume loss: a longitudinal magnetic resonance study of temporal lobe epilepsy. *Ann Neurol* 2002; 51: 641-4.
- Bruton CJ. *The Neuropathology of Temporal Lobe Epilepsy*. Oxford: Oxford University Press, 1988.
- Buckmaster PS, Dudek FE. Neuron loss, granule cell axon reorganization, and functional changes in the dentate gyrus of epileptic kainate-treated rats. *J Comp Neurol* 1997; 385: 385-404.
- Bumanglag AV, Sloviter RS. Minimal latency to hippocampal epileptogenesis and clinical epilepsy after perforant pathway stimulation-induced status epilepticus in awake rats. *J Comp Neurol* 2008; 510: 561-80.
- Cardoso TA, Coan AC, Kobayashi E, Guerreiro CA, Li LM, Cendes F. Hippocampal abnormalities and seizure recurrence after antiepileptic drug withdrawal. *Neurology* 2006; 67: 134-6.
- Cavalheiro EA, Riche DA, Le Gal La Salle G. Long-term effects of intrahippocampal kainic acid injection in rats: a method for inducing spontaneous recurrent seizures. *Electroencephalogr Clin Neurophysiol* 1982; 53: 581-9.
- Cavalheiro EA, Leite JP, Bortolotto ZA, Turski WA, Ikonomidou C, Turski L. Long-term effects of pilocarpine in rats: structural damage of the brain triggers kindling and spontaneous recurrent seizures. *Epilepsia* 1991; 32: 778-82.
- Cavanagh JB, Meyer A. Aetiological aspects of Ammon's Horn Sclerosis associated with temporal lobe epilepsy. *Br Med J* 1956; 2: 1403-7.
- Chang BS, Lowenstein DH. Epilepsy. *N Engl J Med* 2003; 349: 1257-66.
- Chen S, Buckmaster PS. Stereological analysis of forebrain regions in kainate-treated epileptic rats. *Brain Res* 2005; 1057: 141-52.
- Chevret L, Husson B, Nguefack S, Nehlig A, Bouilleret V. Prolonged refractory status epilepticus with early and persistent restricted hippocampal signal MRI abnormality. *J Neurol* 2008; 255: 112-6.
- Cohen I, Navarro V, Clemenceau S, Baulac M, Miles R. On the origin of interictal activity in human temporal lobe epilepsy in vitro. *Science* 2002; 298: 1418-21.
- de Lanerolle NC, Kim JH, Williamson A, Spencer SS, Zaveri HP, Eid T, Spencer DD. A retrospective analysis of hippocampal pathology in human temporal lobe epilepsy: evidence for distinctive patient subcategories. *Epilepsia* 2003; 44: 677-87.
- D'Ambrosio R, Fender JS, Fairbanks JP, Simon EA, Born DE, Doyle DL, Miller JW. Progression from frontal-parietal to mesial-temporal epilepsy after fluid percussion injury in the rat. *Brain* 2005; 128: 174-88.
- DeLorenzo RJ, Hauser WA, Towne AR, Boggs JG, Pellock JM, Penberthy L, et al. A prospective, population-based epidemiologic study of status epilepticus in Richmond, Virginia. *Neurology* 1996; 46: 1029-35.
- Du F, Whetsell WO Jr, Abou-Khalil B, Blumenkopf B, Lothman EW, Schwarcz R. Preferential neuronal loss in layer III of the entorhinal cortex in patients with temporal lobe epilepsy. *Epilepsy Res* 1993; 16: 223-33.
- Dubé C, Richichi C, Bender RA, Chung G, Litt B, Baram TZ. Temporal lobe epilepsy after experimental prolonged febrile seizures: prospective analysis. *Brain* 2006; 129: 911-22.
- Earle KM, Baldwin M, Penfield W. Incisural sclerosis and temporal lobe seizures produced by hippocampal herniation at birth. *AMA Arch Neurol Psychiatry* 1953; 69: 27-42.

- El-Hassar L, Milh M, Wendling F, Ferrand N, Esclapez M, Bernard C. Cell domain-dependent changes in the glutamatergic and GABAergic drives during epileptogenesis in the rat CA1 region. *J Physiol* 2007; 578: 193-211.
- Engel J Jr. Introduction to temporal lobe epilepsy. *Epilepsy Res* 1996; 26: 141-50.
- Engel J Jr. Mesial temporal lobe epilepsy: what have we learned? *Neuroscientist* 2001; 7: 340-52.
- Fabene PF, Merigo F, Galiè M, Benati D, Bernardi P, Farace P, et al. Pilocarpine-induced status epilepticus in rats involves ischemic and excitotoxic mechanisms. *PLoS ONE* 2007; 2(10): e1105.
- Falconer MA, Serafetinides EA, Corsellis JA. Etiology and pathogenesis of temporal lobe epilepsy. *Arch Neurol* 1964; 10: 233-248.
- Farrow TF, Dickson JM, Grünewald RA. A six-year follow-up MRI study of complicated early childhood convulsion. *Pediatr Neurol* 2006; 35: 257-60.
- Fernández G, Effenberger O, Vinz B, Steinlein O, Elger CE, Döhring W, Heinze HJ. Hippocampal malformation as a cause of familial febrile convulsions and subsequent hippocampal sclerosis. *Neurology* 1998; 50: 909-17.
- French JA, Williamson PD, Thadani VM, Darcey TM, Mattson RH, Spencer SS, Spencer DD. Characteristics of medial temporal lobe epilepsy: I. Results of history and physical examination. *Ann Neurol* 1993; 34: 774-80.
- Fuerst D, Shah J, Shah A, Watson C. Hippocampal sclerosis is a progressive disorder: A longitudinal volumetric MRI study. *Ann Neurol* 2003; 53: 413-6.
- Fujikawa DG, Itabashi HH, Wu A, Shinmei SS. Status epilepticus-induced neuronal loss in humans without systemic complications or epilepsy. *Epilepsia* 2000; 41: 981-91.
- Glien M, Brandt C, Potschka H, Voigt H, Ebert U, Loscher W. Repeated low-dose treatment of rats with pilocarpine: low mortality but high proportion of rats developing epilepsy. *Epilepsy Res* 2001; 46: 111-9.
- Goffin K, Nissinen J, Van Laere K, Pitkanen A. Cyclicity of spontaneous recurrent seizures in pilocarpine model of temporal lobe epilepsy in rat. *Exp Neurol* 2007; 205: 501-5.
- Gorter JA, van Vliet EA, Aronica E, Lopes da Silva FH. Progression of spontaneous seizures after status epilepticus is associated with mossy fibre sprouting and extensive bilateral loss of hilar parvalbumin and somatostatin-immunoreactive neurons. *Eur J Neurosci* 2001; 13: 657-69.
- Gorter JA, Gonçalves Pereira PM, van Vliet EA, Aronica E, Lopes da Silva FH, Lucassen PJ. Neuronal cell death in a rat model for mesial temporal lobe epilepsy is induced by the initial status epilepticus and not by later repeated spontaneous seizures. *Epilepsia*. 2003; 44: 647-58.
- Grünewald RA, Farrow T, Vaughan P, Rittey CD, Mundy J. A magnetic resonance study of complicated early childhood convulsion. *J Neurol Neurosurg Psychiatry* 2001; 71: 638-42.
- Hamani C, Mello LE. Spontaneous recurrent seizures and neuropathology in the chronic phase of the pilocarpine and picrotoxin model epilepsy. *Neurol Res* 2002; 24: 199-209.
- Harvey BD, Sloviter RS. Hippocampal granule cell activity and c-Fos expression during spontaneous seizures in awake, chronically epileptic, pilocarpine-treated rats; implications for hippocampal epileptogenesis. *J Comp Neurol* 2005; 488: 441-62.
- Jackson GD, Briellmann RS, Kuzniecky RI. Temporal Lobe Epilepsy. In: Kuzniecky RI, Jackson GD (eds). *Magnetic Resonance in Epilepsy; Neuroimaging Techniques*. Amsterdam: Elsevier, 2004, pp. 99-176.
- Jambaqué I, Hertz-Pannier L, Mikaeloff Y, Martins S, Peudenier S, Dulac O, Chiron C. Severe memory impairment in a child with bihippocampal injury after status epilepticus. *Dev Med Child Neurol* 2006; 48: 223-6.
- Jung S, Jones TD, Lugo JN, Sheerin JH, Miller JW, D'Ambrosio R, et al. Progressive dendritic HCN channelopathy during epileptogenesis in the rat pilocarpine model of epilepsy. *J Neurosci* 2007; 27: 13012-21.
- Kälviäinen R, Salmenperä T, Partanen K, Vainio P, Riekkinen P, Pitkänen A. Recurrent seizures may cause hippocampal damage in temporal lobe epilepsy. *Neurology* 1998; 50: 1377-82.

- Korngut L, Young GB, Lee DH, Hayman-Abello BA, Mirsattari SM. Irreversible brain injury following status epilepticus. *Epilepsy Behav* 2007; 11: 235-40.
- Kuks JB, Cook MJ, Fish DR, Stevens JM, Shorvon SD. Hippocampal sclerosis in epilepsy and childhood febrile seizures. *Lancet* 1993; 342: 1391-4.
- Lehericy S, Semah F, Hasboun D, Dormont D, Clemenceau S, Granat O, et al. Temporal lobe epilepsy with varying severity: MRI study of 222 patients. *Neuroradiology* 1997; 39: 788-96.
- Leite JP, Garcia-Cairasco N, Cavalheiro EA. New insights from the use of pilocarpine and kainate models. *Epilepsy Res* 2002; 50: 93-103.
- Lhatoo SD, Sander JW, Fish D. Temporal lobe epilepsy following febrile seizures: unusually prolonged latent periods. *Eur Neurol* 2001; 46: 165-6.
- Liu RS, Lemieux L, Bell GS, Sisodiya SM, Bartlett PA, Shorvon SD, et al. The structural consequences of newly diagnosed seizures. *Ann Neurol* 2002; 52: 573-80.
- Lowenstein DH, Alldredge BK. Status epilepticus. *N Engl J Med* 1998; 338: 970-6.
- Maher J, McLachlan RS. Febrile convulsions. Is seizure duration the most important predictor of temporal lobe epilepsy? *Brain* 1995; 118: 1518-21.
- Margerison JH, Corsellis JA. Epilepsy and the temporal lobes. A clinical, electroencephalographic and neuropathological study of the brain in epilepsy, with particular reference to the temporal lobes. *Brain* 1966; 89: 499-530.
- Marks DA, Kim J, Spencer DD, Spencer SS. Characteristics of intractable seizures following meningitis and encephalitis. *Neurology* 1992; 42: 1513-8.
- Marks DA, Kim J, Spencer DD, Spencer SS. Seizure localization and pathology following head injury in patients with uncontrolled epilepsy. *Neurology* 1995; 45: 2051-7.
- Mathern GW, Babb TL, Vickrey BG, Melendez M, Pretorius JK. Traumatic compared to non-traumatic clinical-pathologic associations in temporal lobe epilepsy. *Epilepsy Res* 1994; 19: 129-39.
- Mazarati A, Bragin A, Baldwin R, Shin D, Wilson C, Sankar R, et al. Epileptogenesis after self-sustaining status epilepticus. *Epilepsia* 2002; 43 (Suppl 5): 74-80.
- Mikaeloff Y, Jambaque I, Hertz-Pannier L, Zamfirescu A, Adamsbaum C, Plouin P, et al. Devastating epileptic encephalopathy in school-aged children (DESC): a pseudo encephalitis. *Epilepsy Res* 2006; 69: 67-79.
- Mouri G, Jimenez-Mateos E, Engel T, Dunleavy M, Hatazaki S, Paucard A, et al. Unilateral hippocampal CA3-predominant damage and short latency epileptogenesis after intra-amygdala microinjection of kainic acid in mice. *Brain Res* 2008; 1213: 140-51.
- Nadler JV. Kainic acid as a tool for the study of temporal lobe epilepsy. *Life Sci* 1981; 29: 2031-42.
- Natsume J, Bernasconi N, Miyauchi M, Naiki M, Yokotsuka T, Sofue A, Bernasconi A. Hippocampal volumes and diffusion-weighted image findings in children with prolonged febrile seizures. *Acta Neurol Scand* 2007; 186 (Suppl): 25-8.
- Niessen HG, Angenstein F, Vielhaber S, Frisch C, Kudin A, Elger CE, et al. Volumetric magnetic resonance imaging of functionally relevant structural alterations in chronic epilepsy after pilocarpine-induced status epilepticus in rats. *Epilepsia* 2005; 46: 1021-6.
- Nissinen J, Halonen T, Koivisto E, Pitkanen A. A new model of chronic temporal lobe epilepsy induced by electrical stimulation of the amygdala in rat. *Epilepsy Res* 2000; 38: 177-205.
- Parent JM, Yu TW, Leibowitz RT, Geschwind DH, Sloviter RS, Lowenstein DH. Dentate granule cell neurogenesis is increased by seizures and contributes to aberrant network reorganization in the adult rat hippocampus. *J Neurosci* 1997; 17: 3727-38.
- Perez ER, Maeder P, Villemure KM, Vischer VC, Villemure JG, Deonna T. Acquired hippocampal damage after temporal lobe seizures in 2 infants. *Ann Neurol* 2000; 48: 384-7.
- Pisa M, Sandberg PR, Corcoran ME, Fibiger HC. Spontaneous recurrent seizures after intracerebral injections of kainic acid in rats: a possible model of human temporal lobe epilepsy. *Brain Res* 1980; 200: 481-7.

- Pitkänen A, Sutula TP. Is epilepsy a progressive disorder? Prospects for new therapeutic approaches in temporal-lobe epilepsy. *Lancet Neurol* 2002; 1: 173-81.
- Provenzale JM, Barboriak DP, VanLandingham K, MacFall J, Delong D, Lewis DV. Hippocampal MRI signal hyperintensity after febrile status epilepticus is predictive of subsequent mesial temporal sclerosis. *Am J Roentgenol* 2008; 190: 976-83.
- Raol YH, Lund IV, Bandyopadhyay S, Zhang G, Roberts DS, Wolfe JH, et al. Enhancing GABA(A) receptor alpha 1 subunit levels in hippocampal dentate gyrus inhibits epilepsy development in an animal model of temporal lobe epilepsy. *J Neurosci* 2006; 26: 11342-6.
- Sagar HJ, Oxbury JM. Hippocampal neuron loss in temporal lobe epilepsy: correlation with early childhood convulsions. *Ann Neurol* 1987; 22: 334-40.
- Salmenperä T, Kälviäinen R, Partanen K, Pitkänen A. Quantitative MRI volumetry of the entorhinal cortex in temporal lobe epilepsy. *Seizure* 2000; 9: 208-15.
- Salmenperä T, Kononen M, Roberts N, Vanninen R, Pitkanen A, Kalviainen R. Hippocampal damage in newly diagnosed focal epilepsy: a prospective MRI study. *Neurology* 2005; 64: 62-8.
- Schwarcz R, Eid T, Du F. Neurons in layer III of the entorhinal cortex. A role in epileptogenesis and epilepsy? *Ann N Y Acad Sci* 2000; 911: 328-42.
- Schwob JE, Fuller T, Price JL, Olney JW. Widespread patterns of neuronal damage following systemic or intracerebral injections of kainic acid: a histological study. *Neuroscience* 1980; 5: 991-1014.
- Scott RC, Gadian DG, King MD, et al. Magnetic resonance imaging findings within 5 days of status epilepticus in childhood. *Brain* 2002; 125: 1951-9.
- Scott RC, King MD, Gadian DG, Neville BG, Connelly A. Hippocampal abnormalities after prolonged febrile convulsion: a longitudinal MRI study. *Brain* 2003; 126: 2551-7.
- Scott RC, King MD, Gadian DG, Neville BG, Connelly A. Prolonged febrile seizures are associated with hippocampal vasogenic edema and developmental changes. *Epilepsia* 2006; 47: 1493-8.
- Semah F, Picot MC, Adam C, Broglin D, Arzimanoglou A, Bazin B, et al. Is the underlying cause of epilepsy a major prognostic factor for recurrence? *Neurology* 1998; 51: 1256-62.
- Sloviter RS. Decreased hippocampal inhibition and a selective loss of interneurons in experimental epilepsy. *Science* 1987; 235: 73-6.
- Sloviter RS. Permanently altered hippocampal structure, excitability, and inhibition after experimental status epilepticus in the rat: the dormant basket cell hypothesis and its possible relevance to temporal lobe epilepsy. *Hippocampus* 1991; 1: 41-66.
- Sloviter RS. Possible functional consequences of synaptic reorganization in the dentate gyrus of kainate-treated rats. *Neurosci Lett* 1992; 137: 91-6.
- Sloviter RS. On the relationship between neuropathology and pathophysiology in the epileptic hippocampus of humans and experimental animals. *Hippocampus* 1994a; 4: 250-3.
- Sloviter RS. The functional organization of the hippocampal dentate gyrus and its relevance to the pathogenesis of temporal lobe epilepsy. *Ann Neurol* 1994b; 35: 640-4.
- Sloviter RS. The neurobiology of temporal lobe epilepsy: too much information, not enough knowledge. *CR Biol* 2005; 328: 143-53.
- Sloviter RS, Zappone CA, Harvey BD, Frotscher M. Kainic acid-induced recurrent mossy fiber innervation of dentate gyrus inhibitory interneurons: possible anatomical substrate of granule cell hyperinhibition in chronically epileptic rats. *J Comp Neurol* 2006; 494: 944-60.
- Sloviter RS, Zappone CA, Bumanglag AV, Norwood B, Kudrimoti H. On the relevance of prolonged convulsive status epilepticus in animals to the etiology and neurobiology of human temporal lobe epilepsy. *Epilepsia* 2007; 48 (Suppl 8): 6-10.
- Sokol DK, Demyer WE, Edwards-Brown M, Sanders S, Garg B. From swelling to sclerosis: acute change in mesial hippocampus after prolonged febrile seizure. *Seizure* 2003; 12: 237-40.

- Sommer W. Erkrankung des Ammonshorns als aetiologisches Moment der Epilepsien. *Arch Psychiat Nervenkr* 1880; 10: 631-75.
- Spencer SS. Substrates of localization-related epilepsies: biological implications of localizing findings in humans. *Epilepsia* 1998; 39: 114-23.
- Spencer SS. Neural networks in human epilepsy: evidence of and implications for treatment. *Epilepsia* 2002; 43: 219-27.
- Spencer SS. When should temporal-lobe epilepsy be treated surgically? *Lancet Neurol* 2002; 1: 375-82.
- Stables JP, Bertram E, Dudek FE, Holmes G, Mathern G, Pitkanen A, White HS. Therapy discovery for pharmacoresistant epilepsy and for disease-modifying therapeutics: summary of the NIH/NINDS/AES models II workshop. *Epilepsia* 2003; 44: 1472-8.
- Tauck DL, Nadler JV. Evidence of functional mossy fiber sprouting in hippocampal formation of kainic acid-treated rats. *J Neurosci* 1985; 5: 1016-22.
- Teitelbaum JS, Zatorre RJ, Carpenter S, Gendron D, Evans AC, Gjedde A, Cashman NR. Neurologic sequelae of domoic acid intoxication due to the ingestion of contaminated mussels. *N Engl J Med* 1990; 322: 1781-7.
- Turski WA, Cavalheiro EA, Schwarz M, Czuczwar SJ, Kleinrok Z, Turski L. Limbic seizures produced by pilocarpine in rats: behavioural, electroencephalographic and neuropathological study. *Behav Brain Res* 1983; 9: 315-35.
- Van Paesschen W, Duncan JS, Stevens JM, Connelly A. Etiology and early prognosis of newly diagnosed partial seizures in adults: a quantitative hippocampal MRI study. *Neurology* 1997; 49: 753-7.
- VanLandingham KE, Heinz ER, Cavazos JE, Lewis DV. Magnetic resonance imaging evidence of hippocampal injury after prolonged focal febrile convulsions. *Ann Neurol* 1998; 43: 413-26.
- van Vliet EA, Aronica E, Tolner EA, Lopes da Silva FH, Gorter JA. Progression of temporal lobe epilepsy in the rat is associated with immunocytochemical changes in inhibitory interneurons in specific regions of the hippocampal formation. *Exp Neurol* 2004; 187: 367-79.
- Vezzani A, Ravizza T, Balosso S, Aronica E. Glia as a source of cytokines: implications for neuronal excitability and survival. *Epilepsia* 2008; 49 (Suppl 2): 24-32.
- Wennberg R, Arruda F, Quesney LF, Olivier A. Preeminence of extrahippocampal structures in the generation of mesial temporal seizures: evidence from human depth electrode recordings. *Epilepsia* 2002; 43: 716-26.
- White HS. Animal models of epileptogenesis. *Neurology* 2002; 59: S7-S14.
- Wiebe S, Blume WT, Girvin JP, Eliasziw M. A randomized, controlled trial of surgery for temporal-lobe epilepsy. *N Engl J Med* 2001; 345: 311-8.
- Williamson PD, French JA, Thadani VM, Kim JH, Novelly RA, Spencer SS, et al. Characteristics of medial temporal lobe epilepsy: II. Interictal and ictal scalp electroencephalography, neuropsychological testing, neuroimaging, surgical results, and pathology. *Ann Neurol* 1993; 34: 781-7.
- Wuarin JP, Dudek FE. Electrographic seizures and new recurrent excitatory circuits in the dentate gyrus of hippocampal slices from kainate-treated epileptic rats. *J Neurosci* 1996; 16: 4438-48.

Section II:
Clinical characteristics
of mesial temporal lobe epilepsies

Mesial temporal lobe epilepsy: natural history and seizure semiology

Felix Rosenow[1], Soheyl Noachtar[2]

[1] Epilepsy Center Hessen, Department of Neurology, University Hospitals Giessen and Marburg GmbH & Philipps-University Marburg, Marburg, Germany
[2] Epilepsy Center, Department of Neurology, University of Munich, Munich, Germany

■ Natural history

Natural history of a disorder implies the course from onset without intervention until the disorder resolves or death ensues (Last, 1983; Berg, 2008). Mesial temporal lobe epilepsy (MTLE) is a disorder (a syndrome or constellation) defined by spontaneously recurrent seizures of mesial temporal lobe onset caused by different aetiologies. The most frequent and best studied form of MTLE is MTLE associated with hippocampal sclerosis (MTLE-HS). A recent ILAE commission report (Wieser *et al*., 2004) on MTLE-HS summarised the current knowledge of this disorder and came to the conclusion that MTLE-HS was a subtype of a greater syndrome of MTLE, rather than a distinct syndrome. A number of diagnostic features were identified of which only MRI evidence of predominantly unilateral HS was a distinctive clinical feature of MTLE-HS. All other diagnostic criteria were common to different forms of MTLE caused by different aetiologies, including tumours and cavernomas. The criteria of HS based on MRI are now well-defined and applied in clinical practice with excellent sensitivity, specificity and interrater agreement (Menzler *et al*., 2010; Kim *et al*., 1999). A number of features regarding the natural history, including 1) history of an initial precipitating incident (IPI); 2) family history of MTLE; 3) the presence of a latent period; and 4) the presence of a silent period, were considered, in general, to be "potentially distinctive" of MTLE-HS rather than MTLE, however, it was felt that there was insufficient data to form a reliable conclusion (Wieser *et al*., 2004). In contrast, it was acknowledged that the results of clinical investigations, other than MRI, separate MTLE-HS from other forms of MTLE, underlining the relative importance of natural history in the clinical diagnosis of MTLE. Furthermore, several aspects of the history, including the presence of febrile seizures and the time at which an IPI occurs, are reportedly of high prognostic relevance regarding the response to medication and postoperative seizure outcome (French *et al*., 1993; Salanova *et al*., 1994; Stefan *et al*., 2009; Wieser *et al*., 2004). Recent studies suggest that adult-onset MTLE may be caused by a different set of aetiologies which frequently include autoimmune encephalitides, including limbic encephalitis (LE) (Bien *et al*., 2007; Dalmau *et al*., 2008; Malter *et al*., 2010).

Mesial temporal lobe epilepsy with hippocampal sclerosis

Typical case and terminology

Using the presentation of a typical case, the terminology used for the description of the natural history of MTLE is based on the presence of hippocampal sclerosis (similar terms: mesial temporal sclerosis, Ammon's horn sclerosis) is defined.

Illustrative case presentation

A 35-year-old man, referred for presurgical evaluation of epilepsy, reports the following medical history: at the age of 18 months a febrile seizure with hemiconvulsions on the left side occurred at the onset of a febrile illness, not primarily affecting the brain (thus fulfilling the criterion of a previous IPI; a complex febrile seizure). The patient subsequently remained seizure-free for 7.5 years (latent period) before he experienced a rising epigastric sensation, lasting for about 30 seconds and recurring in a stereotypical fashion every one to two months. Over time, this sensation increased in frequency but was only considered to be an ictal symptom when, at the age of 13, this evolved into a seizure characterized by oroalimentary automatisms sometimes associated with reduced responsiveness (epigastric aura → automotor seizure, according to the semiological seizure classification [Lüders *et al.*, 1998], or, when using the ILAE-seizure classification, a simple partial seizure with epigastric sensation evolving into a simple or complex partial seizure with automatisms). Such an evolution in seizure frequency and/or semiology is frequently interpreted as indicative of disease progression.

At this time, carbamazepine treatment was started and the patient became seizure-free for two years (silent period) before seizures recurred, despite good compliance. When the dose of carbamazepine was increased the patient became seizure-free for another six months but subsequently did not regain prolonged seizure freedom, despite several seizure suppressive drugs (SSDs) administered as monotherapy or in combination. The patient had thus developed drug-resistant epilepsy (DRE; refractory or intractable epilepsy), which is frequently interpreted as another sign of progressive epilepsy. Over time, he developed a depressive syndrome as a psychiatric comorbidity which required medication with a selective serotonin reuptake inhibitor (SSRI). He also complained of memory problems, especially regarding a decrease in his ability to remember people's faces. During presurgical diagnosis, his EEG showed right temporal sharp waves, peaking at the sphenoidal electrode and a seizure pattern in the right temporal lobe. The MRI was suggestive of right hippocampal sclerosis *(Figure 1)*. He was rendered seizure-free by right-sided selective amygdalo-hippocampectomy.

Mesial temporal lobe epilepsy with hippocampal sclerosis: onset in childhood and adolescence

MTLE-HS is a syndrome (or constellation) which most frequently starts in childhood or adolescence (French *et al.*, 1993; Wieser, 2004; Berg, 2008). The vast majority of patient cohorts recruited from surgical epilepsy centres had onset of their habitual seizures before the age of 16 (French *et al.*, 1993; Mathern *et al.*, 1995; Wieser, 2004). In the series studied by French *et al.* this was true in 88% of cases and the mean age at onset of non-febrile seizures was nine years. Fifty-four (81%) of the patients had an IPI, of whom 52 (78%) had seizures during febrile illness. Of the patients with these latter seizures, a

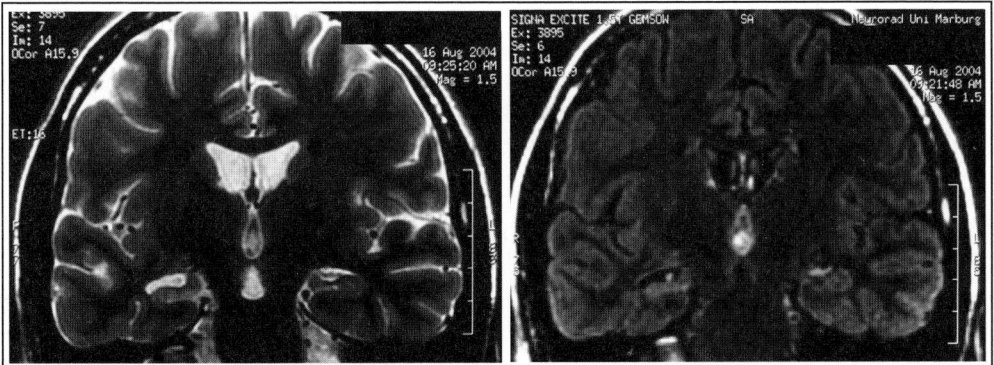

Figure 1. Unilateral hippocampal sclerosis in a patient with MTLE-HS following febrile seizures as initial precipitating incidence (IPI).
Coronal T2-weighted (a) and FLAIR (b) MRI of a 35 year old patient with febrile seizures at age 3-4 years and spontaneous seizures (epigastric aura – automotor seizure – generalized tonic-clonic seizure) since age 7. Video-EEG-findings were concordant with the MRI. The patient was seizure free at last follow-up 5 years after a selective amygdalo-hippocampectomy was performed.

related CNS infection was present in seven and no evidence of a CNS infection in 45 (67%). These febrile seizures lasted longer than 30 minutes in 33 subjects and therefore represented febrile status epilepticus. Frequently, patients with this classic early onset form of MTLE-HS initially respond relatively well to SSDs and experience prolonged seizure-free intervals (silent periods) with, or even without, medication. However, many patients, during the course of the disease, become difficult to treat and frequently become drug-resistant (Berg et al., 2008; Semah et al., 1998). Based on a report of familial MTLE associated with HS following a more benign course (Kobayashi et al., 2003), Labate et al. reported on a benign form of TLE, characterised by rare or no seizures during at least two years and frequently (39%) associated MRI-based evidence of mesial temporal sclerosis (Labate et al., 2006). In line with this, it was reported that seizures spontaneously remit in approximately one third of children with new-onset TLE, however, in this study a lesion on MRI predicted intractable seizures in TLE and the potential need for epilepsy surgery (Spooner et al., 2006). In a prospective trial of 104 patients with MTLE-HS, 25% became seizure-free under medication, and a failure to respond to drugs was predicted by a history of febrile convulsions and epileptiform EEG discharges (Kim et al., 1999).

Therefore, while the majority of patients with MTLE-HS are ultimately difficult to treat with SSDs, a referral bias may have led to an over-estimation of the refractory nature of MTLE-HS in the series reported from tertiary epilepsy centres (French et al., 1993; Mathern et al., 1995; Semah et al., 1998).

Mesial temporal lobe epilepsy with hippocampal sclerosis: onset in adults

Relative to childhood-onset MTLE-HS, where the majority of patients have a history of an IPI which is believed to be causally related, patients with adult-onset MTLE-HS have a significantly different clinical history, aetiology and probably also prognosis. In a recent study of 38 patients with adult-onset MTLE-HS, only 11 (29%) had an IPI followed by a latent period of, on average, 13.5 years or an extrahippocamal epileptogenic lesion (dual pathology), and were therefore considered to have secondary HS (Bien et al., 2007). In seven patients (18%), the cause was unknown while 20 (53%)

were considered to be of immunological aetiology and caused by either definite limbic encephalitis (LE) (9 patients; 24%) or possible LE based on MRI (11 patients; 29%). LE was either related to paraneoplastic onconeuronal autoantibodies (*e.g.* against Hu or Ma) but more frequently to non-paraneoplastic autoantibodies (*e.g.* against VGKC, GAD) (Bien *et al.*, 2007; Malter *et al.*, 2010) or antibodies which occur with or without tumour association (*e.g.* against NMDA-R [with possible ovarian teratomas] and GABAB-R) (Lancaster *et al.*, 2010; Dalmau *et al.*, 2008). Such patients tend to have MRI evidence of bilateral hippocampal hyperintensities evolving over time which may include an initial increase in volume followed by hippocampal atrophy (Bien *et al.*, 2007; Urbach *et al.*, 2006; Malter *et al.*, 2010). *Figure 2* shows the early evolution of LE in a 30-year-old woman presenting with memory deficits, disorientation and seizures, and evolving over time into drug-resistant epilepsy. Frequently, patients present with memory dysfunction and psychiatric or behavioural abnormalities. In the presence of an immunological aetiology, tumour resection, immunomodulation or immunosuppression can be highly effective, underscoring the importance not to overlook such aetiologies (Dalmau *et al.*, 2008; Malter *et al.*, 2010; Lancaster *et al.*, 2010). Considering these relatively recent findings, screening for CSF autoantibodies should be performed in patients with MTLE, especially when adult-onset or bilaterally hippocampal changes are present or when history of an IPI is lacking.

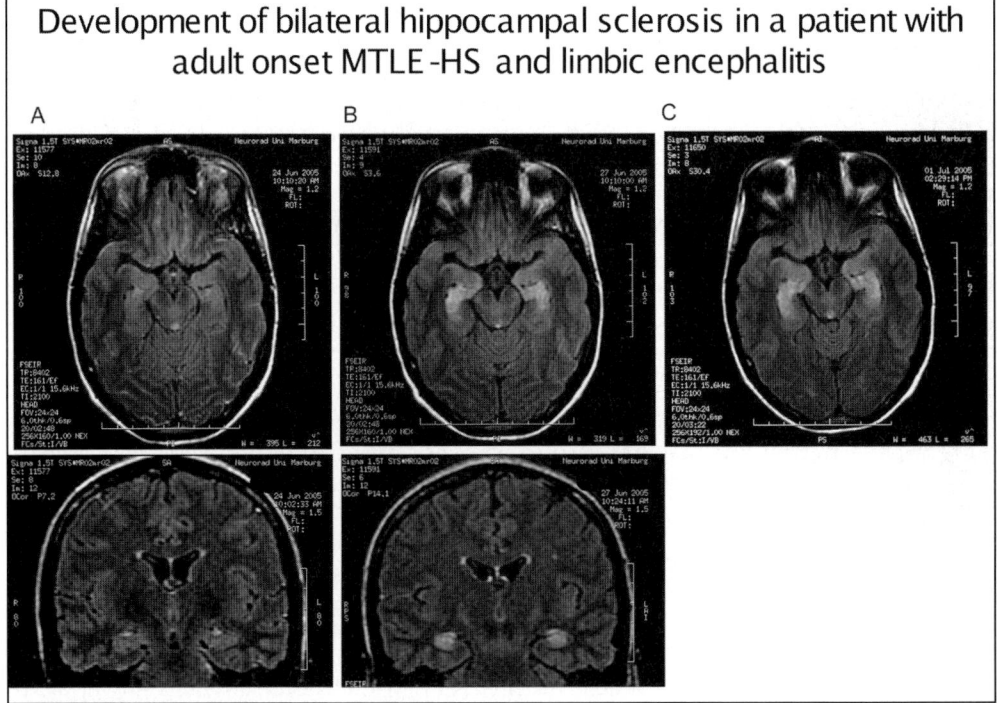

Figure 2. Development of bilateral hippocampal sclerosis in a patient with adult onset MTLE-HS and limbic encephalitis.
Sequential transverse MRIs from June 24th (A), 27th (B) and July 1st (C) 2005, when the 30 years old patient presented with limbic encephalitis. Subsequently she developed a drug-resistant MTLE-HS.

Mesial temporal lobe epilepsies due to other aetiologies

In a recent study of a group of 84 patients with adult-onset MTLE, 23 (27%) had MTLE-HS which was related to LE, 18 (21%) had MTLE-HS unrelated to LE, 18 (21%) had mesial temporal tumours (grade I or II in 12 or all 18), 11(13%) had amygdala lesions (probable dysplasia in 6 of 13) and 14% had other aetiologies, including post-traumatic lesions in five and cavernoma in three (Soeder et al., 2009). Therefore, in lesional (including HS) adult-onset MTLE the likelihood of having HS was less than 50% as compared with tumours *(Figure 3)*, dysplastic lesions, traumatic brain injury and cavernomas *(Figure 4)*, being the most frequent other aetiologies.

The recent report by the ILAE Commission on Classification and Terminology recommends an epilepsy classification with more emphasis on the underlying structural or metabolic cause rather than the localization of the epileptogenic zone (Berg et al., 2010). This is of particular interest when clinical differences are associated with different aetiologies in MTLE. This would appear to be the case for MTLE caused by mesiotemporal cavernomas (MTLE-C), rather than MTLE-HS. By comparing 11 patients with MTLE-C and 33 sex-matched MTLE-HS patients, we were able to identify that patients with MTLE-HS were more frequently drug-resistant (88% vs. 36%), more often had a history of an IPI (70% vs. 27%) and more often presented with automotor seizures (79% vs. 46%). Other

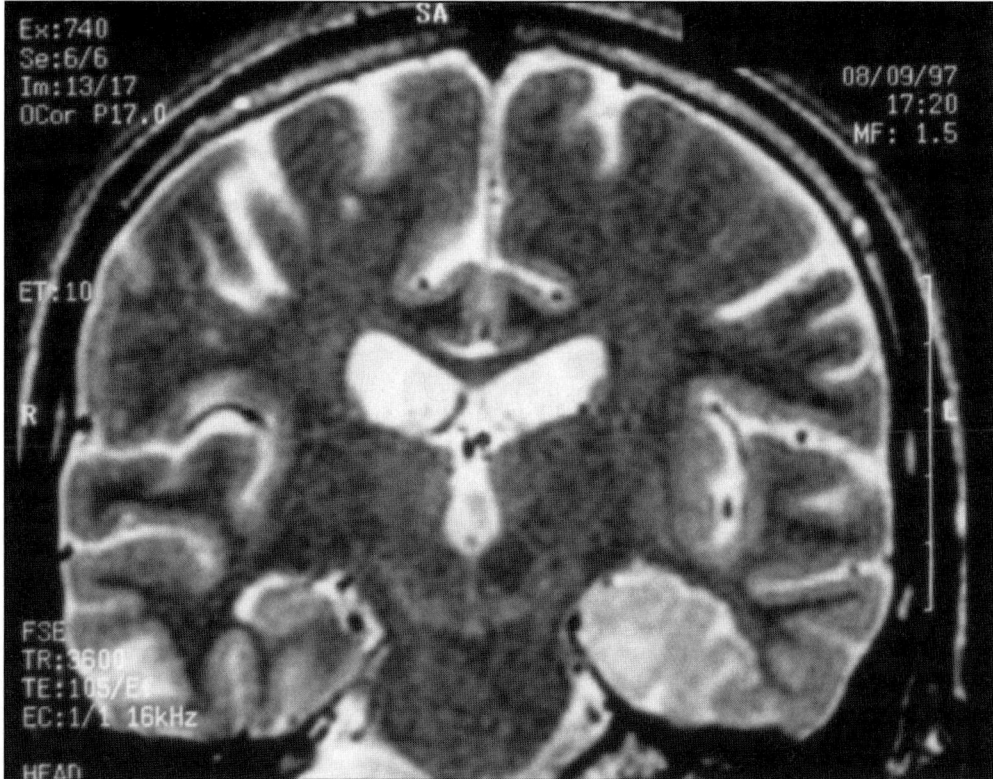

Figure 3. Mesiotemporal ganglioglioma in a patient with drug resistent CT-negative left MTLE since age 8. T2-weighted coronal MRI showing the mesiotemporal ganglioglioma. Interestingly the patient had recurrent episodes of status epilepticus triggered by febrile illnesses. He was rendered seizure free by a left temporal topectomy.

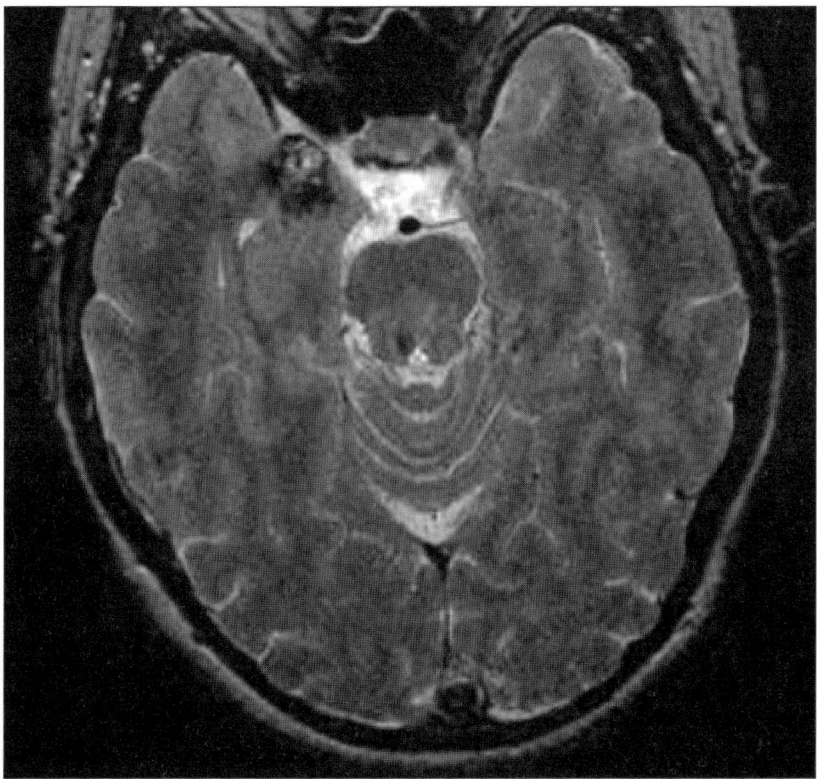

Figure 4. Mesiotemporal cavernoma in a patient with adult onset MTLE.
T2 weighted Neuronavigation MRI of a 51 year old patient with right a cavernoma of the right amygdala with a hemosiderin ring extenting into the head of the hippocampus causing right MTLE. The patient was rendered seizure free by a ECoG-guided topectomy of the epileptogenic lesion.

clinically relevant, but statistically non-significant effects, included seizure semiology, psychiatric comorbidity and cognitive deficits. Furthermore, the postoperative outcome was significantly better in patients with MTLE-C, suggesting that this has a relevant influence on clinical features and prognosis in patients with MTLE (Menzler et al., 2011).

■ Seizure semiology

Localization and lateralization of typical seizure types

The association of seizures, characterized by manual and oral automatisms, with TLE is well established (Jackson & Beevor, 1889; Jackson, 1898; Gibbs et al., 1948) *(Figure 1)*. Typical examples are oroalimentary automatisms such as chewing, swallowing, and lip smacking or hand automatisms such as fumbling (Kotagal, 1991). Generally, consciousness is impaired during these automatisms, although there are well-documented exceptions to this rule in patients with TLE in the non-speech dominant hemisphere (Noachtar et al., 1992; Ebner et al., 1995). The term "psychomotor seizure" refers to seizures characterized by automatisms and lapses of consciousness (Gibbs et al., 1948). An almost motionless "arrest behaviour" (Delgado-Escueta & Walsh, 1985) (dialeptic phase) is often observed at the onset of typical automotor seizures (Lüders et al., 1998). Automotor seizures occur most frequently in patients with TLE epilepsies, but they may also less commonly occur in patients with frontal lobe epilepsies (Manford et al., 1996), especially those of orbitofrontal origin (Bancaud & Talairach, 1992) *(Figure 5)*. When automotor seizures result from spread into one of the temporal lobes, they are often preceded by other seizure types. The symptomatogenic zone of automotor seizure onset is not clearly defined, but there is some evidence that epileptic activation of the anterior cingulate gyrus leads to distal automatisms (Talairach et al., 1973).

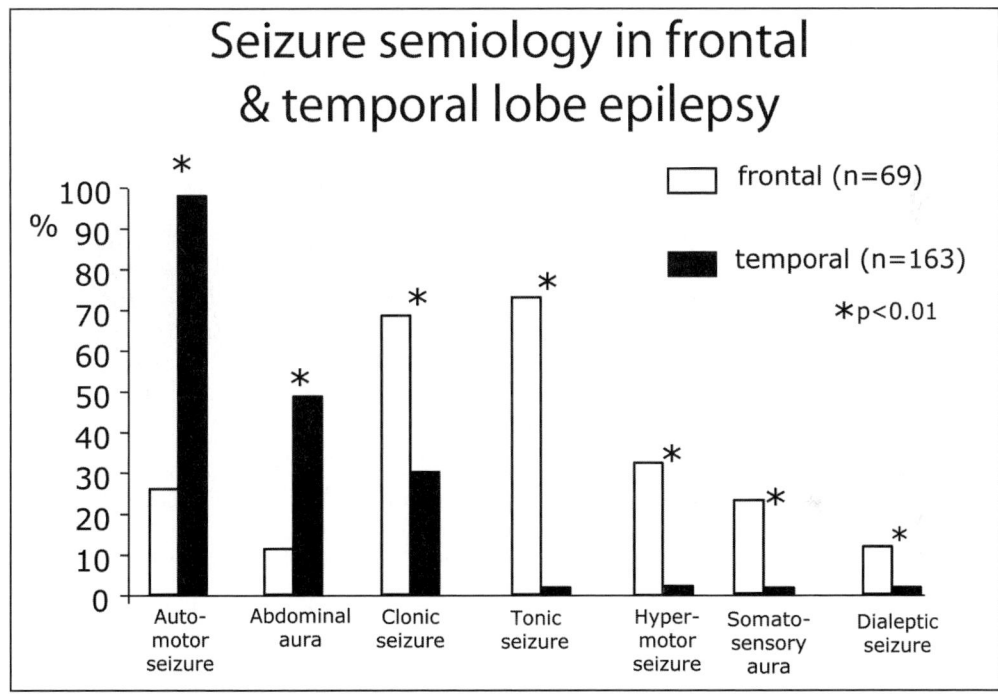

Figure 5. Seizure semiology in frontal and temporal lobe epilepsy.
Frequency of different seizure types in temporal and frontal lobe epilepsy at the University of Munich Epilepsy Monitoring Unit.

TLE patients frequently show periictal lateralizing phenomena such as dystonic hand posturing, head version, ictal vomiting, unilateral clonic seizures, postictal aphasia, and preserved responsiveness during automatisms. Dystonic hand posturing and forced head version reliably indicate seizure onset in the contralateral hemisphere (Wyllie et al., 1986; Kotagal et al., 1989; Chee et al., 1993). However, some have challenged the lateralizing significance of head version (Robillard et al., 1983; Ochs et al., 1984). This controversy was resolved by a quantitative analysis of head version in TLE patients (O'Dwyer et al., 2007). The evolution over time is important; at seizure onset, ipsilateral head turning is followed by contralateral head version prior to secondary generalisation (O'Dwyer et al., 2007). Unilateral manual automatisms are associated with ipsilateral seizure onset in TLE (Wada, 1982). This observation probably, at least partly, reflects dystonia of the contralateral hand and seems to be of lateralizing significance only when there is dystonia of the contralateral hand (Kotagal, 1991). Predominantly ipsilateral upper limb automatisms are more common than predominantly contralateral automatisms (Mirzadjanova et al.,

2010). The duration of ictal ipsilateral upper limb automatisms is significantly longer than the duration of contralateral automatisms. Patients with ipsilateral upper limb automatisms have more often exclusively unitemporal interictal epileptiform discharges (IED) (84.2%) than patients with contralateral automatisms (11.1%; $p < 0.001$). The positive predictive value (PPV) of the combination of these parameters was 84.2%. Excellent surgical seizure outcome is more likely in patients with ipsilateral upper limb automatisms (77.8%) compared to those with contralateral automatisms (20%) (Mirzadjanova et al., 2010). The lateralization of upper limb automatisms in TLE has good lateralizing value only when the lateralization of interictal epileptiform discharges are also taken into consideration (Mirzadjanova et al., 2010). The hand used to perform postictal nose wiping is reported to be ipsilateral to the side of seizure origin in 97% of TLE patients (Leutmezer et al., 1998; Wennberg, 2000), a finding that may be due to neglect of the contralateral arm. Postictal aphasia is suggestive of seizure onset in the speech dominant hemisphere (Gabr et al., 1989). Preserved responsiveness during ictal automatisms is seen only in patients with TLE of the non-speech dominant hemisphere (Ebner et al., 1995; Noachtar et al., 1992).

Several other seizure phenomena have been described, pointing to seizure onset in the typically right non-dominant hemisphere. Ictal vomiting lateralizes seizure onset to the right hemisphere in patients with TLE (Kramer et al., 1988) and ictal urinary urge is associated with non-dominant temporal seizure onset based on a series of six patients (Baumgartner et al., 2000). Ictal spitting points to seizure onset in the non-dominant temporal lobe (Voss et al., 1999). Postictal coughing occurs with seizure onset in the non-dominant hemisphere (Wennberg, 2001).

Ipsilateral eye blinking is a rare phenomenon (1.5%) which is mostly observed in TLE patients, but is highly suggestive of ipsilateral seizure onset (Wada, 1980; Benbadis et al., 1996; Henkel et al., 1999). The positive predictive value of the above-mentioned lateralizing seizure phenomena was shown to be correct in 80%-100% of such patients.

Several studies have looked at differences in the seizure semiology of patients with mesial *versus* lateral neocortical TLE (Gil-Nagel & Risinger, 1997; Dupont et al., 1999; Pfänder et al., 2002). The combination of ipsilateral hand automatisms and contralateral hand dystonia is reported only in patients with MTLE (Dupont et al., 1999). Although, strictly speaking, these were not distinguished by any single seizure type or seizure phenomenon, abdominal auras and unilateral hand dystonia are more commonly observed in seizures of patients with MTLE, whereas non-specific or psychic auras and unilateral clonic seizures following automatisms are more frequent in lateral neocortical TLE (Gil-Nagel & Risinger, 1997; Pfänder et al., 2002).

In summary, seizure semiology provides a wealth of localizing information. Even a very subtle seizure type, such as pure ictal tachycardia, *i.e.* a vegetative seizure type, provides localizing information since it occurs more frequently in TLE than extratemporal epilepsy (Weil et al., 2005) (Figure 6).

The role of seizure evolution

Epileptic seizures frequently evolve from one seizure type into another. Initial seizure symptoms such as abdominal aura and psychic aura are typical of TLE. An abdominal aura which is followed by an automotor seizure is very typically, though not exclusively, seen in patients with TLE (Henkel et al., 2002). The sensation of *déjà vu* is frequently described in TLE. Early clonic seizures following manual hand automatisms occur

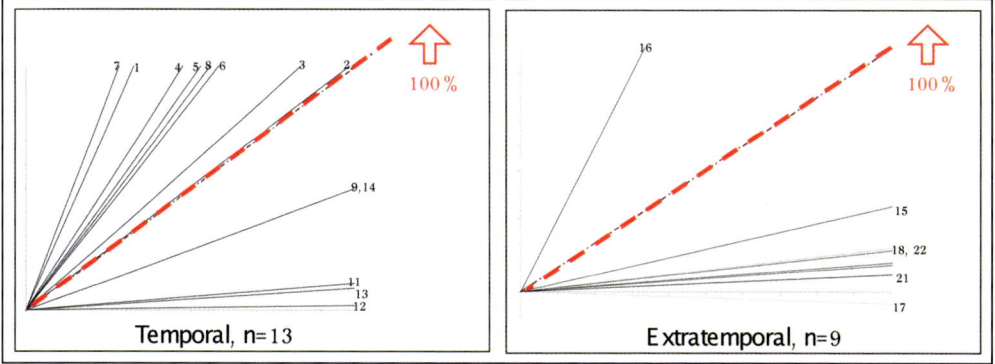

Figure 6. Families of slope lines in the point of maximum increase of heart rate replaced to zero. Only one patients with extratemporal seizure onset showed pure ictal tachycardia whereas this was the case in 8 of 13 TLE patients (from Weil *et al.*, 2005).

significantly more frequently in patients with neocortical TLE than in patients with MTLE. In contrast, patients with MTLE present hand dystonia significantly more often in the course of their seizures than patients with neocortical TLE (Pfänder *et al.*, 2002). Typical seizure evolution in TLE includes: (1) abdominal auras to automotor seizures to generalised tonic-clonic seizures and (2) psychic auras to automotor seizures to generalised tonic-clonic seizures.

References

- Bancaud J, Talairach J. Clinical semiology of frontal lobe seizures. In: Chauvel P, Delgado-Escueta AV, Halgren E, Bancaud J (eds.). *Frontal Lobe Seizures and Epilepsies*. Vol. 57. New York: Raven Press, 1992, pp. 3-58.
- Baumgartner C, Groppel G, Leutmezer F, Aull-Watschinger S, Pataraia E, Feucht M, *et al*. Ictal urinary urge indicates seizure onset in the nondominant temporal lobe. *Neurology* 2000; 55: 432-4.
- Benbadis SR, Kotagal P, Klem GH. Unilateral blinking: a lateralizing sign in partial seizures. *Neurology* 1996; 46: 45-8.
- Berg AT. The natural history of mesial temporal lobe epilepsy. *Curr Opin Neurol* 2008; 21: 173-8.
- Berg AT, Berkovic SF, Brodie MJ, Buchhalter J, Cross JH, van Emde BW, *et al*. Revised terminology and concepts for organization of seizures and epilepsies: report of the ILAE Commission on Classification and Terminology, 2005-2009. *Epilepsia* 2010; 51: 676-85.
- Bien CG, Urbach H, Schramm J, Soeder BM, Becker AJ, Voltz R, *et al*. Limbic encephalitis as a precipitating event in adult-onset temporal lobe epilepsy. *Neurology* 2007; 69: 1236-44.
- Chee MW, Kotagal P, Van Ness PC, Gragg L, Murphy D, Lüders HO. Lateralizing signs in intractable partial epilepsy: blinded multiple-observer analysis. *Neurology* 1993; 43: 2519-25.
- Cohen-Gadol AA, Bradley CC, Williamson A, Kim JH, Westerveld M, Duckrow RB, Spencer DD. Normal magnetic resonance imaging and medial temporal lobe epilepsy: the clinical syndrome of paradoxical temporal lobe epilepsy. *J Neurosurg* 2005; 102: 902-9.
- Dalmau J, Gleichman AJ, Hughes EG, Rossi JE, Peng X, *et al*. Anti-NMDA-receptor encephalitis: case series and analysis of the effects of antibodies. *Lancet Neurol* 2008; 7: 1091-8.
- Delgado-Escueta AV, Walsh GO. Type I complex partial seizures of hippocampal origin: excellent results of anterior temporal lobectomy. *Neurology* 1985; 35: 143-54.

- Dupont S, Semah F, Boon P, Saint-Hilaire JM, Adam C, Broglin D, et al. Association of ipsilateral motor automatisms and contralateral dystonic posturing: a clinical feature differentiating medial from neocortical temporal lobe epilepsy. *Arch Neurol* 1999; 56: 927-32.
- Ebner A, Dinner DS, Noachtar S, Lüders H. Automatisms with preserved responsiveness: a lateralizing sign in psychomotor seizures. *Neurology* 1995; 45: 61-4.
- Falconer MA. Genetic and related aetiological factors in temporal lobe epilepsy. A review. *Epilepsia* 1971; 12: 13-31.
- Falconer MA, Serafetinides EA, Corsellis JA. Aetiology and pathogenesis of temporal lobe epilepsy. *Arch Neurol* 1964; 10: 233-48.
- French JA, Williamson PD, Thadani M, Darcey TM, Mattson RH, Spencer SS, Spencer DD. Characteristics of medial temporal lobe epilepsy: I. Results of history and physical examination. *Ann Neurol* 1993; 34: 774-80.
- Gabr M, Lüders H, Dinner D, Morris H, Wyllie E. Speech manifestations in lateralization of temporal lobe seizures. *Ann Neurol* 1989; 25: 82-7.
- Gibbs EL, Gibbs FA, Fuster B. Psychomotor epilepsy. *Arch Neurol Psychiatry* 1948; 60: 331-9.
- Gil-Nagel A, Risinger MW. Ictal semiology in hippocampal *versus* extrahippocampal temporal lobe epilepsy. *Brain* 1997; 120: 183-92.
- Hattemer K, Thiel P, Haag A, Chen X, Benes L, Hamer HM, et al. Drug resistance of mesial temporal lobe epilepsy depends on aetiology and is less frequent with cavernomas as compares to hippocampal sclerosis. *Epilepsia* 2009; 50 (Suppl 11): S414.
- Henkel A, Noachtar S, Pfander M, Lüders HO. The localizing value of the abdominal aura and its evolution: a study in focal epilepsies. *Neurology* 2002; 58: 271-6.
- Henkel A, Winkler PA, Noachtar S. Ipsilateral blinking: a rare lateralizing seizure phenomenon in temporal lobe epilepsy. *Epileptic Disord* 1999; 1: 195-7.
- Jackson JH. Case of epilepsy with tasting movements and "dreamy state" – very small patch of softening in the left uncinate gyrus. *Brain* 1898; 21: 580-90.
- Jackson JH, Beevor CE. Case of tumor of the right temporo-sphenoidal lobe bearing on the localization of the sense of smell and on the interpretation of a particular variety of epilepsy. *Brain* 1889; 12: 346-57.
- Jensen I, Klinken L. Temporal lobe epilepsy and neuropathology. Histological findings in resected temporal lobes correlated to surgical results and clinical aspects. *Acta Neurol Scand* 1976; 54(5): 391-414.
- Kim WJ, Park SC, Lee SJ, Lee JH, Kim JY, Lee BI, Kim DI. The prognosis for control of seizures with medications in patients with MRI evidence for mesial temporal sclerosis. *Epilepsia* 1999; 40(3): 290-3.
- Kobayashi E, D'Agostino MD, Lopes-Cendes I, Berkovic SF, Li ML, Andermann E, et al. Hippocampal atrophy and T2-weighted signal changes in familial mesial temporal lobe epilepsy. *Neurology* 2003; 60: 405-9.
- Kotagal P. Seizure symptomatology of temporal lobe epilepsy. In: Lüders HO (ed.). *Epilepsy Surgery*. New York: Raven Press, 1991: 143-56.
- Kotagal P, Lüders H, Morris HH, Dinner DS, Wyllie E, Godoy J, et al. Dystonic posturing in complex partial seizures of temporal lobe onset: a new lateralizing sign. *Neurology* 1989; 39: 196-201.
- Kramer RE, Lüders H, Goldstick LP, Dinner DS, Morris HH, Lesser RP, et al. Ictus emeticus: an electroclinical analysis. *Neurology* 1988; 38: 1048-52.
- Labate A, Ventura P, Gambardella A, Le Piane E, Colosimo E, Leggio U, et al. MRI evidence of mesial temporal sclerosis in sporadic "benign" temporal lobe epilepsy. *Neurology* 2006; 66(4): 562-5.
- Lancaster E, Lai M, Peng X, Hughes E, Constantinescu R, Raizer J, et al. Antibodies to the GABA(B) receptor in limbic encephalitis with seizures: case series and characterization of the antigen. *Lancet Neurol* 2010; 9(1): 67-76.

- Leutmezer F, Serles W, Lehrner J, Pataraia E, Zeiler K, Baumgartner C. Postictal nose wiping: a lateralizing sign in temporal lobe complex partial seizures. *Neurology* 1998; 51: 1175-7.
- Lüders H, Acharya J, Baumgartner C, Benbadis S, Bleasel A, Burgess R, et al. Semiological seizure classification. *Epilepsia* 1998; 39: 1006-13.
- Malter MP, Helmstaedter C, Urbach H, Vincent A, Bien CG. Antibodies to glutamic acid decarboxylase define a form of limbic encephalitis. *Ann Neurol* 2010; 67(4): 470-8.
- Manford M, Fish DR, Shorvon SD. An analysis of clinical seizure patterns and their localizing value in frontal and temporal lobe epilepsies. *Brain* 1996; 119: 17-40.
- Mathern GW, Babb TLVickrey BG, Melendez M, Pretorius JK. The clinical-pathogenic mechanisms of hippocampal neuron loss and surgical outcomes in temporal lobe epilepsy. *Brain* 1995; 118: 105-18.
- Mathern GW, Pretorius JK, Babb TL. Influence of the type of initial precipitating injury and at what age it occurs on course and outcome in patients with temporal lobe seizures. *J Neurosurg* 1995; 82: 220-7.
- Menzler K, Iwinska-Zelder J, Shiratori K, Jaeger RK, Oertel WH, Hamer HM, Rosenow F, Knake S. Evaluation of MRI criteria (1.5 T) for the diagnosis of hippocampal sclerosis in healthy subjects. *Epilepsy Res* 2010; 89: 349-54.
- Menzler K, Thiel P, Hermsen A, Chen X, Benes L, Miller D, et al. The role of underlying structural cause for epilepsy classification: clinical features and prognosis in mesial temporal lobe epilepsy caused by hippocampal sclerosis versus cavernoma. *Epilepsia* 2011; 52: 707-11.
- Mirzadjanova Z, Peters AS, Remi J, Bilgin C, Silva Cunha JP, Noachtar S. Significance of lateralization of upper limb automatisms in temporal lobe epilepsy: A quantitative movement analysis. *Epilepsia* 2010; 51: 2140-6.
- Noachtar S, Ebner A, Dinner DS. Das Auftreten von Automatismen bei erhaltenem Bewusstsein. Zur Frage der Bewusstseinsstörung bei komplex-fokalen Anfällen. In: Scheffner D (ed.). *Epilepsie 91*. Reinbek: Einhorn-Presse Verlag, 1992: 82-7.
- O'Brien TJ, Kilpatrick C, Murrie V, Vogrin S, Morris K, Cook MJ. Temporal lobe epilepsy caused by mesial temporal sclerosis and temporal neocortical lesions. A clinical and electroencephalographic study of 46 pathologically proven cases. *Brain* 1996; 119: 2133-41.
- O'Dwyer R, Silva Cunha JP, Vollmar C, Mauerer C, Feddersen B, Burgess RC, et al. Lateralizing significance of quantitative analysis of head movements before secondary generalization of seizures of patients with temporal lobe epilepsy. *Epilepsia* 2007; 48: 524-30.
- Ochs R, Gloor P, Quesney F, Ives J, Olivier A. Does head-turning during a seizure have lateralizing or localizing significance? *Neurology* 1984; 34: 884-90.
- Pfänder M, Arnold S, Henkel A, Weil S, Werhahn KJ, Eisensehr I, et al. Clinical features and EEG findings differentiating mesial from neocortical temporal lobe epilepsy. *Epileptic Disord* 2002; 4: 189-95.
- Robillard A, Saint-Hilaire JM, Mercier M, Bouvier G. The lateralizing and localizing value of adversion in epileptic seizures. *Neurology* 1983; 33: 1241-2.
- Salanova V, Markand ON, Worth R. Clinical characteristics and predictive factors in 98 patients with complex partial seizures treated with temporal resection. *Arch Neurol* 1994; 51: 1008-13.
- Semah F, Picot MC, Adam C, Broglin D, Arzimanoglou A, Bazin B, et al. Is the underlying cause of epilepsy a major prognostic factor for recurrence? *Neurology* 1998; 51: 1256-62.
- Soeder BM, Gleissner U, Urbach H, Clusmann H, Elger CE, Vincent A, Bien CG. Causes, presentation and outcome of lesional adult onset mediotemporal lobe epilepsy. *J Neurol Neurosurg Psychiatry* 2009; 80: 894-9.
- Spooner CG, Berkovic SF, Mitchell LA, Wrennall JA, Harvey AS. New-onset temporal lobe epilepsy in children: lesion on MRI predicts poor seizure outcome. *Neurology* 2006; 67: 2147-53.
- Stephen LJ, Kwan P, Brodie MJ. Does the cause of localization-related epilepsy influence the response to antiepileptic drug treatment? *Epilepsia* 2001; 42: 357-62.

- Stefan H, Hildebrandt M, Kerling F, Kasper BS, Hammen T, Dörfler A, Weigel D, Buchfelder M, Blümcke I, Pauli E, et al. Clinical prediction of postoperative seizure control: structural, functional findings and disease histories. *J Neurol Neurosurg Psychiatry* 2009; 80: 196-200.
- Talairach J, Bancaud J, Geier S, Bordas-Ferrer M, Bonis A, Szikla G, et al. The cingulate gyrus and human behaviour. *Electroencephalogr Clin Neurophysiol* 1973; 34: 45-52.
- Voss NF, Davies KG, Boop FA, Montouris GD, Hermann BP. Spitting automatism in complex partial seizures: a nondominant temporal localizing sign? *Epilepsia* 1999; 40: 114-6.
- Wada JA. Unilateral blinking as a lateralizing sign of partial complex seizure of temporal lobe origin. In: Wada JA and Penry JK (eds.). *Advances in Epileptology, 10th Epilepsy International Symposium*. New York: Raven Press, 1980: 533.
- Wada JA. Cerebral lateralization and epileptic manifestations. In: Akimoto H, Kazamatsuri H, Seino M and Ward A (eds). *Advances in Epileptology: 13th Epilepsy International Symposium*. New York: Raven Press, 1982, pp. 365-72.
- Wallace SJ. Spontaneous fits after convulsions with fever. *Arch Dis Child* 1977; 52: 192-6.
- Weil S, Arnold S, Eisensehr I, Noachtar S. Heart rate increase in otherwise subclinical seizures is different in temporal *versus* extratemporal seizure onset: support for temporal lobe autonomic influence. *Epileptic Disord* 2005; 7: 199-204.
- Wennberg R. Electroclinical analysis of postictal noserubbing. *Can J Neurol Sci* 2000; 27: 131-6.
- Wennberg R. Postictal coughing and noserubbing coexist in temporal lobe epilepsy. *Neurology* 2001; 56: 133-4.
- Wieser HG, for the ILAE commission on Neurosurgery of Epilepsy. ILAE Commission Report. Mesial temporal lobe epilepsy with hippicampal sclerosis. *Epilepsia* 2004; 45: 695-714.
- Wyllie E, Lüders H, Morris HH, Lesser RP, Dinner DS. The lateralizing significance of versive head and eye movements during epileptic seizures. *Neurology* 1986; 36: 606-11.

Cognitive and psychiatric symptoms and their treatment in temporal lobe epilepsy: the role of the mesiotemporal structures

Bettina Schmitz[1], Marco Mula[2], Michael Trimble[3]

[1] Department of Neurology, Vivantes Humboldt-Klinikum, Berlin, Germany
[2] Department of Neurology, Amedeo Avogadro University, Novara, Italy
[3] Institute of Neurology, Queen Square, London, UK

Mesial temporal lobe epilepsy (MTLE) is a good example of the rediscovered concept that epilepsy syndromes are complex neuropsychiatric disorders and should not simply be defined by seizure type and aetiology. Temporal lobe epilepsy (TLE) affects neuronal networks which are most relevant to the patient's emotional state, perception and communication. This chapter summarises the links between MTLE and major psychiatric disorders such as psychosis, depression and personality disorders, but also introduces modern cognitive concepts such as theory of mind (ToM) and emotional recognition, both of which are crucial for satisfying interpersonal relationships.

Some patients with TLE have significant difficulties in specific areas of social behaviour and these problems contribute to often poor social prognosis and reduced quality of life for themselves and their families, sometimes also to the frustration of their doctors. The behavioural peculiarities in patients with TLE were formerly often summarised under the term "epileptic personality disorder", a psychiatric diagnosis which is difficult for neurologists to interpret, hard for patients to accept, and regularly triggers therapeutic pessimism. Recent neuropsychological research has demonstrated that some of these behavioural deficits can be explained by neuronal network dysfunction linked to the epileptogenic focus, which is highly interesting both from a theoretical and a practical point of view.

The relationship between seizures, treatment and psychiatric comorbidity in TLE is complex, and optimal treatment and adequate support requires that patients are viewed from a comprehensive neuropsychiatric perspective, and ideally within a multidisciplinary setting.

■ Depression, dysphoria and suicide

Epilepsy is a chronic disorder, which, like many chronic neurological disorders, is associated with an increased risk of depressive disorders. There are a number of psychological factors which contribute to this comorbidity, which include: demoralisation and a negative outlook on life, financial disadvantages, stigma and social discrimination, and the unpredictable risk of becoming unconscious, falling and damaging one's self, and, in public, of social embarrassment. As well as the epileptogenic focus itself, other physiological risk factors for epilepsy include for, example, depressogenic antiepileptic drugs (AEDs) and epilepsy surgery, which is often followed by a transitory depressive reaction. A finding which has been replicated and which stresses the clinical relevance of depression in epilepsy is the association between depressive symptoms and quality of life (QOL) in people with epilepsy. Gilliam et al. (1997) noted depression to be the most important predictor of QOL, being a more powerful predictor than actual seizure frequency. Perrine et al. (1995) and Boylan et al. (2004) reported similar findings. Moreover, people with epilepsy and depression are more likely to experience side effects of AEDs (Cramer et al., 2003; Kanner, 2007), are more often drug-refractory (Hitiris et al., 2007), and have a poorer outcome after epilepsy surgery (Kanner, 2008).

Epidemiology

Several community studies have shown that the prevalence of depression is increased in unselected populations suffering from epilepsy. For example, Edeh and Toone (1987) carried out a general practice study in the UK and reported that 22% of unselected patients with epilepsy were diagnosed with a depressive disorder. A Canadian Community Health Survey examined 253 people with epilepsy using a rating scale to identify a history of depression. The authors noted a 22% lifetime prevalence of depression which was much higher than the 12% prevalence rate reported in the general population (Tellez-Zenteno et al., 2005). More recently, Ettinger et al. (2004) assessed depression in 775 subjects with epilepsy and compared prevalence rates with those of patients with asthma, as well as healthy controls. In this study a rating scale assessment was again used (Centers of Epidemiological Studies - Depression Instrument). Symptoms of depression were significantly more frequent in the epilepsy group (36.5%), when compared to those with asthma (27.8%) and controls (11.8%).

In selected patient groups, such as tertiary referral centres, or centres for epilepsy surgery, the frequency of depression seems to be even higher. Victoroff et al. (1994) evaluated 60 patients with intractable complex partial seizures using a structured clinical interview for DSM-IIIR, and observed that 58% had a lifetime diagnosis of depressive disorders. Jones et al. (2005a) examined 199 patients from five epilepsy centres, again using a structured clinical interview, namely the MINI, and noted that 34% met the diagnostic criteria for a mood or anxiety disorder, and 19% met the criteria for major depression. Ring et al. (1998) examined 60 patients awaiting TLE surgery, and reported, at preoperative assessment, that a major depressive disorder was present in 21%. These data probably reflect the severity of the seizure disorder, however, it is tempting to speculate that the data also reflect the degree of underlying brain dysfunction and shared neurobiology between epilepsy and depression. In this regard, an interesting finding, which has been replicated by different authors, is the observation that the relationship between epilepsy and depression is not necessarily unidirectional and patients with comorbidity may not always present with a seizure disorder prior to the emergence of depression. In fact, it has been noted, in epidemiological studies, that having a prior mood disorder can be associated with an increased risk of epilepsy (Forsgren & Nystrom, 1990; Hesdorffer et al., 2000). There may be a number of reasons for this including, perhaps, the use of proconvulsive antidepressants and the development of epilepsy following suicidal attempts, drug abuse or other kinds of trauma, such as head trauma. However, these findings may also reflect common underlying pathogenesis, which may relate to some, as yet unknown, genetic factor or a link with neurotransmitter function (for example, related to transmitters which are known to play a role in both epilepsy and depression such as serotonin, glutamate or GABA).

The link with temporal lobe epilepsy

There has been considerable debate regarding the association between epilepsy syndromes and depression. Patients with lesional TLE are more likely to have intractable seizures and take more extensive medication than those with extratemporal lobe epilepsy. They may, therefore, be at an increased risk of developing depression. Thus, some studies have shown patients with TLE to be more prone to depression than other groups, although other investigations have failed to confirm this observation. By examining the relationship between depression and type of TLE, Quiske et al. (2000) found that patients with TLE who had mesial temporal sclerosis were more likely to report symptoms of depression than patients with neocortical temporal lobe pathology. It would appear that patients with complex partial seizures are more likely to have a depressive disorder (Robertson, 1998). With regards to the temporal lobe association with depression, there are, interestingly, a number of studies outside the field of epilepsy in the psychiatric literature which suggest an association between hippocampal volume loss and affective disturbances (Bremner et al., 2000; Frodl et al., 2002). Thus, although further research in this area is needed, neuroimaging studies reveal an underlying brain network of depression in psychiatric patients without a neurological disorder, which includes the hippocampus, thus in keeping with the findings in patients with epilepsy.

Studies have been reported which link frontal lobe dysfunction to the development of depression in epilepsy. The latter have emerged from investigations using brain imaging (PET or SPECT), and neuropsychological batteries. Hermann et al. (1991) noted that patients with TLE and depression were more likely to perform poorly in frontal lobe neuropsychological tasks, especially with a left-sided seizure focus. Schmitz et al. (1997) noted similar frontal changes and localizations using SPECT, and Bromfield et al. (1990) using PET reported that patients with TLE and associated depression revealed bilateral reduction of frontal lobe metabolism, a phenomenon also called "hypo-frontality". Although these studies were necessarily restricted to a limited number of patients, the concordance between the findings supports an anatomical association between TLE, depression, and frontal lobe dysfunction.

Depression and antiepileptic drugs

Several AEDs are extensively used in psychiatric practice as mood stabilisers (Melvin et al., 2008) or anti-anxiety agents (Mula et al., 2007). In patients with epilepsy, however, some may precipitate depression (*Table I*). The pathogenesis of such a paradoxical effect is clearly multifactorial with some variables related to the drug (e.g. high dosage and rapid titration schedule, ability to reduce folate levels, and potentiation of GABAergic neurotransmission) and several other variables related to the epilepsy itself (e.g. presence of hippocampal sclerosis [HS] and the forced normalization phenomenon) (Mula & Sander,

Table I. Psychotropic properties of antiepileptic drugs

Antiepileptic drug	Negative	Positive
Barbiturates	Depression, hyperactivity	Anxiolytic, hypnotic
Carbamazepine Oxcarbazepine	Irritability	Mood stabilizing, antimanic
Ethosuximide	Behavioural abnormalities, psychosis	–
Felbamate	Depression, anxiety, irritability	(Increased attention and concentration)
Gabapentin	Behavioural problems in children, depression	(Anxiolytic)
Lamotrigine	Insomnia, agitation	Mood stabilizing, antidepressant
Levetiracetam	Irritability, emotional lability, psychosis	–
Phenytoin	Encephalopathy	Antimanic?
Pregabalin	?	Anxiolytic
Tiagabine	Depression (non-convulsive status epilepticus)	–
Topiramate	Depression, psychomotor slowing, psychosis	–
Valproate	Encephalopathy	Mood stabilizing, antimanic (anxiolytic)
Vigabatrin	Depression, aggression, psychosis	–
Zonisamide	Agitation, depression, psychosis	–

2007). In this regard, what is striking is the involvement of the limbic structures in the development of treatment-emergent depressive symptoms. In fact, a particular subgroup of drug refractory TLE patients is at high risk whenever an antiepilepileptic drug is introduced; these are subjects with a family and personal history of mood disorders and a previous history of febrile convulsions (Mula et al., 2007), indicating that abnormally functional limbic structures are much more determinant than structurally abnormal functional limbic structures.

The AEDs most often associated with the occurrence of depressive symptoms seem to be those which act at the benzodiazepine-GABA receptor complex, and include barbiturates, tiagabine, topiramate, and vigabatrin. Since, in psychiatric practice, it is known that benzodiazepines and other GABA agonists are associated clinically with depression, and that abnormalities of cerebrospinal fluid GABA have been reported in patients with depression (Trimble, 1996), the link between sudden cessation of seizures, GABAergic agents and the onset of depression seems reasonably secure.

In conclusion, taking all these data together, it is possible to speculate that GABAergic potentiation may precipitate depression in patients with a fertile background (*i.e.* a genetic predisposition to mood disorders exemplified by previous functional abnormalities in the limbic system and family history).

Dysphoria in epilepsy

Debate is ongoing regarding the phenomenology of depressive disorders in epilepsy. Some authors observed that up to 22% of patients who were consecutively assessed for the occurrence of depression could be classified as having atypical features (Mendez et al., 1986) and this percentage could be as much as 71% among subjects with drug-resistant epilepsy (Kanner et al., 2000; 2004). At this point, it is important to state that a number of potential causes may account for the atypical nature of depressive symptoms in epilepsy, such as behavioural periictal symptoms, psychotropic effects of antiepileptic drugs, high rates of comorbid anxiety disorders or symptoms, and the spectrum of subclinical and subsyndromic forms of depression which represent, to some degree, an important cause of atypical presentations of primary mood disorders in psychiatric practice. In any case, the possibility that mood disorders associated with epilepsy have unique characteristics is plausible. Classic reports on psychiatry, by authors such as Kraepelin and Bleuler, have described a pleomorphic pattern of symptoms, including affective symptoms with prominent irritability intermixed with euphoric moods, fear and anxiety, as well as anergia, pain and insomnia, typical of patients with epilepsy. Gastaut confirmed such observations (Gastaut et al., 1955) and, later, Blumer coined the term "interictal dysphoric disorder" (IDD) to refer to this type of somatoform-depressive disorder seen in patients with epilepsy (Blumer, 2000). Blumer used the term "dysphoria" to emphasise the periodicity of mood changes and the presence of outbursts of irritability and aggressive behaviour as key symptoms.

Although there is no clear evidence that IDD is linked to TLE, it is becoming apparent that TLE patients present with a number of periictal behavioural manifestations which actually account for the atypical phenomenology of mood disorders in epilepsy (Mula et al., 2010).

Suicide

The relationship between epilepsy and suicide has been investigated in a few studies using a case-control design, mostly in Scandinavia (Mula et al., 2010). A recent meta-analysis estimated the overall standardised mortality ratio (SMR) for suicide in epilepsy as 3.3 (95% CI 2.8, 3.7). The SMR, however, ranges between 2.1 for people with newly diagnosed epilepsy in the community and 13.9 for those following temporal lobe resections (Bell et al., 2009). The cause of the increased risk of suicide associated with epilepsy is not entirely clear. In the past, it was linked to socio-economic deprivation associated with epilepsy (Matthews & Barabas, 1981; Harris & Barraclough, 1997) and a specific association with TLE had been suggested (1980). However, recent studies show that epilepsy-related variables are not as relevant as psychiatric comorbidities (Christensen et al., 2007). It is clear that more data are warranted and well-designed studies are needed to identify and isolate relevant variables.

The issue of suicide in epilepsy has been recently revitalised by the Food and Drug Administration (FDA) warning on suicidal risk with AEDs (FDA, 2008). Many authors have noted numerous concerns about the methodology of the FDA analysis (Bell et al., 2009; Hesdorffer & Kanner, 2009), however, it has, at least, emphasised the importance of screening people with epilepsy for suicidality, depression or anxiety disorders (Hesdorffer & Kanner, 2009). Consideration should be given as to the choice of AED, taking into account both the seizure type and the risk of AED-induced depressive symptoms. People with epilepsy should be warned that there is a small increased risk of suicidality associated with some AEDs, but that the risk of not taking AEDs is more substantial. They should also be encouraged to report any symptoms to their physician.

Psychosis

Compared to affective disorders, psychoses are rare complications in epilepsy, affecting about 4%-6% of patients in clinical case series. The issue of epilepsy-related psychosis was a popular theme in psychiatric literature in the middle of the last century, focussing on interictal schizophrenia-like psychoses. Interest in these psychoses has waned and over recent decades postictal psychoses have been studied more extensively. However, postictal psychoses are of short duration and psychotic patients are difficult to investigate, leaving many questions unanswered in terms of exact underlying pathophysiology.

Classification

For pragmatic reasons, it remains convenient to group psychoses in epilepsy according to the temporal relationship with seizures. *Ictal psychoses* are more likely to be linked to simple or complex partial seizure status than to absence status but have never been examined in any detail. In clinical practice, ictal psychoses are most frequently seen with seizures of temporal lobe origin but some are secondary to frontal lobe seizures. Simple focal status or aura continua may cause complex hallucinations, thought disorders, and affective symptoms. Continuous epileptic activity is restricted and may escape scalp EEG recordings *(Table II)*.

Table II. Clinical characteristics of psychoses in relation to seizure activity

	Interictal	Ictal	Postictal	Alternative
Relative frequency	~20%	~10%	~50%	~10%
Consciousness	Normal	Impaired	Impaired or normal	Normal
Typical features	Schizophrenia-like psychopathology	Mild motor symptoms	Lucid interval	Initial symptom insomnia
Duration	Months	Hours to days	Days to weeks	Weeks
EEG	Unchanged	Status epilepticus	Increased slowing, increased epileptiform activity	Normalized
Treatment	Antipsychotics	Antiepileptic drugs i.v.	Benzodiazepines, seizure control	Sleep regulation, reduction of antiepileptic drugs

Among the various types of psychoses, those which are directly related to seizures are most common. The most common type of psychosis in epilepsy is *postictal psychosis*. Psychoses without any clear relationship to seizures, so called "interictal psychoses", may develop after several years of active epilepsy, and are most often of the temporal lobe type. Despite some psychopathological peculiarities, these psychoses resemble chronic schizophrenia-like illness and recent findings suggest subtle underlying limbic pathology analogous to similar observations in "endogenous" schizophrenia.

Psychoses can also be triggered by AEDs and particularly those which have strong anti-convulsive properties may trigger psychotic reactions. Some of these psychoses may be considered toxic as they are often dose-related. Psychoses which are associated with seizure freedom and EEG normalisation are covered by the term "forced normalisation" and *"alternative psychosis"*. Seizure control is often associated with milder behavioural problems, emotional instability, or insomnia, and psychotic reactions are relatively rare.

Interictal psychoses occur between seizures or, more often, independently of seizures and cannot directly be linked to the ictus. They are less frequent than periictal psychoses and account for 10%-30% of diagnoses in unselected case series (Schmitz et al., 1999). Interictal psychoses are, however, clinically more significant in terms of severity and duration than periictal psychoses which usually are brief and self-limiting.

Epidemiology *(Table III)*

In a case control study, Stefansson et al. compared the prevalence of non-organic psychiatric disorders between patients with epilepsy and patients with other somatic diseases, taken from a disability register in Iceland (Stefansson et al., 1998). Although the difference in psychiatric diagnoses overall was not significant, there was a higher rate of psychoses, particularly schizophrenia and paranoid states, amongst males with epilepsy.

In a study from Denmark, Qin et al. confirmed the increased risk of schizophrenia and schizophrenia-like psychoses in epilepsy and further identified that a family history of psychoses or epilepsy was a significant risk factor for psychosis (Qin et al., 2005). Based on a record linkage study, Bredkjaer et al. looked for associations between epilepsy from the national patient register of Denmark and the equivalent psychiatric register (Bredkjaer et al., 1998). The incidence of non-organic, non-affective psychoses, which included schizophrenia and schizophrenia spectrum disorders, was significantly increased in epilepsy, even when patients with learning disability or substance misuse were excluded.

Higher prevalence rates for psychoses were found in studies using more highly selected populations, such as hospital cases series. Gureje (1991) studied patients attending a neurological clinic and noted that 37% of patients were psychiatric cases and 29% of these were psychotic. In a retrospective investigation, Mendez et al. reported that interictal psychotic disorders were found in over 9% of a large cohort of patients with epilepsy, in contrast to just over 1% in patients with migraines (Mendez et al., 1993). Studies from Japan examining new referrals for epilepsy quoted a 6% prevalence of psychoses in patients with normal intelligence (in contrast to 24% in patients with learning disabilities) (Matsuura et al., 2005).

Table III. Epidemiology of postictal psychosis

Investigated cohort	Prevalence	Reference
Unselected outpatients	2%	Schmitz, 1995
Pharmacoresistant TLE	9%	Kanemoto, 1996
TLE + hippocampus sclerosis	15%	Kanemoto, 1996
TLE + HS + atrophy	56%	Kanemoto, 1996
Video-EEG-monitoring	6-10%	Kanner, 1996; 2004

The link with temporal lobe epilepsy

Compared to mood disorders, where the association with the temporolimbic structures is still a matter of debate, the link between thought disorders and epilepsy seems more evident. There is a clear predominance of TLE in almost all case series of patients with epilepsy and psychosis; among the pooled data from 10 studies, 217 (76%) of 287 patients suffered from TLE (Trimble, 1991). Furthermore, there is evidence from several studies that focal seizure symptoms, which indicate ictal mesial temporal or limbic involvement, are over-represented in patients with psychosis. Hermann and Chabria noted a relationship between ictal fear and high scores on paranoia and schizophrenia scales of the Minnesota Multiphasic Personality Inventory (MMPI) (Chabria, 1988). Kristensen and Sindrup found an excess of dysmnesic and epigastric auras in their psychotic group (Kristensen & Sindrup, 1978) and also reported a higher rate of ictal amnesia. In another controlled study, ictal impairment of consciousness was related to psychosis, but simple seizure symptoms indicating limbic involvement were unrelated (Schmitz & Wolf, 1995). Mula et al. investigated dimensions of schizotypy in patients with epilepsy (Mula et al., 2008). The term "schizotype" was introduced to identify a clinical phenotype biologically correlated to schizophrenia (Siever & Davis, 2004). A strong association between TLE and core elements of schizophrenia related to First Rank Schneiderian symptoms has been identified, suggesting that the link between epilepsy and schizophrenia has a strong biological component, and temporal lobe dysfunction represents fertile ground for the development of thought disorders.

Laterality

Left lateralization of temporal lobe dysfunction or temporal lobe pathology as a risk factor for schizophreniform psychosis was originally suggested by Flor-Henry (1969). Studies supporting the laterality hypothesis have been made using surface EEG, depth electrode recordings, computed tomography, neuropathology, neuropsychology, positron-emission tomography (PET), and more recently, MRI. Earlier literature has been summarised by Trimble (1991). In a synopsis of 14 studies with 341 patients, 43% had left, 23% right, and 34% bilateral abnormalities. This is a striking bias towards left lateralization. Trimble pointed out that a specific group with hallucinations and delusions, defined by Schneider and referred to as "First Rank Symptoms", which usually (but by no means exclusively) signifies schizophrenia (Trimble, 1991), may be relevant. He suggested that these may be signifiers of temporal lobe dysfunction, representing disturbances of language and symbolic representation. In this sense, he equated them to a Babinski sign for the neurologist, i.e. pointing to a location and lateralization of an abnormality in the central nervous system.

These laterality findings have received support from brain imaging studies, especially SPECT and MRI. Using a verbal fluency activation paradigm and HMPAO SPECT, Mellers et al. compared patients with schizophrenia-like psychoses of epilepsy (n = 12), with schizophrenia (n = 11), and epilepsy and no psychoses (n = 16) (Mellers et al., 1998). The psychotic epilepsy patients showed lower blood flow in the superior temporal gyrus during activation than the other two groups. Using MR spectroscopy, Maier et al. were able to compare hippocampal-amygdala volumes and hippocampal N-acetyl aspartate (NAA) levels in patients with TLE and schizophrenia-like psychoses of epilepsy (n = 12), TLE and no psychoses (n = 12), schizophrenia and no epilepsy (n = 26) and matched normal controls (n = 38). The psychotic patients showed significant left-sided reduction of NAA, and this was more pronounced in the psychotic epilepsy group. Regional volume reductions were noted bilaterally in this group, and in the left hippocampus-amygdala in the schizophrenic group (Maier et al., 2000).

Flugel et al. examined 20 psychotic and 20 non-psychotic cases with TLE using Magnetisation Transfer Imaging. They reported significant reductions in the magnetization transfer ratio (an index of signal loss) in the left superior and middle temporal gyri in psychotic patients. This was unrelated to volume changes and was best revealed in a subgroup with no focal MRI lesions (Flugel et al., 2006).

Structural lesions

The literature on brain damage and epileptic psychosis is very controversial. Some authors have suggested a higher rate of pathological neurological examinations, diffuse slowing on EEG, and mental retardation (Kristensen et al., 1978a; 1978b), while others could find no association with psychosis (Jensen 1979). Neuropathological studies of resected temporal lobes from patients with TLE have suggested a link between psychosis and the presence of cerebral malformations such as hamartomas and gangliogliomas, compared with mesial temporal sclerosis (Taylor, 1971). These findings are consistent with those of structural abnormalities in the brains of schizophrenic patients without epilepsy arising during foetal development.

Bruton et al. noted enlarged ventricles, periventricular gliosis, and an excess of acquired focal damage in the brains of institutionalized psychotic epileptic patients, compared with non-psychotic controls. They also reported that schizophrenia-like psychoses were distinguished by an excess of perivascular white matter softening (Bruton et al., 1988).

In a study which specifically examined hippocampal and amygdala volumes, Tebartz van Elst and colleagues examined 26 patients with epileptic psychoses, 24 with TLE and no psychosis, and 20 healthy controls (Tebartz van Elst et al., 2002). The psychotic patients had significantly increased amygdala sizes in comparison with the other two groups, which were bilateral and unrelated to the laterality of the focus or length of epilepsy history. No hippocampal differences were noted in this study. In a complementary study on the same groups, Rusch et al. were unable to find any neocortical volumetric differences (Rusch et al., 2004).

Although the underlying pathology may be different, the absence of gliosis in the hippocampus and related structures characterizing schizophrenia, the site of the pathology, the timing of the lesions, and the consequent functional changes in the brain may all be crucial to the later development of any behavioural changes in both epilepsy and schizophrenia. Thus, behavioural changes which manifest in some patients should be viewed as an integral part of the process of epilepsy. However, the recent evidence, especially from brain imaging studies suggests that Slater's original hypothesis was only partly correct. Thus, interictal psychoses appear to be different from schizophrenia, especially with regards to the admixture of affective symptoms and long-term prognosis. While hippocampal changes may relate to both disorders, the increased bilateral amygdala size (of about 17%-20%), and the lesser volumetric changes in the hippocampus, suggest the two psychopathological states are biologically quite different. While the laterality findings, with regards to the functioning of the left hemisphere, appear to hold up, the data point away from fundamentally cortical abnormalities in these psychoses, and bring the amygdala and related structures to the forefront of pathogenesis.

Psychosis following surgery

Temporal lobectomy is an established treatment for patients with intractable epilepsy. However, ever since the early series, the possibility that surgery itself may be associated with the development of psychiatric disturbance, in particular psychosis, has been discussed. Some of the best evidence was based on the Maudsley series, initially described by Taylor in 1975 and more recently by Bruton in 1988. In most centres, surgery is no longer performed on floridly psychotic patients, based on the observation that psychoses generally do not improve postsurgically. A few centres, however, regularly include psychiatric screening as part of their preoperative assessment, but postoperative psychiatric follow-up is often nonexistent. Assessment of psychosocial adjustment is rarely performed, in contrast to the often scrupulous recording of neuropsychological deficits.

The Maudsley series demonstrated that some patients developed new psychosis postoperatively with increased reports of depression. Bruton (1988) has suggested that the development of postoperative psychoses may be more common with certain pathologies (gangliogliomas). Patients with right-sided temporal lobectomies may be more prone to these psychiatric disturbances (Trimble, 1991). In some cases, the sudden relief of seizures, which occurs following surgery, may suggest a mechanism similar to forced normalisation, although no persistent clear relationship emerges between the success of the operation and the development of psychotic postoperative states. In recent times, several small series of patients with psychoses were reported with successful surgery without worsening of their psychosis but with marked improvement in seizure control (Reutens et al., 1997).

■ Personality and cognition

In our clinical experience, some patients are unable to resolve epilepsy-related social problems even with optimal treatment and multi-disciplinary counselling, support and time-consuming rehabilitation programmes. This may seem difficult to understand, particularly when seizures are well-controlled, there are no deficits based on standard psychometric tests, and there is no evidence of major psychiatric disorders based upon psychiatric evaluations. Why is it that some patients are not well-integrated into the workplace, have difficulties finding partners, or prefer to live alone? Talking to our patients in the clinic provides us with a good opportunity to observe communicative peculiarities or disorders. There are some patients who take a lot of time to describe their symptoms in much detail, but are not really interested in our advice. In these cases, patient-doctor communication does not run smoothly and is "desynchronized" (quote from Martin Schöndienst). Some patients have problems understanding our non-verbal signals when time has run out (such as closing a file, looking at the time, *etc.*). Doctors may then react irritably and it may become difficult to close the session. In such cases, both doctor and patient may be left with a sense of annoyance and frustration.

The psychiatric diagnoses for these patients is often a personality disorder, described as *"epileptische Wesensänderung"* in early reports or "personality disorder cluster A" according to recent classification systems. This diagnosis is often used to explain why psychiatric treatments and social rehabilitation do not work. For a patient, this diagnosis is hard to accept and most neurologists have difficulties understanding the concept of a personality disorder. They may associate this with a poor prognosis and react with therapeutic nihilism. Nevertheless, based on epidemiologicial data, there is evidence that personality disorders are frequent in epilepsy, and in presurgical patients with TLE prevalence rates in the order of 60% to 80% have been described (*Table IV*).

Table IV. Personality disorders (PD) in epilepsy epidemiology

Investigated cohort	Prevalence	Reference
PDs in community surveys	5-13%	Coid, 2003
Juvenile myoclonic epilepsy	23%	Trinka *et al.*, 2006
PDs in presurgical populations with TLE	80% 61%	Serafetinides, 1975 Koch-Stoecker, 2002
"Organic PD" in surgically treated TLE (irreversible following surgery, predictor of poor outcome, only one patient became seizure-free)	10%	Koch-Stoecker, 2002

Interestingly, communication skills or styles are linked to epilepsy syndromes. In a controlled study comparing patients with juvenile myoclonic epilepsy (JME) and TLE, with respect to personality features, there were no differences when using standardised personality questionnaires (Neo Five). There was, however, a significant difference with respect to professional preference. Of JME patients, 70% worked in professions which required communicative skills, while 70% TLE patients preferred jobs which were more theoretical and did not involve much communication (Pung *et al.*, 2006). These findings confirm syndrome-related tendencies or weaknesses which were empirically described in an earlier report (Janz, 1969).

Communicative and emotional problems were described early on to be some of the typical personality features of patients with epilepsy in general and, in particular, patients with TLE. Stauder mentioned an egocentric, self-complacent attitude (1935). Tellenbach noted that patients were unable to express empathy (Tellenbach, 1965). Landolt (1960) (quoted from Janz, 1969) observed patients with a strange lack of awareness to themselves and their environment, and concluded "intelligence has no relevance for success in life".

With the description of the Geschwind syndrome, a discussion was started on the role of the limbic system in the formation of personality. According to Bear, TLE is an example of a sensory-limbic-hyperconnectivity syndrome, the opposite of the disconnection syndrome described by Kluver-Bucy (Bear, 1979) (*Figure 1*).

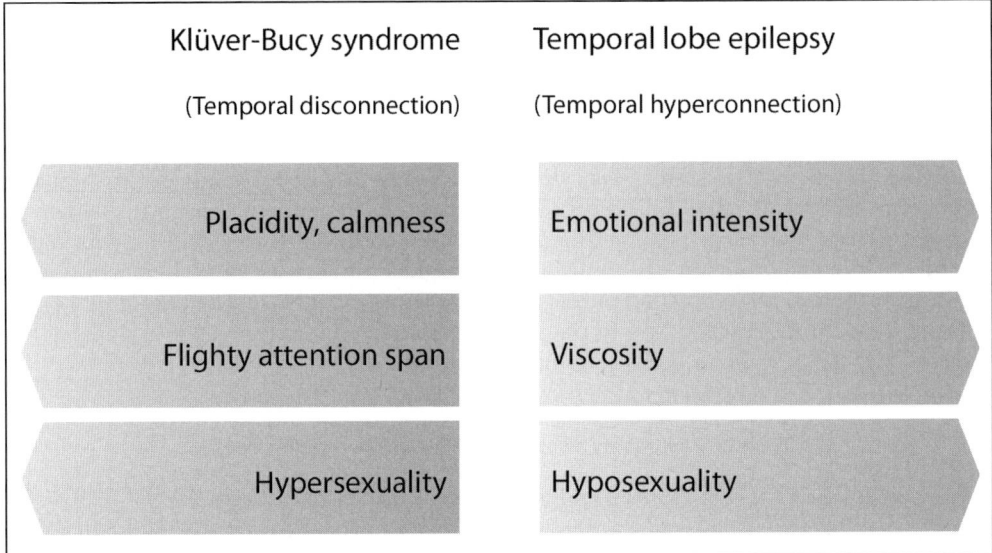

Figure 1. Personality type in temporal lobe epilepsy.
Adapted from Gastaut et al., 1955; Waxman & Geschwind, 1975

The affective features associated with Geschwind syndrome include emotionality, euphoria, sad mood, change of sexuality, anger, aggression, lack of humour and feelings of guilt. Important key symptoms of this syndrome are hypergraphia and religiosity. As mentioned above, affective disorders are significantly more common in TLE, compared to non-epileptic controls or patients with other epilepsy syndromes. Patients with TLE not only suffer from transient and sometimes severe postictal depression but also interictal chronic dysthymia. Endogenous-type depression is rare, a more typical disorder is chronic fluctuating affective disorder with emotional lability and paroxysmal mood swings, including euphoric spells. This syndrome, extensively described by Dietrich Blumer, has been systematically studied and, using standardised rating scales, may be linked to bipolar disorder (Blumer et al., 1998), although again, clinically speaking, endogenous-type bipolar disorder is rare in epilepsy (Ettinger et al., 2005). Summarising the earlier psychiatric literature on personality and the more recent data on affective disorders in epilepsy, there is evidence for a disorder in emotional regulation in patients with epilepsy, particularly when the focus is localized in the mesial temporal lobe. An affective disorder is, however, not only relevant to the patient's emotional state, but also to emotional perception and, therefore, interpersonal communication.

The limbic system plays a key role in the perception and processing of emotional stimuli, which are presented via mimics, gestures or speech prosody. From an ontological perspective, this is a highly relevant function which allows the quick and correct interpretation of whether somebody is friendly or potentially dangerous. This is extremely relevant for survival in nature. Affected animals behave without anxiety and they explore their environment based on oral and olfactory senses because visual perceptions can no longer be interpreted. In nature, monkeys cannot survive following amygdalectomy; they are isolated from members of their own species, sometimes even attacked, or become victims to animals of prey (Dicks et al., 1969). The Kluver-Bucy-syndrome, after bilateral amygdalectomy, is associated with "emotional agnosia".

Several studies have demonstrated that patients with epilepsy have problems with respect to emotional perception (*e.g.* recognition of emotional expressions) and that these deficits are linked to amygdala dysfunction. Houghton *et al.* (2000) showed that deficits correlate with reduced amygdala volume. Patients with ictal fear (an aura associated with epileptic activity in the amygdala) have a greater impairment of fearful expression recognition than patients with other types of epilepsy (Reynders *et al.*, 2005). The recognition of anxiety-related expressions may be more affected than other emotional qualities such as sadness, disgust, or positive emotions (Meletti *et al.*, 2003). Interestingly, as well as the phenomenon of impaired recognition, misinterpretation is also reported (Shaw *et al.*, 2007). Patients with lateralized epilepsies to the right and febrile seizures during childhood are more impaired (Meletti *et al.*, 2003; Benuzzi *et al.*, 2004). Furthermore, age at onset of epilepsy may play a role; patients with earlier onset of epilepsy were shown to display greater deficits (Meletti *et al.*, 2003). These studies suggest that normal emotional perception requires normal amygdala function (McClelland *et al.*, 2006) and that early damage (before the age of five) cannot be compensated through plastic processes.

The influence of epilepsy surgery is, as yet, unclear but several studies suggest that laterality may play an important role. Sanz-Martin *et al.* (2006) described a case with deterioration of emotional perception following right-sided temporal lobe resection. Yamada *et al.* (2005) reported a patient with left TLE with postsurgical improvement. A prospective study with 19 patients undergoing temporal lobe resections for epilepsy (Shaw *et al.*, 2007) confirmed that improvements in tests on emotional perception were only observed following left-sided resections.

Another function which is crucial for social communication is described by ToM. ToM relates to the ability to empathize with other people and recognise that another person has feelings and intentions similar to oneself. This function depends on an extensive neuronal network including the amygdala and the orbitofrontal cortex (Shaw *et al.*, 2004). ToM can be tested by presenting stories (*e.g.* using cartoons) which can only be understood when the thoughts and intentions of the people in the cartoons are correctly interpreted. In addition to these classic ToM tests, there are a number of other tests which can be used in order to investigate various aspects of social cognition, such as the Faux Pas Test, the Mind in the Eyes Test, the Cheating Test as well as tests for sense of humour. ToM tests were initially developed for autism research, but are increasingly used for other neurological conditions and deficits have, for example, been found in frontotemporal dementia.

In the field of epilepsy, the use of ToM tests for social cognition deficits was described in patients with frontal lobe epilepsies and TLE (Schacher *et al.*, 2006). There are possibly subtle differences depending on the type of epilepsy. Farrant *et al.* (2005) described problems in understanding jokes in patients with frontal lobe epilepsy, but the interpretation of ToM stories was not impaired in comparison to the controls. Unfortunately, TLE patients were not included in this study.

Treatment

Depression

It is important to state that there is only one reported controlled trial of the effects of an intervention for mood disorders in epilepsy, and the evidence for treatment strategies relies heavily on clinical experience (Mula et al., 2008). An expert US panel comprising members from the Epilepsy Foundation's Mood Disorders Initiative composed a Consensus Statement (Barry et al., 2008).

Psychiatric symptoms temporally-related to the occurrence of seizures (preceding or following a seizure or a cluster of seizures, occurring when the patient achieves sudden and complete seizure control or when seizures worsen) do not need any specific psychotropic treatment and better seizure control is often the best solution.

In the case of a mood disorder characterised by symptoms occurring independently of seizures, psychopharmacotherapy can be required but evidence in favour of any particular drug is lacking. The only published controlled trial involved nomifensine, an antidepressant which is no longer available (Robertson & Trimble, 1985). Selective serotonin reuptake inhibitors (SSRIs) have become the first-line drug treatment for primary major depression and dysthymic disorder in psychiatric practice. However, studies addressing efficacy and safety in epilepsy are lacking. During recent years, a number of authors have approached the clinical problem of treating mood disorders in epilepsy from different points of view (Mula et al., 2004; Kanner & Balabanov, 2005; Prueter & Norra, 2005). A few open studies have been published on the use of sertraline (Kanner et al., 2000; Thomè-Souza et al., 2007), citalopram (Specchio et al., 2004; Khun et al., 2003; Hovorka et al., 2000), reboxetine (Khun et al., 2003), mirtazapine (Khun et al., 2003), and fluoxetine (Thomè-Souza et al., 2007). The study by Thomè-Souza et al. (2007) is of particular interest since this is the only published study to date which involves children and adolescents with epilepsy and depression.

In general, all presented studies have shown antidepressant drug treatment to be well tolerated, but the reported response rates were highly variable, for example, citalopram, response rates varied from 38% (Khun et al., 2003) to 65% (Hovorka et al., 2007) after treatment for eight weeks. It is evident that the reported variability is influenced by a number of factors which include: the selection of patients, the lack of rigorous psychiatric assessment for correct diagnosis (dysthymia, major depression, bipolar depression, and interictal dysphoric disorder), the presence of other comorbid axis I disorders, the presence of brain damage, cognitive impairment, a family history of mood disorders, and so on. All of these variables are very rarely taken into consideration in these studies, although they are essential for the correct interpretation of results.

If studies on psychoactive drugs in epilepsy are rare, studies on psychological therapy for mood disorders in epilepsy are exceptionally so. We are aware of only two papers, one involving adult patients (Tan & Bruni, 1986) and the other involving children (Martinovic et al., 2006), both of which show that cognitive behavioural therapies play a role in the management of mood disorder symptoms in epilepsy.

The issue of psychotropic drug treatment for depression in epilepsy is interlinked with that of the "proconvulsant" or "anticonvusant" effects of antidepressants *(Figure 1)*. Tricyclic antidepressants developed a clinical reputation for convulsant liability soon after their introduction (Dailey & Naritoku, 1996). The concept that antidepressant medications are more likely to produce convulsions in patients with epilepsy than in patients without this disorder is intuitively appealing, and is seemingly compatible with the concept that seizure predisposition is fundamental to the definition of epilepsy. However, it is clear that the biology of seizure predisposition is complex, moreover, it is not clear whether the risk of seizure expression arises from seizure liability itself or from a more complex predisposition inherent in the mechanisms of comorbidity between affective disorders and epilepsies (Jobe & Browing, 2005). A recent meta-analysis of controlled trials comparing seizure risk of antidepressants in psychiatric patients demonstrated lower seizure rates in patients using more recent antidepressants compared to patients in the placebo groups, suggesting that some of the more recent antidepressants may have anticonvulsant properties. This has been demonstrated in experimental studies (Alper et al., 2007).

Psychosis

Therapeutic strategies for psychoses in epilepsy are very different depending on the individual situation. In the majority of cases, patients require treatment with antipsychotic medication, although these, like most antidepressants, can lower seizure threshold.

Ictal psychoses may only occasionally require treatment with neuroleptic drugs, as they usually settle rapidly with intravenous AED treatment. Postictal psychoses often do not require psychotropic medication, resolving themselves in a few hours. However, it is important to stress how dangerous these cases can be, and it is essential to note any command hallucinations or delusions of harm which may affect the patient or others, and protect accordingly. In the first instance, treatment with a benzodiazepine is helpful, since there is a risk of precipitating further seizures and exacerbating the psychosis with other drugs, especially some antipsychotic drugs. Regular benzodiazepine treatment for perhaps 48 hours is often sufficient. In the longer term, it is important to realize that postictal psychoses have a tendency to recur. It is therefore important to warn patients of this and prevent clusters of seizures with an effective antiepileptic drug. Sometimes, it is possible to prevent such a cluster and hence subsequent psychosis by administering a benzodiazepine (e.g. 3×10 mg clobazam or 3×2 mg lorazepam) and/or an antipsychotic drug (e.g. 3×2 mg risperidone) following the first seizure and subsequently for a few days. However, sometimes all these measures fail, in which case intermittent or even continuous antipsychotic treatment becomes important.

Interictally, the paranoid or schizophrenia-like states need to be evaluated in terms of their relationship to seizure frequency. Thus, in patients who stop having seizures in association with the onset of psychosis, a first procedure may be to lower antiepileptic drugs in order to allow a seizure to reoccur. When neuroleptic drugs are used a drug may be chosen which decreases the seizure threshold.

When patients with epilepsy have no alteration of seizure frequency, or when psychosis occurs in the context of increased seizure frequency, a neuroleptic drug which is less likely to precipitate seizures, such as a recent atypical antipsychotic, is recommended. Olanzapine and risperidone have been used most frequently in epilepsy, and both drugs are associated with a relatively low risk of seizures, particularly risperidone (Amann et al., 2003).

It should be recalled that patients who take anticonvulsants, which increase hepatic metabolism, will have lower serum levels of neuroleptics and may therefore require somewhat higher doses, compared to patients who do not take such anticonvulsants, in order to achieve a similar clinical effect. The side-effects of long-term treatment should be considered, particularly in patients taking AEDs with similar side-effect profiles. Olanzapine is more sedating than risperidone and is associated with a risk of reduced glucose intolerance which is relevant to elderly patients, however, extrapyramidal side effects are less common compared to risperidone. Weight gain should also be considered when prescribing olanzapine, particularly in combination with an AED which also induces weight gain, such as valproate or pregabaline. Potential cardiotoxic effects of antipsychotics (QT prolongation with, for example, pimozide and ziprosidone) should be considered in elderly patients, particularly when they take carbamazepine or phenytoin. Clozapine is only exceptionally prescribed for epilepsy because of the well-known epileptogenic risks. Clozapine also causes weight again and salivation, and due to its haematotoxicity, combination with carbamazepine should be avoided.

Treatment strategies for personality disorders/deficits of emotional recognition and social cognition

The pharmacological and psychological treatment options for personality disorders are limited and there are no controlled studies focusing on personality disorders in epilepsy. However, recent findings on distinct neuropsychological deficits with respect to social cognition and emotional recognition may allow more specific treatment strategies to be developed. For patients and their relatives this may be helpful simply in terms of reflecting their deficits. By understanding the nature of certain weaknesses, acceptance may become easier and it may be possible to develop better coping strategies. The early identification of specific neuropsychological deficits is, furthermore, important in order to counsel patients with respect to more or less suitable professional aims, and also to predict the prognosis of social rehabilitation programmes. Whether specific behavioural treatments are able to improve deficits related to social and emotional cognition is a clinically important question which deserves further research.

■ Conclusion

MTLE is a syndrome with a typical course over time, involving neuronal networks which are crucial for emotional regulation and social behaviour. There is evidence that psychiatric disorders are over-represented in patients with epilepsy in general, and the link between specific psychiatric disorders and TLE is strong, both clinically and theoretically. The link between the limbic system and the modulation of emotional and social behaviour is well accepted. Thus, affected emotional states and behaviour are not unexpected in a disorder such as MTLE, which is often associated with lesions in the medial temporal structures that tend to be present from an early phase in life. In clinical practice it is not rare to encounter clinical syndromes which bridge classic neurology and psychiatry and this seems to be even more frequent when patients present a complex and polymorphic psychiatric syndrome with clear EEG temporal lobe abnormalities but without any evidence or history of epileptic seizures. In such cases, antiepileptic drugs often induce a dramatic clinical improvement. It is tempting to speculate that "para-epileptic" mechanisms may be relevant for the phenomenology of the behavioural syndrome (Mula, 2009). Finally, and referring to a quote by Bear, it should be stressed that epilepsy is not synonymous with seizures, and the latter are but one manifestation of the disordered cerebral function of patients with epilepsy.

"If the temporal lobe is a meeting place for sensory stimuli and biological drives [...] then aberrantly firing neurons or those with a lowered threshold for discharge could [...] produce cumulative errors of emotional association. This pathophysiological mechanism may be independent of [...] the process resulting in seizures, providing the basis for interictal behaviour changes." (Bear, 1986)

References

- Alper KK, Schwartz KA, Kolts RL, Khan A. Seizure incidence in psychopharmacological clinical trials: an analysis of Food and Drug Administration (FDA) summary basis of approval reports. *Biol Psychiatry* 2007; 62: 345-5.
- Amann BL, Pogarell O, Mergl R, Juckel G, Grunze H, Mulert C, Hegerl U. EEG abnormalities associated with antipsychotics: a comparison of quetiapine, olanzapine, haloperidol and healthy subjects. *Hum Psychopharmacol* 2003; 18: 641-6.
- Barry JJ, Ettinger AB, Friel P, Gilliam FG, Harden CL, Hermann B, *et al*. Consensus statement: the evaluation and treatment of people with epilepsy and affective disorders. *Epilepsy Behav* 2008; 13 (Suppl 1): S1-29.
- Bear DM. Temporal lobe epilepsy-a syndrome of sensory-limbic hyperconnection. *Cortex* 1979; 15: 357-84.
- Bell GS, Mula M, Sander JW. Suicidality in people taking antiepileptic drugs: What is the evidence? *CNS Drugs* 2009; 23: 281-92.
- Bell GS, Gaitatzis A, Bell CL, Johnson AL, Sander JW. Suicide in people with epilepsy: how great is the risk? *Epilepsia* 2009; 50: 1933-42.
- Benuzzi F, Meletti S, Zamboni G, Calandra-Buonaura G, Serafini M, Lui F, *et al*. Impaired fear processing in right mesial temporal sclerosis: a fMRI study. *Brain Res Bull* 2004; 63: 269-81.
- Blumer D. Dysphoric disorders and paroxysmal affects: recognition and treatment of epilepsy-related psychiatric disorders. *Harv Rev Psychiatry* 2000; 8: 8-17.
- Blumer D, Altshuler LL. *Affective disorders*. In: Engel J, Pedley TA. *Epilepsy. A Comprehensive Textbook*. Philadelphia: Lippincott, Raven, 1998, pp. 2083-99.
- Boylan LS, Flint LA, Labovitz DL, Jackson SC, Starner K, Devinsky O. Depression but not seizure frequency predicts quality of life in treatment-resistant epilepsy. *Neurology* 2004; 62: 258-61.
- Bredkjaer SR, Mortensen PB, Parnas J Epilepsy and non-organic non-affective psychosis. National epidemiologic study. *Br J Psychiatry* 1998; 172: 235-8.
- Bremner JD, Narayan M, Anderson ER, Staib LH, Miller HL, Charney DS. Hippocampal volume reduction in major depression. *Am J Psychiatry* 2000; 157: 115-8.
- Bromfield E, Altschuler L, Leiderman D. Cerebral metabolism and depression in patients with complex partial seizures. *Epilepsia* 1990; 31: 625.
- Bruton CJ *The Neuropathology of Temporal Lobe Epilepsy*. Oxford: Oxford University Press, 1988, Maudsley Monograph No 31.
- Christensen J, Vestergaard M, Mortensen PB, Sidenius P, Agerbo E. Epilepsy and risk of suicide: a population-based case-control study. *Lancet Neurol* 2007; 6: 693-8.
- Coid JW. Personality disorders in prisoners and their motivation for dangerous and disruptive behaviour. *Crim Behav Ment Health* 2002; 12: 209-26.
- Cramer JA., Blum D, Reed M, Fanning K, *et al*. The influence of comorbid depression on quality of life for people with epilepsy. *Epilepsia* 2003; 44: 1578-84.

- Dailey JW, Naritoku DK. Antidepressants and seizures: clinical anecdotes overshadow neuroscience. *Biochem Pharmacol* 1996; 52: 1323-9.
- Dicks D, Myers R, Kling AS. Uncus and Amygdala lesions: effects on social behaviour in the free-ranging rhesus monkey. *Science* 1969; 165: 69-71.
- Edeh J, Toone B. Relationship between interictal psychopathology and type of epilepsy. Results of a survey in general practice. *Br J Psychiatry* 1987; 151: 95-101.
- Ettinger A, Reed M, Cramer J. Epilepsy Impact Project Group Depression and comorbidity in community-based patients with epilepsy or asthma. *Neurology* 2004; 63: 1008-14.
- Ettinger AB, Reed ML, Goldberg JF, Hirschfeld RM. Prevalence of bipolar symptoms in epilepsy vs. other chronic health disorders. *Neurology* 2005; 65: 535-40.
- Farrant A, Morris RG, Russell T, Elwes R, Akanuma N, Alarcón G, Koutroumanidis M. Social cognition in frontal lobe epilepsy. *Epilepsy Behav* 2005; 7: 506-16.
- Flor Henry P. Psychosis and temporal lobe epilepsy. A controlled investigation. *Epilepsia* 1969; 10: 363-95.
- Flugel D, Cercignani M, Symms MR, Koepp MJ, Foong JA. Magnetization transfer imaging study in patients with temporal lobe epilepsy and interictal psychosis. *Biol Psychiatry* 2006; 59: 560-7.
- Forsgren L, Nystrom L. An incident case-referent study of epileptic seizures in adults. *Epilepsy Res* 1990; 6: 66-81.
- Frodl T, Meisenzahl EM, Zetzsche T, Born C, Groll C, Jager M. Hippocampal changes in patients with a first episode of major depression. *Am J Psychiatry* 2002; 159: 1112-8.
- Gastaut HG, Morin G, Lesevre N. Behavior of psychomotor epileptics between seizures; disorders of general activity and sociability. *Ann Med Psychol* 1955; 113: 1-27.
- Gilliam F, Kuzniecky R, Faught E, Black L, Carpenter G, Schrodt R. Patient validated content of epilepsy specific quality of life measurement. *Epilepsia* 1997; 38: 233-6.
- Gureje O. Interictal psychopathology in epilepsy – Prevalence and pattern in a Nigerian clinic. *Br J Psychiatry* 1991; 158: 700-5.
- Harris EC, Barraclough B. Suicide as an outcome for mental disorders. A meta-analysis. *Br J Psychiatry* 1997; 170: 205-28.
- Herrman BP, Chabria S. Interictal psychopathology in patients with ictal fear. *Arch Neurol* 1980; 37: 667-8.
- Hermann BP, Seidenberg M, Haltiner A, Wyler AR. Mood state in unilateral temporal lobe epilepsy. *Biol Psychiatry* 1991; 30: 1205-18.
- Hesdorffer DC, Hauser WA, Annegers JF, Cascino G. Major depression is a risk factor for seizures in older patients. *Ann Neurol* 2000; 47: 246-9.
- Hesdorffer DC, Kanner AM. The FDA alert on suicidality and antiepileptic drugs: Fire or false alarm? *Epilepsia* 2009; 50: 978-86.
- Hitiris N, Mohanraj R, Norrie J, Sills GJ, Brodie MJ. Predictors of pharmacoresistant epilepsy. *Epilepsy Res* 2007; 75: 192-6.
- Houghton JM, Brooks P, Wing A, Eldridge P, Walsh R, Davies P, *et al.* Does TLE impair the ability to recognise cues to the emotional state of others? *Epilepsia* 2000; 41 (S7): 249.
- Hovorka J, Herman E, Nemcova ILI. Treatment of interictal depression with citalopram in patients with epilepsy. *Epilepsy Behav* 2000; 1: 444-7.
- Janz D. *Die Epilepsien. Spezielle Pathologie und Therapie.* 2nd edition. Stuttgart: Thieme, 1969, 1998.
- Jensen I, Larsen JK. Mental aspects of temporal lobe epilepsy. *J Neurol Neurosurg Psychiatry* 1979; 42: 256-65.
- Jobe PSC, Browning RS. The serotonergic and noradrenergic effects of antidepressant drugs are anticonvulsant, not proconvulsant. *Epilepsy Behav* 2005; 7: 602-19.

- Jones JE, Hermann BP, Barry JJ, Gilliam F, Kanner AM, Meador KJ. Clinical Assessment of Axis 1. Psychiatric morbidity in chronic epilepsy: a multicentre investigation. *J Neuropsychiatry Clin Neurosci* 2005; 17: 172-9.
- Kanemoto K, Kawasaki J, Kawai I. Postictal psychosis: a comparison with acute interictal and chronic psychoses. *Epilepsia* 1996; 37: 551-6.
- Kanner AM. Depression and epilepsy: a new perspective on two closely related disorders. *Epilepsy Curr*. 2006; 6: 141-6.
- Kanner AM. Epilepsy and mood disorders. *Epilepsia* 2007; 48 (Suppl 9): 20-2.
- Kanner AM. Depression in epilepsy: a complex relation with unexpected consequences. *Curr Opin Neurol* 2008; 21: 190-4.
- Kanner AM, Balabanov A. Depression and epilepsy: how closely related are they? *Neurology* 2002; 58 (Suppl 5): S27-39.
- Kanner AM, Balabanov AJ. Pharmacotherapy of mood disorders in epilepsy: the role of newer psychotropic drugs. *Curr Treat Options Neurol* 2005; 7: 281-90.
- Kanner AM, Kozak AM, Frey M. The Use of sertraline in patients with epilepsy: Is it safe? *Epilepsy Behav* 2000; 1: 100-5.
- Kanner AM, Soto A, Gross-Kanner H. Prevalence and clinical characteristics of postictal psychiatric symptoms in partial epilepsy. *Neurology* 2004; 62: 708-13.
- Kanner AM, Stagno S, Kotagal P, Morris HH. Postictal psychiatric events during prolonged video-electroencephalographic monitoring studies. *Arch Neurol* 1996: 53: 258-63.
- Koch-Stoecker S. Personality disorders as predictors of severe postsurgical psychiatric complications in epilepsy patients undergoing temporal lobe resections. *Epilepsy Behav* 2002; 3: 526-31.
- Kristensen O, Sindrup HH. Psychomotor epilepsy and psychosis. I. Physical aspects. *Acta Neurol Scand* 1978a; 57: 361-9.
- Kristensen O, Sindrup HH. Psychomotor epilepsy and psychosis. II. Electroencephalographic findings. *Acta Neurol Scand* 1978b; 57: 370-9.
- Kuhn KU, Quednow BB, Thiel M, Falkai P, Maier W, Elger CE. Antidepressive treatment in patients with temporal lobe epilepsy and major depression: a prospective study with three different antidepressants. *Epilepsy Behav* 2003; 4: 674-9.
- Maier M, Mellers J, Toone B, Trimble M, Ron MA. Schizophrenia, temporal lobe epilepsy and psychosis: an *in vivo* magnetic resonance spectroscopy and imaging study of the hippocampus/amygdala complex. *Psychol Med* 2000; 30: 571-81.
- Martinovic Z, Simonovic P, Djokic R Preventing depression in adolescents with epilepsy. *Epilepsy Behav* 2006; 9: 619-24.
- Matsuura M, Adachi N, Muramatsu R, Kato M, Onuma T, Okubo Y, et al. Intellectual disability and psychotic disorders of adult epilepsy. *Epilepsia* 2005; 46 (Suppl 1): S11-4.
- Matthews WS, Barabas G. Suicide and epilepsy: a review of the literature. *Psychosomatics* 1981; 22: 515-24.
- McClelland S, Garcia RE, Peraza DM, Shih TT, Hirsch LJ, Hirsch J, Goodman RR. Facial emotion recognition after curative nondominant temporal lobectomy in patients with mesial temporal sclerosis. *Epilepsia* 2006; 47: 1337-42.
- Meletti S, Benuzzi F, Rubboli G, Cantalupo G, Stanzani Maserati M, et al. Impaired facial emotion recognition in early-onset right mesial temporal lobe epilepsy. *Neurology* 2003; 60: 426-31.
- Mellers JD, Adachi N, Takei N, Cluckie A, Toone BK, Lishman W. A SPET study of verbal fluency in schizophrenia and epilepsy. *Br J Psychiatry* 1998; 173: 69-74.
- Melvin CL, Carey TS, Goodman F, Oldham JM, Williams JW Jr, Ranney LM. Effectiveness of antiepileptic drugs for the treatment of bipolar disorder: findings from a systematic review. *J Psychiatr Pract*. 2008; 14 (Suppl 1): S9-14.

- Mendez MF, Grau R, Doss RC, Taylor JL. Schizophrenia in epilepsy: seizure and psychosis variables. *Neurology* 1993; 43: 1073-7.
- Mendez MF, Cummings JL, Benson DF. Depression in epilepsy. Significance and phenomenology. *Arch Neurol* 1986; 43(8): 766-70.
- Mula M, Monaco F, Trimble MR. Use of psychotropic drugs in patients with epilepsy: interactions and seizure risk. *Expert Rev Neurother* 2004; 4: 953-64.
- Mula M, Pini S, Cassano GB. The role of anticonvulsant drugs in anxiety disorders: a critical review of the evidence. *J Clin Psychopharmacol* 2004; 27: 263-72.
- Mula M. Report on autoscopic or mirror hallucinations and altruistic hallucinations. *Epilepsy Behav* 2009; 16: 212-3.
- Mula M, Trimble MR, Sander JW. Are psychiatric adverse events of antiepileptic drugs a unique entity? A study on topiramate and levetiracetam. *Epilepsia* 2007: 48: 2322-6.
- Mula M, Sander JW Effects of antiepileptic drugs on mood in patients with epilepsy. *Drug Saf* 2007; 30: 555-67.
- Mula M, Schmitz B, Sander JW. The pharmacological treatment of depression in adults with epilepsy. *Expert Opin Pharmacother* 2008; 9: 3159-68.
- Mula M, Bell GS, Sander JW. Suicidality in epilepsy and possible effects of antiepileptic drugs. *Curr Neurol Neurosci Rep* 2010; 10: 327-32.
- Mula M, Trimble MR, Lhatoo SD, Sander JW. Topiramate and psychiatric adverse events in patients with epilepsy. *Epilepsia* 2003; 44: 659-63.
- Mula M, Trimble MR, Yuen A, Liu RS, Sander JW. Psychiatric adverse events during levetiracetam therapy. *Neurology* 2003; 61: 704-6.
- Mula M, Cavanna AL, Viana M, Barbagli D, Tota G, Cantello R, Monaco F. Clinical correlates of schizotypy in patients with epilepsy. *J Neuropsychiatry Clin Neurosci* 2008; 20: 441-6.
- Mula M, Jauch Cavanna A, Gaus V, Kretz R, Collimedaglia L, Barbagli D, et al. Interictal dysphoric disorder and periictal dysphoric symptoms in patients with epilepsy. *Epilepsia* 2010; 51: 1139-45.
- Perrine K, Hermann BP, Meador KJ, Vickrey BG, Cramer JA, Hays RD. The relationship of neuropsychological functioning to quality of life in epilepsy. *Arch Neurol* 1995; 52: 997-1000.
- Prueter C, Norra C Mood disorders and their treatment in patients with epilepsy. *J Neuropsychiatry Clin Neurosci* 2005; 17: 20-8.
- Pung T, Schmitz B. Circadian rhythm and personality profile in juvenile myoclonic epilepsy. *Epilepsia* 2006; 47 (Suppl 2): S111-4.
- Qin P, Xu H, Laursen TM, Vestergaard M, Mortensen PB. Risk for schizophrenia and schizophrenia-like psychosis among patients with epilepsy: population based cohort study. *BMJ* 2005; 331: 23.
- Quiske A, Helmstaedter C, Lux S, Elger CE. Depression in patients with temporal lobe epilepsy is related to mesial temporal sclerosis. *Epilepsy Res* 2000; 39: 121-5.
- Reutens DC, Savard G, Andermann F, Dubeau F, Olivier A. Results of surgical treatment in temporal lobe epilepsy with chronic psychosis. *Brain* 1997; 120 (Pt 11): 1929-36.
- Reynders HJ, Broks P, Dickson JM, Lee CE, Turpin G. Investigation of social and emotion information processing in temporal lobe epilepsy with ictal fear. *Epilepsy Behav* 2005; 7: 419-29.
- Ring HA, Moriarty J, Trimble MR. A perspective Study of the early post surgical psychiatric associations of epilepsy surgery. *J Neurol Neurosurg Psychiatry* 1998; 64: 601-4.
- Robertson MM, Trimble MR. The treatment of depression in patients with epilepsy. A double-blind trial. *J Affect Disord* 1985; 9: 127-36.
- Rusch N, Tebartz van Elst L, Baeumer D, Ebert D, Trimble MR. Absence of cortical gray matter abnormalities in psychosis of epilepsy: a voxel-based MRI study in patients with temporal lobe epilepsy. *J Neuropsychiatry Clin Neurosci* 2004; 16: 148-55.

- Sanz-Martin A, Guevara MA, Corsi-Cabrera M, Ondarza-Rovira R, Ramos-Loyo J. Differential effect of left and right temporal lobectomy on emotional recognition and experience in patients with epilepsy. *Rev Neurol* 2006; 42: 391-8.
- Schacher M, Winkler R, Grunwald T, Kraemer G, Kurthen M, Reed V, Jokeit H. Mesial temporal lobe epilepsy impairs advanced social cognition. *Epilepsia* 2006; 47: 2141-6.
- Schmitz B. Psychosen bei Epilepsie. Eine epidemiologische Untersuchung. [Thesis] FU Berlin, 1988.
- Schmitz B, Wolf P. Psychosis with epilepsy: frequency and risk factors. *Journal of Epilepsy* 1995; 8: 295-305.
- Schmitz B, Robertson M, Trimble MR. Depression and schizophrenia in epilepsy: social and biological risk factors. *Epilepsy Research* 1999; 35: 59-68.
- Schmitz EB, Moriarty J, Costa DC, Ring HA, Ell PJ, Trimble MR. Psychiatric profiles and patterns of cerebral blood flow in focal epilepsy: interactions between depression, obsessionality, and perfusion related to the laterality of the epilepsy. *J Neurol Neurosurg Psychiatry* 1997; 62: 458-63.
- Serafetinides EA. Psychosocial aspects of neurosurgical management of epilepsy. *Adv Neurol* 1975; 8: 323-31.
- Shaw P, Lawrence E, Bramham J, Brierley B, Radbourne C, David AS. A prospective study of the effects of anterior temporal lobectomy on emotion recognition and theory of mind. *Neuropsychologia* 2007; 45: 2783-90.
- Shaw P, Lawrence EJ, Radbourne C, Bramham J, Polkey CE, David AS. The impact of early and late damage to the human amygdala on "theory of mind" reasoning. *Brain* 2004; 127, 1535-48.
- Siever LJ, Davis KL. The pathophysiology of schizophrenia disorders: perspectives from the spectrum. *Am J Psychiatry* 2004; 161: 398-413.
- Specchio LM, Iudice A, Specchio N, La Neve A, Spinelli A, Galli R, et al. Citalopram as treatment of depression in patients with epilepsy. *Clin Neuropharmacol* 2004; 27: 133-6.
- Stefansson SB, Olafsson E, Hauser WA. Psychiatric morbidity in epilepsy: a case controlled study of adults receiving disability benefits. *J Neurol Neurosurg Psychiatry* 1998; 64: 238-41.
- Tan SY, Bruni J. Cognitive-behavior therapy with adult patients with epilepsy: a controlled outcome study. *Epilepsia* 1986; 27: 225-33.
- Taylor DC. Ontogenesis of chronic epileptic psychoses. A reanalysis. *Psychol Med* 1971; 1: 247-53.
- Taylor DC. Factors influencing the occurrence of schizophrenia-like psychosis in patients with temporal lobe epilepsy. *Psychol Med* 1975; 5: 249-54.
- Tebartz Van Elst L, Baeumer D, Lemieux L, Woermann FG, Koepp M, Krishnamoorthy S, et al. Amygdala pathology in psychosis of epilepsy: A magnetic resonance imaging study in patients with temporal lobe epilepsy. *Brain* 2002; 125: 140-9.
- Tellenbach H. Epilepsie als Anfallsleiden und als Psychose. Über alternative Psychosen paranoider Prägung bei "forcierter Normalisierung" (Landolt) des Elektroencephalogramms Epileptischer. *Nervenarzt* 1965; 36: 190-202.
- Tellez-Zenteno JF, Patten SB, Jetté N, Williams J, Wiebe S. Psychiatric comorbidity in epilepsy: a population-based analysis. *Epilepsia* 2007; 48: 2336-44.
- Thomè-Souza MS, Kuczynski E, Valente KD. Sertraline and fluoxetine: safe treatments for children and adolescents with epilepsy and depression. *Epilepsy Behav* 2007; 10: 417-25.
- Trimble M. *The Psychoses of Epilepsy*. New York: Raven Press, 1991.
- Trimble MR. *Biological Psychiatry*. 2nd ed. Chichester: John Wiley & Sons, 1995.
- Trinka E, Kienpointner G, Unterberger I, Luef G, Bauer G, Doering LB, Doering S. Psychiatric comorbidity in juvenile myoclonic epilepsy. *Epilepsia* 2006; 47: 2086-91.

- US Department of Health and Human Services, Food and Drug Administration, Center for Drug Evaluation and Research, Office of Translational Sciences, Office of Biostatistics. *Statistical Review and Evaluation: Antiepileptic Drugs and Suicidality*. May 21, 2008.
- Victoroff JI, Benson F, Grafton ST, Engel J Jr, Mazziotta JC. Depression in complex partial seizures. Electroencephalography and cerebral metabolic correlates. *Arch Neurol* 1994; 51: 155-163.
- Yamada M, Murai T, Sato W, Namiki C, Miyamoto T, Ohigashi Y. Emotion recognition from facial expressions in a temporal lobe epileptic patient with ictal fear. *Neuropsychologia* 2005; 43: 434-41.

The clinical syndrome of mesial temporal lobe epilepsy in children

Andras Fogarasi[1], Alexis Arzimanoglou[2]

[1] *Bethesda Children's Hospital, Budapest, Hungary*
[2] *Pediatric Epileptology, University Hospitals, Lyon, France*

Mesial temporal lobe epilepsy (MTLE) is described as a discrete syndrome in adults with temporal lobe epilepsy (TLE) and associated hippocampal sclerosis (HS) (French, 1993; Williamson, 1993; 1998; Wieser, 2004). Early diagnosis of MTLE can be especially important in medically refractory cases when anteromesial temporal lobectomy may eliminate seizures (Wieser, 1993; Rosenow, 2001). Epileptic seizures of MTLE patients typically start at the end of the first decade of life, and these seizures initially respond well to antiepileptic drug (AED) treatment during the first years of the syndrome (Blume, 2006). Thus, the characteristic clinical picture of MTLE is rarely observed in children. In the report by Murakami *et al.* (1996), 19 patients (0.8%) of a total of 2,319 children with epilepsy were identified to have MTLE syndrome. In this chapter, we describe not only the typical features of childhood MTLE, its prognosis in children, and impact on the developing brain, but also assess the presence of hippocampal abnormalities in children without MTLE. Childhood TLE due to mesial temporal lesions other than HS (*e.g.* dysplasia, tumours) is more frequent than the classic MTLE syndrome of adults.

■ Aetiology: impact of early precipitating injuries on the hippocampus

Several studies have stirred a debate regarding the role of early precipitating injuries, especially febrile seizures (FSs), in the development of HS (Fisher, 1998; Van Landingham, 1998; Szabo, 1999; Berg, 1999; Dube, 2000; Schulz, 2001; Grunewald, 2002). The particular importance of focal prolonged febrile convulsions (PFCs) in the history of patients with HS is well recognized (Maher, 1995; Lewis, 2002). Seventy percent of patients with MTLE due to HS were shown to have a history of childhood FSs (French, 1993; Wieser, 2004).

According to the most widely held theory, FSs cause HS which is responsible for the appearance of TLE some years later. There are presumably additional genetic or developmental factors which determine why some individuals develop HS after FSs and others do not. Sodium channel defects can cause HS in mice (Kearney, 2001) and severe FSs in humans (Abou-Khalil, 2001; Wieser, 2004; Ceulemans, 2004), thus the same gene defect may lead to both FSs and HS.

One study analyzed qualitative and quantitative MRI data taken within five days of status epilepticus in 35 children (Scott, 2002). Status epilepticus, in the form of prolonged febrile convulsions, rather than febrile status epilepticus, resulted in hippocampal oedema, a phenomenon that can lead to HS (Sokol, 2003).

According to another theory, a hippocampal abnormality (probably dysgenesis) may generate FSs which cause HS in the already affected hippocampus (Fernandez, 1998; Barsi, 2000). This theory is supported by an MRI study which found significant hippocampal atrophy in half of the children within two weeks after their first FS (Grunewald, 2001). These data suggest that, in some patients, the early FS is the result of pre-existing brain abnormalities. According to longitudinal studies, not only PFCs but other early precipitating injuries (*e.g.* trauma, hypoxia, CNS infection) may lead to HS later on (Mathern, 2002).

■ Seizure semiology

Early studies on TLE found that patients over six years have similar seizures to those of adults (Yamamoto, 1987; Wyllie, 1993; Brockhaus, 1995; Mohamed, 2001; Terra-Bustamante, 2005) and only infants and young children show different seizure semiology (Duchowny, 1992; Wyllie, 1995; Bourgeois, 1998). Infants with TLE can also have special seizures such as infantile spasms (Kellaway, 1979; Dulac, 1999) or apnoeic attacks (Akaike, 2008).

Our research group completed a video analysis of 605 archived seizures from 155 consecutive patients (aged 10 months to 49 years) who had seizure freedom after temporal lobectomy. Eighty patients (52%) had HS. Age-dependency of several axes of seizure semiology was assessed: aura, number of different lateralizing signs, occurrence of ictal emotional signs, autonomic symptoms, automatisms and secondary generalisation, as well as the ratio of motor seizure components (Fogarasi, 2007). Our findings support the notion that brain maturation significantly influences the evolution of some important aspects of TLE seizure semiology. As the presence of motor components decreased with patient age, the number of lateralizing signs, automatisms and secondary generalised seizures increased. In other studies run by our research group, some of the lateralizing signs also showed age-dependent appearance (Fogarasi, 2006a) while the autonomic symptoms were strongly associated with TLE in children (Fogarasi, 2006b). Conversely, other characteristics (aura, emotional and autonomic signs) were independent of the maturation process. The increased frequency of automatisms, lateralizing signs and secondary generalised tonic-clonic seizures (SGTCS) supports the notion that temporal lobe seizures undergo a gradual development, becoming more complex in the older population (Fogarasi, 2002; Ray, 2005). Seizure semiology, but also HS aetiology, was importantly age-dependent in this group (*Figure 1*). To identify age-dependent, HS-independent variables, we performed general linear models for the association of semiological axes with age while controlling for HS. A linear analysis adjusted for the presence of HS showed that the frequency of automatisms and SGTCS, as well as the number of different lateralizing signs, increased with age independently of aetiology, while the ratio of motor seizure component was dependent on not only age but also the aetiology of HS.

Animal studies investigating the ontogenetic expression of drug-induced limbic epilepsy in immature young rats showed a comparable age-dependent ictal behaviour. By investigating kainic acid and pilocarpine-induced seizures in young rats during the first two

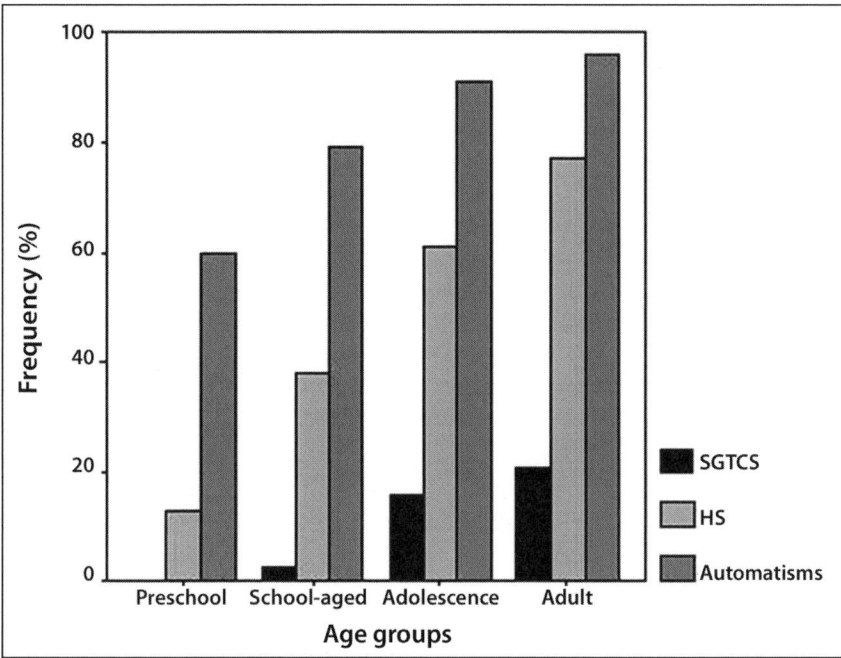

Figure 1. Positive correlation between age and semiological axes (frequency of automatisms and secondary generalised seizures) and aetiology (frequency of hippocampal sclerosis) in patients with temporal lobe epilepsy.

postnatal weeks, corresponding to a maturational age of human infants, rat pups were shown to develop hyperactivity, scratching, hyperextension of the limbs, tremor, head bobbing, and myoclonic movements (Cherubini, 1983; Cavalheiro, 1987; Moshe, 1993; Holmes, 1997). More mature rats aged over two weeks produced limbic seizures consisting of rearing, akinesia, and masticatory movements, in addition to prominent motor signs. Further studies in hippocampal-kindled rat pups demonstrated that the afterdischarge thresholds (the lowest current intensity necessary to elicit an afterdischarge) are greatest during the second to third postnatal week, suggesting resistance of the limbic system to synchronization (Moshe, 1981).

■ EEG studies

As for other focal epilepsies, children with TLE frequently show bilateral, generalised or mislocalizing epileptiform discharges on EEG (Wyllie, 1993). Harvey *et al.* comprehensively analyzed the EEG data of 63 children with TLE and found generalised or extratemporal slow-wave and interictal epileptiform discharges (IEDs) in 10 (16%). Two of these children had centrotemporal IEDs with characteristic morphology and field topography of Rolandic epilepsy (Harvey, 1997). Fontana *et al.* assessed electroclinical characteristics of 77 children with TLE (including 23 due to HS) and found that two thirds of these patients had IEDs outside the temporal region (Fontana 2006). Ebner *et al.* compared a childhood and adult HS database in the Bethel Epilepsy Center (Ebner, 1999) and found that children frequently had IEDs with maximal amplitude over extratemporal electrodes and identified a relatively small percentage of children (19%) with EEG seizure patterns confined to the temporal region, compared to 58% in the adult group. A research group from

Toronto reported a nine-year-old boy with intractable TLE and histologically proven HS. Not only did the scalp EEG show fronto-centro-temporal spike and waves, but magnetoencephalography also demonstrated interictal dipoles in the bilateral Rolandic regions (RamachandranNair, 2007). This patient became seizure-free after an anteromesial temporal lobectomy, proving that the seizure onset zone was much more localized than the irritative zone.

Impact of mesial temporal lobe epilepsy on the developing brain

While there have been extensive neuropsychological studies on adults with TLE, much less work in this field has considered children with MTLE, which suggests that children and adults with TLE frequently suffer from similar cognitive deficits. Specific deficits affect language, verbal and figural memory, socioperceptive competence, and executive functions resulting in difficulties in school performance (Laurent, 2006).

As previously demonstrated 40 years ago, children with TLE need more time to learn, have a poorer recall for verbal material as well as significantly poorer performance regarding non-verbal tasks, such as visual-spatial memory and non-verbal attention (Fedio, 1969).

In a study by Oxbury et al., verbal and non-verbal memory was assessed as part of a broader neuropsychological assessment battery in children with TLE due to HS (Oxbury, 1998). The authors concluded that longer duration of TLE was not associated with a decline in full scale IQ and memory. However, arithmetic tests in patients with seizure onset at less than six years showed that those with shorter epilepsy duration do better than those with longer duration. Assessment of school performance of children with MTLE revealed that spelling and mathematics are often more difficult for these individuals. Comparing laterality, children with right-sided temporal focus had fewer difficulties with mathematics but could present perceptual deficits affecting reading and writing.

In a recent study memory deficits in children with mesial (n = 31) and lateral (n = 12) TLE were compared (Gonzalez, 2007). Memory deficits were not lateralized (with the exception of facial recognition) in these children. Assessment of intratemporal location revealed clear differences in arbitrary associative learning and complex figure recall. Because only the mesial subgroup displayed memory dysfunction relative to normative standards, their data supported an associative model of hippocampal function for childhood memory. According to their data, the nature of memory impairment experienced by children with TLE cannot be extrapolated from adult models.

Lendt et al. evaluated neuropsychological patterns in 52 children with unilateral TLE and compared this data with that of adults (Lendt et al., 1999). Their research showed that low memory performance in children was more rare and less specific to the site of seizure onset zone than in adults. Nevertheless, poor language performance was strongly associated with left-sided TLE. Although parents reported frequent difficulties in several domains such as memory, attention, language, and school problems, memory deficits are known to cause more pronounced symptoms in adults. They suggested that these differences might arise from the different aetiology and shorter duration of epilepsy in children.

Prognosis of childhood mesial temporal lobe epilepsy

Based on longitudinal studies, typical MTLE syndrome starts with seizure onset in the first and second decade of life followed later by pharmacoresistant epilepsy (Wieser, 1993). Outcome and prognostic factors of epilepsy surgery in adolescents and adults with MTLE have been studied extensively, however, less is known about childhood surgical cases. Smyth et al. conducted a multi-institutional analysis of prognostic indicators of TLE surgery in 49 preadolescent (< 14 years) patients, including 26 children with MTLE (Smyth, 2007), with results which differ from previous adult TLE studies. Excellent surgical outcome was significantly associated with only one seizure type and lack of developmental delay, while a trend of bilateral or extratemporal EEG findings and high preoperative seizure frequency (daily seizures) was associated with worse outcome. Age at seizure onset, age at surgery, and duration of epilepsy were not significantly related to postoperative outcome. Interestingly, in only 46% of children with histologically confirmed HS was the condition prospectively diagnosed by preoperative MR imaging.

Mohamed et al. assessed a group of children (four to 12 years of age) and adolescents (13 to 20 years of age) who underwent temporal lobe resection due to MTLE (Mohamed, 2001). Postoperative follow-up showed that 28% of patients were seizure-free with a tendency of lower seizure-free outcome in individuals with bilateral temporal IEDs or bilateral HS, based on MRI. They concluded that postsurgical seizure outcome in children and adolescents is similar to that in adult MTLE series.

Hippocampal sclerosis without mesial temporal lobe epilepsy in children

According to different studies, HS may develop in children without the classic electroclinical characteristics of MTLE. Based on an assessment of 101 patients with sporadic benign TLE (who after two years of follow-up had either rare seizures or no seizures), 39 were shown to have unilateral HS (Labate, 2006). The side of HS correlated well with the epileptiform activity and early febrile convulsions were more frequent in patients with benign TLE and HS, based on MRI.

Riney et al. analyzed MRI data of the hippocampus in 29 children with resective surgery for extrahippocampal epilepsy (Riney, 2006). Interestingly, 21 of 29 (72%) patients were found to have a hippocampal abnormality consistent with HS, although they never had MTLE. In addition, the duration of epilepsy did not correlate with the presence of hippocampal abnormality. They concluded that HS was the result of seizures from the focus which was remote from the hippocampus in these children.

Auer et al. assessed hippocampal voxel-based volumetry and T2 relaxation time in eight highly-educated healthy college students with a history of childhood simple FSs and no epilepsy (Auer, 2008). Mean volume of the hippocampi was smaller while T2 relaxation time was higher in subjects with FSs, relative to the control group. This recent study suggests that even simple FSs may cause HS which may not necessarily cause epilepsy.

Siegler et al. reported on the MRI data of 14 children with Dravet syndrome (severe myoclonic epilepsy of infancy; SMEI) (Siegler, 2006). This is a malignant epilepsy syndrome with early prolonged unilateral or generalised tonic-clonic FSs, therapy-resistant epilepsy, and psychomotor delay. None of the seizure types (atypical absence, myoclonic and clonic seizures) or EEG signs (generalized IEDs, photoparoxysmal reaction) associated with Dravet syndrome are typical of MTLE; however, 10 of these 14 children developed

HS during the course of the disease (Figure 2). Hippocampal sclerosis was detected on MRI as early as 14 months of age and, interestingly, three children with well-documented seizure laterality showed HS ipsilateral to the seizure onset zone in unilateral prolonged clonic febrile seizures. Children with HS and Dravet syndrome had neither complex partial seizures nor temporal spikes on EEG.

These cases suggest a role of early precipitating injury in this special subgroup of patients with HS development without resulting MTLE. These data also raise the possibility that, besides HS, other factors or individual sensitivity may play a role in the development of MTLE syndrome. It is well known that only a proportion of children with PFCs develop HS later in life. It is thus feasible that these patients carry some form of resistance against (or the lack of sensitivity to) the development of HS. One explanation for this individual sensitivity may be an inherited abnormal cytokine reaction, as previously described (Kanemoto, 2000).

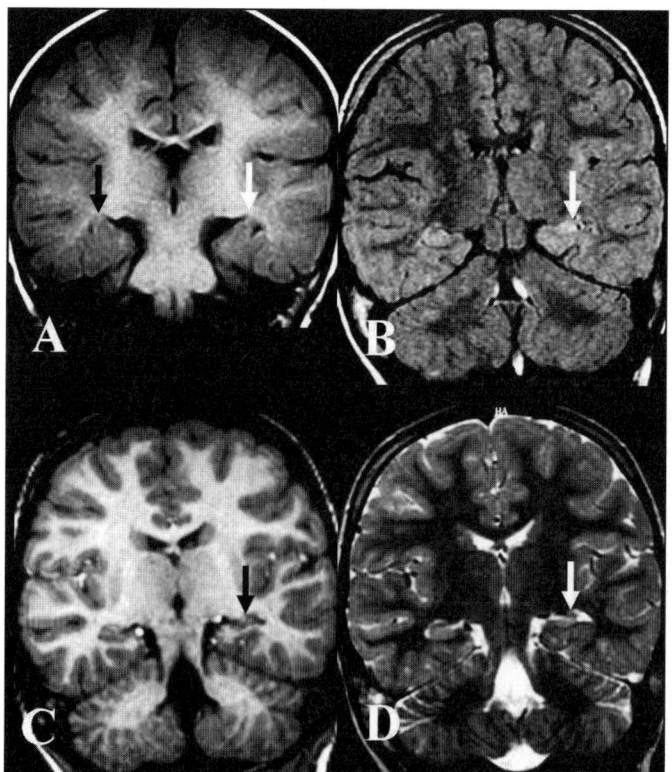

Figure 2. Patient with severe myoclonic epilepsy in infancy and hippocampal sclerosis.
A. Coronal T1-weighted image at six months of age shows the left (white arrow) and right (black arrow) hippocampus are of equal size. **B.** Coronal thin slice reconstruction from 3D-MPRAGE sequence. **C.** Coronal T1. **D.** Coronal T2-weighted images at three years of age show that the left hippocampus (arrows) is smaller, with higher T2 signal intensity, than the right hippocampus, confirming left hippocampal sclerosis.

■ Temporal *versus* extratemporal lobe epilepsies in children

In contrast to adults, extratemporal lobe epilepsies are more frequent than TLE in children (Farmer, 1998). Our study group systematically analyzed 177 seizures from 35 children with seizure-free outcome after extratemporal (frontal or occipital) resection (Fogarasi, 2005). These data showed that typical temporal lobe ictal elements (Chee, 1993; Leutmezer, 1998; Delgado-Escueta, 1998; Kotagal, 1999; Escueta, 1977), psychomotor seizures, version, dystonic posturing, oral and manual automatisms, as well as post-ictal nose wiping, appeared frequently in children with extratemporal, especially occipital lobe epilepsies. Similarly, interictal spikes were seen to be located outside the lobe with lesion in 49% of patients and typical remote IEDs consisted of temporal lobe spikes in the occipital lobe group. Although it is known that both the frontal (Lieb, 1991) and occipital (Schulz, 1998) lobes have functional connections with temporal structures, it seems that clinical manifestation of occipito-temporal networks is more prominent in children. This may explain the more accelerated maturation of the posterior region (Chugani, 1987). These electroclinical similarities between temporal and extratemporal lobe epilepsies make the identification of TLE very difficult in children, in contrast to adults who demonstrate much more distinct entities of partial epilepsies arising in different lobes (Salanova, 1992; Laskowitz, 1995; Manford, 1996).

■ Case report: typical mesial temporal lobe epilepsy in childhood

We report a 10-year-old girl without epilepsy in her family. After an inconclusive perinatal history, she had two febrile seizures at the age of 12 and 17 months. Epilepsy started at the age of six years with short psychomotor seizures consisting of epigastric aura, staring, oral automatisms and unresponsiveness. She was seizure-free on carbamazepine monotherapy for three years. Despite several AED trials including carbamazepine, valproate, clobazam, vigabatrin, phenytoin and benzodiazepine, seizures became more and more

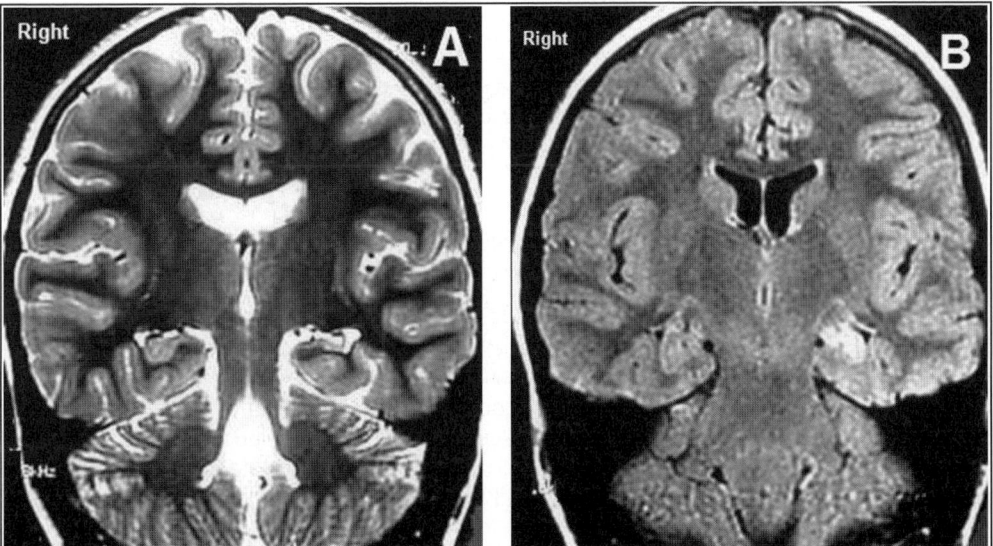

Figure 3. 11-year-old girl with left hippocampal atrophy and sclerosis.
A. Coronal T2-weighted image. **B.** Coronal FLAIR image.

frequent. At the age of 11 years, she had three to five seizures a day. MRI demonstrated left hippocampal atrophy and sclerosis *(Figure 3)*, while EEG showed left anterior temporal spikes as well as left temporal slowing *(Figure 4)*. During long-term video-EEG monitoring, habitual psychomotor seizures were recorded exclusively with left temporal seizure pattern on ictal EEG *(Figure 5)*. During the first year after left anteromesial temporal lobectomy, some epigastric aura appeared but she has remained aura and seizure-free for five years. Her psychomotor development is excellent.

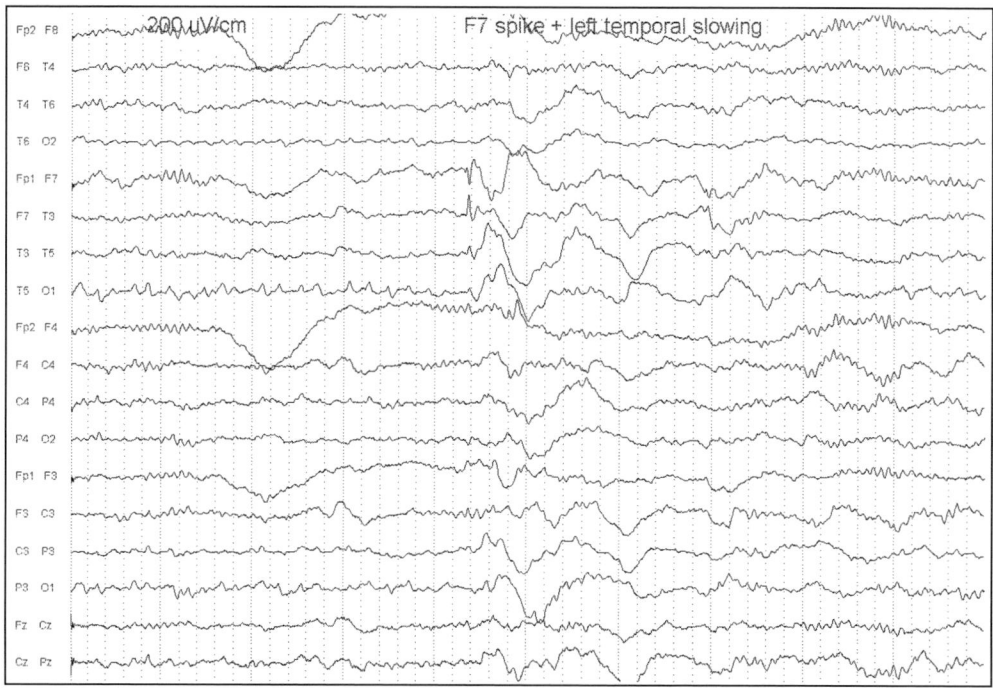

Figure 4. Left anterior temporal spike followed by slowing over the left temporal region (sleep EEG).
This case shows that typical MTLE syndrome may appear in children. Characteristics of MTLE included early febrile seizures, epilepsy onset during the first decade, psychomotor seizures, gradual development of drug resistance, as well as typical and concordant EEG and neuroimaging data.

■ Conclusion

According to extensive research, childhood and adult MTLE share similarities, however, there are important characteristics which are specific to childhood MTLE. While HS is the typical aetiological factor of TLE in adults, this phenomenon is more rarely observed in childhood. Both human and animal studies support the notion that although the immature brain is highly sensitive to seizures, it can be relatively resistant to the development of seizure-induced HS. Nevertheless, early seizures may harm hippocampal function and anatomy due to specific factors such as age, aetiology, prior neurological abnormality or genetic predisposition, resulting in either MTLE or other epilepsy syndromes later in life.

The clinical syndrome of mesial temporal lobe epilepsy in children

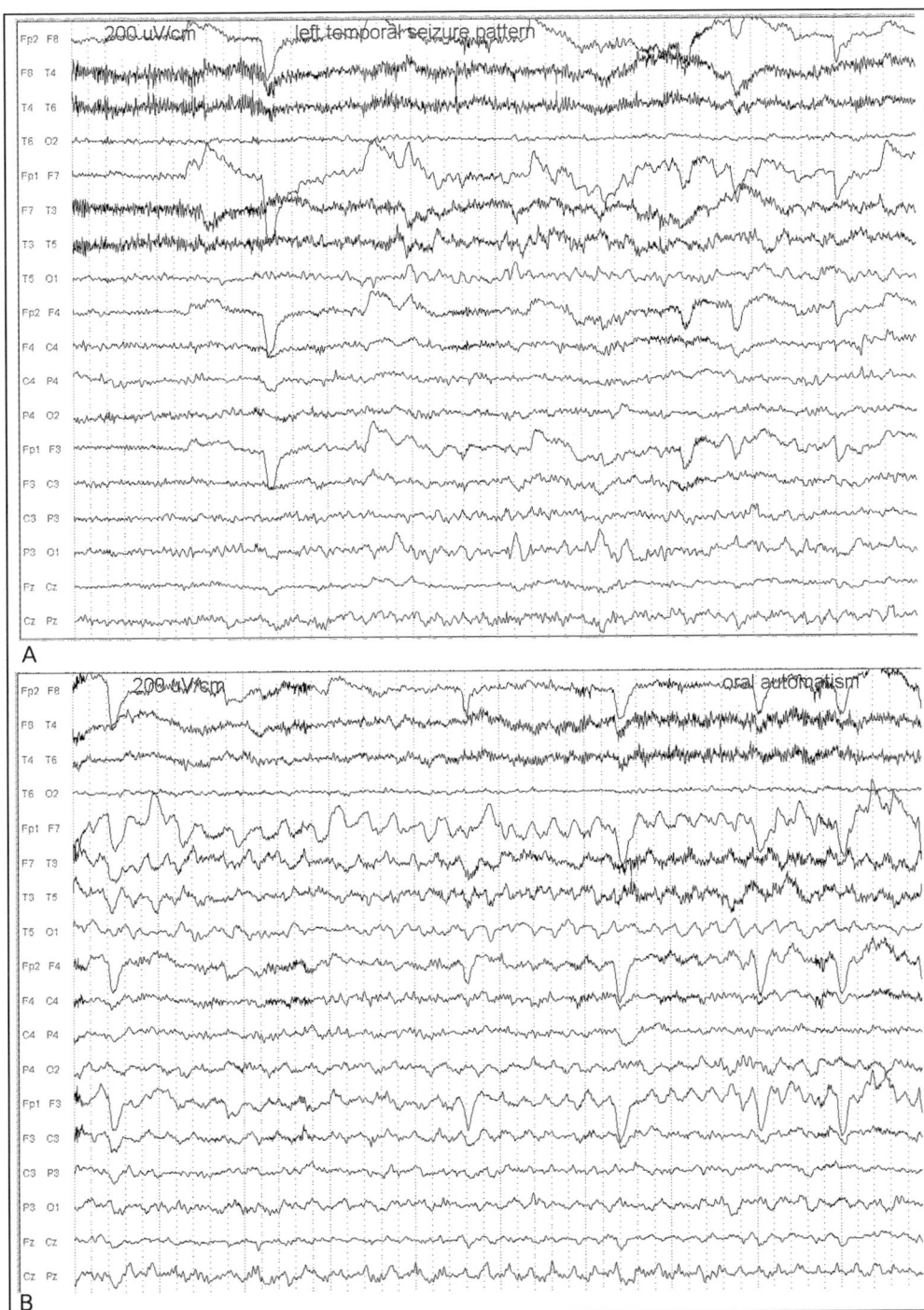

Figure 5. Seizure pattern with onset **(A)** and evolution **(B)** in the left temporal region.

References

- Abou-Khalil B, Ge Q, Desai R, Ryther R, Bazyk A, Bailey R, et al. Partial and generalized epilepsy with febrile seizures plus and a novel *SCN1A* mutation. *Neurology* 2001; 57: 2265-72.
- Akaike H, Nakagawa E, Sugai K, Fujikawa Y, Komaki H, Ohtsuki T, Sasaki M. Three infantile cases of temporal lobe epilepsy presenting as apnea. *No To Hattatsu* 2008; 40: 33-7.
- Auer T, Barsi P, Bone B, Angyalosi A, Aradi M, Szalay C, et al. History of simple febrile seizures is associated with hippocampal abnormalities in adults. *Epilepsia* 2008; 49: 1562-9.
- Barsi P, Kenéz J, Solymosi D, Kulin A, Halasz P, Rasonyi G, et al. Hippocampal malrotation with normal corpus callosum: a new entity? *Neuroradiology* 2000; 42: 339-45.
- Berg AT, Shinnar S, Levy SR, Testa FM. Childhood-onset epilepsy with and without preceding febrile seizures. *Neurology* 1999; 53: 1742-8.
- Blume WT. The progression of epilepsy. *Epilepsia* 2006; 47 (Suppl 1): 71-8.
- Bourgeois BF. Temporal lobe epilepsy in children. *Brain Dev* 1998; 20: 135-41.
- Brockhaus A, Elger CE. Complex partial seizures of temporal lobe origin in children of different age groups. *Epilepsia* 1995; 36: 1173-81.
- Cavalheiro EA, Silva DF, Turski WA, Calderazzo-Filho LS, Bortolotto ZA, Turski L. The susceptibility of rats to pilocarpine-induced seizures is age-dependent. *Dev Brain Res* 1987; 37: 43-58.
- Ceulemans BPGM, Claes LRF, Lagae LG. Clinical correlation of mutations in the *SCN1A* gene: from febrile seizures to severe myoclonic epilepsy in infancy. *Ped Neurol* 2004; 30: 236-43.
- Chee MW, Kotagal P, Van Ness PC, Gragg L, Murphy D, Lüders HO. Lateralizing signs in intractable partial epilepsy: blinded multiple-observer analysis. *Neurology* 1993; 43: 2519-25.
- Cherubini E, De Feo MR, Mecarelli O, Ricci GF. Behavioral and electrographic patterns induced by systemic administration of kainic acid in developing rats. *Dev Brain Res* 1983; 9: 69-77.
- Chugani HT, Phelps ME, Mazziotta JC. Positron emission tomography study of human brain development. *Ann Neurol* 1987; 22: 487-97.
- Delgado-Escueta AV, Bascal FE, Treimann DM. Complex partial seizures on closed-circuit television and EEG: a study of 691 attacks in 79 patients. *Ann Neurol* 1982; 11: 292-300.
- Dube C, Chen K, Eghbal-Ahmadi M, Brunson K, Soltesz I, Baram TZ. Prolonged febrile seizures in the immature rat model enhance hippocampal excitability long term. *Ann Neurol* 2000; 47: 336-44.
- Duchowny MS, Levin B, Jayakar P, Resnick T, Alvarez L, Morrison G, Dean P. Temporal lobectomy in early childhood. *Epilepsia* 1992; 33: 298-303.
- Dulac O, Chiron C, Robain O, Plouin P, Jambaque I, Pinard JM. Infantile spasms: a pathophysiological hypothesis. In: Nehlig A, ed. *Childhood Epilepsies and Brain Development*. London: John Libbey, 1999, pp. 93-102.
- Ebner A. EEG in temporal lobe epilepsy children *versus* adults: are there age specific differences? *Temporal lobe epilepsy in children* – EUREPA Teaching Course 1999, Bethel, Germany.
- Escueta AV, Kunze U, Waddell G, Boxley J, Nadel A. Lapse of consciousness and automatisms in temporal lobe epilepsy: a videotape analysis. *Neurology* 1977; 27: 144-55.
- Farmer JP. Operative strategies in the management of extratemporal epilepsy of childhood. In: Tuxhorn I, Holthausen H, Boenigk H, eds. *Pediatric Epilepsy Syndromes and their Surgical Treatment*. London: John Libbey, 1998, pp. 691-5.
- Fedio P, Mirsky AF. Selective intellectual deficits in children with temporal lobe or centrencephalic epilepsy. *Neuropsychology* 1969; 7: 287-300.
- Fernández G, Effenberger O, Vinz B, Steinlein O, Elger CE, Döhring W, Heinze HJ. Hippocampal malformation as a cause of familial febrile convulsions and subsequent hippocampal sclerosis. *Neurology* 1998; 50: 909-17.

- Fisher PD, Sperber EF, Moshe SL. Hippocampal sclerosis revisited. *Brain Dev* 1998; 20: 563-73.
- Fogarasi A, Jokeit H, Faveret E, Janszky J, Tuxhorn I. The effect of age on seizure semiology in childhood temporal lobe epilepsy. *Epilepsia* 2002; 43: 638-43.
- Fogarasi A, Tuxhorn I, Hegyi M, Janszky J. Predictive clinical factors for the differential diagnosis of childhood extratemporal seizures. *Epilepsia* 2005; 46: 1280-5.
- Fogarasi A, Janszky J, Tuxhorn I. Peri-ictal lateralizing signs in children: blinded multiobserver study of 100 children ⩽ 12 years. *Neurology* 2006; 66: 271-4.
- Fogarasi A, Janszky J, Tuxhorn I. Autonomic symptoms during childhood partial epileptic syndromes. *Epilepsia* 2006; 47: 584-8.
- Fogarasi A, Tuxhorn I, Janszky J, Janszky I, Rásonyi G, Kelemen A, Halász P. Age-dependent seizure semiology in temporal lobe epilepsy. *Epilepsia* 2007; 48: 1697-702.
- Fontana E, Negrini F, Francione S, Mai R, Osanni E, Menna E, *et al*. Temporal lobe epilepsy in children: electroclinical study of 77 cases. *Epilepsia* 2006; 47 (Suppl 5): 26-30.
- Friedland RJ, Bronen RA. Magnetic resonance imaging of neoplastic, vascular, and indeterminate substrates. In.: Cascino GD, Jack CR, eds. *Neuroimaging in Epilepsy: Principles and Practice*. Boston: Butterworth-Heinemann, 1996, pp. 29-50.
- Gonzalez LM, Anderson VA, Wood SJ, Mitchell LA, Harvey AS. The localization and lateralization of memory deficits in children with temporal lobe epilepsy. *Epilepsia* 2007; 48: 124-32.
- Grunewald RA, Farrow T, Vaughan P, Rittey CD, Mundy J. A magnetic resonance study of complicated early childhood convulsion. *J Neurol Neurosurg Psychiatry* 2001; 71: 638-42.
- Grunewald R. Childhood seizures and their consequences for the hippocampus. *Brain* 2002; 125: 135-6.
- Harvey AS, Berkovic SF, Wrennall JA, Hopkins IJ. Temporal lobe epilepsy in childhood: clinical, EEG, and neuroimaging findings and syndrome classification in a cohort with new-onset seizures. *Neurology* 1997; 49: 960-8.
- Holmes GL. Epilepsy in the developing brain: lessons from the laboratory and clinic. *Epilepsia* 1997; 38: 12-30.
- Kanemoto K, Kawasaki J, Miyamoto T, Obayashi H, Nishimura M. Interleukin (IL)-1beta, IL-1alpha, and IL-1 receptor antagonist gene polymorphisms in patients with temporal lobe epilepsy. *Ann Neurol* 2000; 47: 571-4.
- Kearney JA, Plummer NW, Smith MR, Kapur J, Cummins TR, Waxman SG, *et al*. A gain-of-function mutation in the sodium channel gene *Scn2a* results in seizures and behavioral abnormalities. *Neuroscience* 2001; 102: 307-17.
- Kellaway P, Hrachovy RA, Frost JD Jr, Zion T. Precise characterization and quantification of infantile spasms. *Ann Neurol* 1979; 6: 214-8.
- Kotagal P. Significance of dystonic posturing with unilateral automatisms. *Arch Neurol* 1999; 56: 912-3.
- Labate A, Ventura P, Gambardella A, Le Piane E, Colosimo E, Leggio U, *et al*. MRI evidence of mesial temporal sclerosis in sporadic "benign" temporal lobe epilepsy. *Neurology* 2006; 66: 562-5.
- Laskowitz DT, Sperling MR, French JA, O'Connor MJ. The syndrome of frontal lobe epilepsy: characteristics and surgical management. *Neurology* 1995; 45: 780-7.
- Laurent A, Arzimanoglou A. Cognitive impairments in children with non-idiopathic temporal lobe epilepsy. *Epilepsia* 2006; 47 (Suppl 2): 99-102.
- Lendt M, Helmstaedter C, Elger CE. Pre- and postoperative neuropsychological profiles in children and adolescents with temporal lobe epilepsy. *Epilepsia* 1999; 40: 1543-50.
- Leutmezer F, Serles W, Lehrner J, Pataraia E, Zeiler K, Baumgartner C. Postictal nose wiping: a lateralizing sign in temporal lobe complex partial seizures. *Neurology* 1998; 51: 1175-7.

- Lewis DV, Barboriak DP, MacFall JR, Provenzale JM, Mitchell TV, Van Landingham KE. Do prolonged febrile seizures produce medial temporal sclerosis? Hypotheses, MRI evidence and unanswered questions. *Prog Brain Res* 2002; 135: 263-78.
- Lieb JP, Dasheiff RM, Engel J. Role of the frontal lobes in the propagation of mesial temporal lobe seizures. *Epilepsia* 1991; 32: 822-37.
- Maher J, McLachlan RS. Febrile convulsions. Is seizure duration the most important predictor of temporal lobe epilepsy? *Brain* 1995; 118: 1521-8.
- Manford M, Fish DR, Shorvon SD. An analysis of clinical seizure patterns and their localizing value in frontal and temporal lobe epilepsies. *Brain* 1996; 119: 17-40.
- Mathern GW, Adelson PD, Cahan LD, Leite JP. Hippocampal neuron damage in human epilepsy: Meyer's hypothesis revisited. *Prog Brain Res* 2002; 135: 237-51.
- Mohamed A, Wyllie E, Ruggieri P, Kotagal P, Babb T, Hilbig A, et al. Temporal lobe epilepsy due to hippocampal sclerosis in pediatric candidates for epilepsy surgery. *Neurology* 2001; 56: 1643-9.
- Moshe SL. The effects of age on the kindling phenomenon. *Dev Psychobiol* 1981; 14: 75-81.
- Moshe SL. Intractable seizures in infancy and early childhood. *Neurology* 1993; 43 (Suppl 5): 2-7.
- Murakami N, Ohno S, Oka E, Tanaka A. Mesial temporal lobe epilepsy in childhood. *Epilepsia* 1996; 37 (Suppl 3): 52-6.
- Oxbury SM, Campbell L, Baxendale SA, Oxbury JM. Cognitive function in relation to duration of temporal lobe epilepsy due to Ammon's horn sclerosis. *Epilepsia* 1998; 39 (Suppl 2): 120.
- RamachandranNair R, Ochi A, Benifla M, Rutka JT, Snead OC 3rd, Otsubo H. Benign epileptiform discharges in Rolandic region with mesial temporal lobe epilepsy: MEG, scalp and intracranial EEG features. *Acta Neurol Scand* 2007; 116: 59-64.
- Ray A, Kotagal P. Temporal lobe epilepsy in children: overview of clinical semiology. *Epileptic Disord* 2005; 7: 299-307.
- Riney CJ, Harding B, Harkness WJ, Scott RC, Cross JH. Hippocampal sclerosis in children with lesional epilepsy is influenced by age at seizure onset. *Epilepsia* 2006; 47: 159-66.
- Rosenow F, Lüders H. Presurgical evaluation of epilepsy. *Brain* 2001; 124: 1683-1700.
- Salanova V, Andermann F, Olivier A, Rasmussenn T, Quesney LF. Occipital lobe epilepsy: electroclinical manifestations, electrocorticography, cortical stimulation and outcome in 42 patients treated between 1930 and 1991. Surgery of occipital lobe epilepsy. *Brain* 1992; 115: 1655-80.
- Schulz R, Holthausen H, Tuxhorn I, Pieper T, Ebner A. The localizing value of elementary visual auras in occipital lobe epilepsy. In: Tuxhorn I, Holthausen H, Boenigk H, eds. *Pediatric Epilepsy Syndromes and their Surgical Treatment*. London: John Libbey, 1998: 405-16.
- Schulz R, Ebner A. Prolonged febrile convulsions and mesial temporal lobe epilepsy in an identical twin. *Neurology* 2001; 57: 318-20.
- Scott RC, Gadian DG, King MD, Chong WK, Cox TC, Neville BG, Connelly A. Magnetic resonance imaging findings within 5 days of status epilepticus in childhood. *Brain* 2002; 125: 1951-9.
- Siegler Z, Barsi P, Neuwirth M, Jerney J, Kassay M, Janszky J, et al. Hippocampal sclerosis in severe myoclonic epilepsy in infancy: a retrospective MRI study. *Epilepsia* 2005; 46: 704-8.
- Smyth MD, Limbrick DD Jr, Ojemann JG, Zempel J, Robinson S, O'Brien DF, et al. Outcome following surgery for temporal lobe epilepsy with hippocampal involvement in preadolescent children: emphasis on mesial temporal sclerosis. *J Neurosurg* 2007; 106 (Suppl 3): 205-10.
- Sokol DK, Demyer WE, Edwards-Brown M, Sanders S, Garg B. From swelling to sclerosis: acute change in mesial hippocampus after prolonged febrile seizure. *Seizure* 2003; 12: 237-40.

- Szabo CA, Wyllie E, Siavalas EL, Najm I, Ruggieri P, Kotagal P, Lüders H. Hippocampal volumetry in children 6 years or younger: assessment of children with and without complex febrile seizures. *Epilepsy Res* 1999; 33: 1-9.
- Terra-Bustamante VC, Inuzuca LM, Fernandes RM, Funayama S, Escorsi-Rosset S, Wichert-Ana L, et al. Temporal lobe epilepsy surgery in children and adolescents: clinical characteristics and post-surgical outcome. *Seizure* 2005; 14: 274-81.
- Van Landingham KE, Heinz ER, Cavazos JE, Lewis DV. Magnetic resonance imaging evidence of hippocampal injury after prolonged focal febrile convulsions. *Ann Neurol* 1998; 43: 413-26.
- Wieser HG, Engej J Jr, Williamson PD, Babb TL, Gloor P. Surgically remediable temporal lobe syndromes. In: Engel J Jr, ed. *Surgical Treatment of the Epilepsies*. New York: Raven Press; 1993, pp. 49-63.
- Wieser HG and the ILAE Commission on Neurosurgery of Epilepsy. Mesial temporal lobe epilepsy with hippocampal sclerosis. *Epilepsia* 2004; 45: 695-714.
- Williamson PD, French JA, Thadani VM, Kim JH, Novelly RA, Spencer SS, et al. Characteristics of medial temporal lobe epilepsy: II. Interictal and ictal scalp electroencephalography, neuropsychological testing, neuroimaging, surgical results, and pathology. *Ann Neurol* 1993; 34: 781-7.
- Williamson PD, Thadani VM, French JA, Darcey TM, Mattson RH, Spencer SS, Spencer DD. Medial temporal lobe epilepsy: videotape analysis of objective clinical seizure characteristics. *Epilepsia* 1998; 39: 1182-8.
- Wyllie E, Chee M, Granstrom ML, DelGiudice E, Estes M, Comair Y, et al. Temporal lobe epilepsy in early childhood. *Epilepsia* 1993; 34: 859-68.
- Wyllie E. Developmental aspects of seizure semiology: problems in identifying localized-onset seizures in infants and children. *Epilepsia* 1995; 36: 1170-2.
- Yamamoto N, Watanabe K, Negoro T, Takaesu E, Aso K, Furune S, Takahashi I. Complex partial seizures in children: ictal manifestations and their relation to clinical course. *Neurology* 1987; 37: 1379-82.

Mesial *versus* neocortical temporal lobe epilepsy

Nancy Foldvary-Schaefer

Cleveland Clinic, Neurological Institute, Cleveland, USA

While the syndrome of mesial temporal lobe epilepsy (MTLE) due to hippocampal sclerosis has fairly stereotyped manifestations, the clinical, electrophysiological, and neuroradiological manifestations of epilepsies arising from the neocortical temporal lobe (NTLE) are much more heterogeneous and consequently, less syndromatic. Differentiating between patients with neocortical temporal seizures and those with MTLE during non-invasive evaluation is important because many patients with NTLE, particularly non-lesional cases, require intracranial monitoring and more extensive or tailored resections to optimize surgical outcome and minimize morbidity. While the prevalence of neocortical temporal seizures is unknown, they are believed to be much rarer than those originating from the mesial temporal structures. This chapter reviews the clinical and electrophysiological features of NTLE from studies comparing carefully selected groups of patients with neocortical and mesial temporal epilepsies based on invasive EEG evaluation, seizure freedom after resective surgery or a combination of the two.

■ Clinical characteristics of neocortical lobe epilepsy

Because the pathological substrates are more diverse in NTLE than in MTLE, the age of onset of NTLE is variable, with seizures sometimes beginning in the third decade of life, or later (O'Brien, 1996). In a study comparing seizure-free patients after neocortical temporal resection and preservation of mesial structures with those after anteromesial temporal resection for MTLE due to hippocampal sclerosis (HS), the mean age of habitual seizure onset was significantly later for NTLE patients; 18.5 *vs.* 8.4 years (Foldvary, 1997). This difference was confirmed in a series comparing mesial and neocortical temporal epilepsy based on stereoelectroencephalographic recordings (Maillard, 2004). Mean age at the onset of epilepsy was significantly older for neocortical temporal patients (11.2 years) and patients with seizure onset involving both mesial and lateral structures (12.8 years), compared to those with mesial onset (7.9 years). However, others have found no significant difference in age at seizure onset between groups (Gil-Nagel, 1997; Pfänder, 2002).

There are significantly less risk factors for NTLE than MTLE, and febrile seizures in infancy or early childhood, as well as a history of significant cerebral insults prior to four years of age, are relatively rare (Cendes, 2000; Foldvary, 1997; Gil-Nagel, 1997; Maillard, 2004; O'Brien, 1996; Pacia, 1995). One series found head trauma, birth injury, and CNS infection to be more common in NTLE than MTLE (O'Brien, 1996).

■ Seizure semiology of neocortical lobe epilepsy

Ictal activation of identical structures may render the clinical symptoms of neocortical temporal seizures indistinguishable from those observed in patients with MTLE. This is largely due to the fact that, as demonstrated by depth electrode recordings, neocortical seizures tend to spread to the mesial structures. Therefore, seizure semiology may not reliably differentiate the two. However, some differences have been observed which, in combination with a given clinical setting and EEG, may suggest neocortical onset.

In a detailed video-EEG analysis investigation, the duration of clinical seizure was significantly shorter in NTLE than MTLE (43 *vs.* 69 seconds) and the onset and offset of clinical seizure was more ambiguous (Foldvary, 1996). The incidence of auras was found to be higher in MTLE (79-85%) than NTLE (58-84%), based on several series, although not significant (Foldvary, 1997; Gil-Nagel, 1997; Maillard, 2004; O'Brien, 1996; Phänder, 2002). Psychic phenomena, including *déjà vu*, *jamais vu* and depersonalization, and nonspecific auras are most commonly reported by patients with NTLE (Foldvary, 1997; Gil-Nagel, 1997; Pacia, 1996). Although abdominal auras have also been described in patients with neocortical temporal seizures, they are significantly more common in patients with MTLE (Ebner, 1994; Gil-Nagel, 1997; Maillard, 2004; Pfänder, 2002). In another series, fear and subjective dreamy states were reported exclusively by patients with mesial temporal seizures (Maillard, 2004), while much rarer auditory, vestibular and visual phenomena, due to activation of Heschl's gyrus and visual and auditory association cortices, reliably predicted temporal neocortical origin (Ebner, 1994; Maillard, 2004).

Several ictal behaviours have been found which differentiate mesial and neocortical temporal seizures. In general, studies have shown that NTLE seizures lack features commonly exhibited in MTLE. Oral and manual automatisms are more common in MTLE (58-75%) than NTLE (11-47%), and when present in NTLE are often subtle and observed late in the semiology sequence (Duchowny, 1994; Foldvary, 1996; Gil-Nagel, 1997; Maillard, 2004; Mihara, 1993). Contralateral dystonic posturing is significantly more common in MTLE, observed exclusively in mesial temporal seizures in one series (Foldvary, 1996; Mihara, 1993; O'Brien, 1996; Pfänder, 2002). Other behaviours observed more often in mesial temporal seizures include hyperventilation, body shifting, post-ictal coughing, repetitive leg movements, and side-to-side head movements (Foldvary, 1996). Early clonic activity of the contralateral upper extremity or facial grimacing/clonus, particularly in the absence of automatisms, is highly suggestive of a neocortical temporal origin (Duchowny, 1994; Gil-Nagel, 1997; Mihara, 1993; O'Brien, 1996; Pfänder, 2002). No difference has been found in the occurrence of behavioural arrest, vocalization, ictal speech, bilateral tonic posturing, reactivity, post-ictal aphasia, or occurrence of secondary generalisation during video-EEG monitoring (Foldvary, 1996; Gil-Nagel, 1997; Maillard, 2004; Mihara, 1993; Pfänder, 2002). It is not surprising that many behaviours do not reliably distinguish between mesial and neocortical temporal onset, as the symptoms of partial seizures reflect activation of cortical areas which may be distant from the ictal onset zone.

■ Surface EEG findings in neocortical lobe epilepsy

The electrophysiological manifestations of NTLE vary somewhat with the location and type of epileptogenic lesion and in many cases, will be indistinguishable from those of MTLE. In most studies comparing the type and distribution of interictal EEG abnormalities, no significant differences have been reported (Foldvary, 1997; O'Brien, 1996). However, in one of the largest series, patients with NTLE were significantly more likely to have discharges maximum at T7/8, TP7/8 or P7/8, whereas, SP1/2 or FT9/10 maximum discharges characterized the interictal EEG of those with MTLE (Pfänder, 2002). No difference between NTLE and MTLE in the rate of bitemporal (0% vs. 2%), extratemporal (6% vs. 2%) or contralateral mesial or diffuse temporal (3-8% vs. 1-5%) discharges was found.

Using source modelling, Ebersole et al. found differences in voltage topography of spikes in patients with NTLE and MTLE (Ebersole, 2000). In patients with MTLE (hippocampal atrophy, intracranial EEG mesial temporal seizure onset and seizure freedom following anteromesial temporal resection), frontotemporal negative maximum discharges had a corresponding positive maximum near the vertex. Conversely, patients with frontotemporal negative maximum spikes and corresponding contralateral temporal positivity were less likely to have hippocampal atrophy, more likely to have extramesial temporal onset on intracranial EEG and less likely to be seizure-free postoperatively, suggestive of NTLE. The same investigators found that MTLE spikes resulted in dipoles with an elevated, vertical orientation while those characteristic of NTLE resulted in dipoles with a horizontal and radial orientation. The voltage field of basal temporal spikes was often similar to that of MTLE. Spikes arising from the temporal pole resulted in dipoles with a horizontal, anteroposterior orientation, in contrast to lateral temporal spikes which most often produced horizontal and radial dipoles with maximum negativity in the lateral temporal region and positivity over the contralateral temporal lobe.

In contrast to the interictal EEG, surface ictal patterns of neocortical temporal seizures have been more extensively studied. The first, and among the most detailed, study categorized surface ictal EEGs of 93 epilepsy surgery candidates who underwent intracranial EEG evaluation or were referred directly for temporal lobectomy (Ebersole, 1996). An initial, regular 5 to 9 Hz rhythm, localized to the temporal region and not preceded by any other pattern, was most specific for seizures arising from the hippocampus. Less often, a similar vertex/parasagittal positive rhythm, or combination of the two, was seen in seizures of mesial temporal origin. Temporal neocortical seizures were most often characterized by irregular, polymorphic 2 to 5 Hz lateralized activity, commonly followed by rhythmic 5 to 9 Hz activity, as seen in MTLE or preceded by repetitive or periodic sharp waves. Seizures with non-lateralized ictal patterns, such as diffuse slowing or background attenuation, were most often seen in NTLE. Of note, both ictal and interictal discharges restricted to the hippocampus, based on depth recordings, are generally not discernable on surface EEG or produce non-lateralized ictal patterns only (Ebersole, 2000; Pacia & Ebersole, 1997). The rhythmic theta-alpha pattern, characteristic of MTLE, is observed only after the hippocampal seizure propagates to the adjacent inferolateral temporal neocortex (Pacia & Ebersole, 1997).

Similar findings have been reported in most subsequent studies comparing surface ictal EEG characteristics in NTLE and MTLE. Most notably, the presence of bilateral ictal patterns, early appearance of bilateral EEG changes, lower incidence of rhythmic sharp activity > 4 Hz, and hemispheric (rather than temporal) rhythmic activity are suggestive of seizures arising from the neocortical temporal region (Foldvary, 1997; O'Brien, 1996). In one series, the mean maximal frequency of lateralized rhythmic activity (LRA) was significantly lower in NTLE (5.5 Hz) than MTLE (6.7 Hz) (Foldvary, 1997). Others have found no differences in ictal patterns between neocortical and mesial temporal seizures, with temporal rhythmic theta or alpha activity, irregular, polymorphic 2 to 5 Hz hemispheric or temporal patterns, and non-lateralized arrhythmic activity observed relatively equally in both groups (Gil-Nagel & Risinger, 1997; Pfänder, 2000).

■ Predictive models of neocortical lobe epilepsy

Multiple logistic regression modelling has been used to determine whether subjects with NTLE and MTLE can be correctly classified given the presence or absence of certain clinical, semiological, and electrographic attributes (Foldvary, 1997; Pfänder, 2002). In the first of these studies (Foldvary, 1997), the estimated sensitivities, specificities, and predictive values for those variables which significantly differed between the MTLE and NTLE groups were analysed *(Table I)*. For continuous variables, a cutpoint for maximizing sensitivity and specificity was determined using receiver operating characteristic (ROC) curves. Reasonably high sensitivities and specificities were estimated for age at seizure

Table I. Estimated sensitivity, specificity and positive and negative predictive values for selected variables which differ between MTLE and NTLE groups
Significant difference was considered at $p < 0.05$. Sensitivity: the probability that a patient with MTLE possessed an attribute; Specificity: the probability that a patient with NTLE did not possess the attribute; PPV (positive predictive value): the probability that a patient had MTLE given the presence of an attribute; NPV (negative predictive value): the probability of NTLE given its absence.
Adapted from Foldvary (1997)

Variable	Sensitivity	Specificity	PPV	NPV
CLINICAL				
Age of onset ≤ 13 years	0.80 (.56-.94)	0.88 (.47-1.0)	0.94 (.73-.99)	0.64 (.35-.85)
Any risk factor	0.85 (.62-.97)	0.75 (.35-.97)	0.90 (.67-.99)	0.67 (.30-.93)
SEMIOLOGICAL				
Oral automatisms	0.58 (.39-.77)	0.85 (.63-1.0)	0.91 (.77-1.0)	0.43 (.16-.70)
Dystonic posturing	0.19 (.002-.37)	1.00 (.87-1.0)	1.00 (.79-1.0)	0.30 (.10-.51)
Manual automatisms	0.70 (.54-.86)	0.85 (.61-1.0)	0.93. 82-1.0)	0.50 (.20-.80)
Leg movements	0.41 (.20-.61)	0.96 (.88-1.0)	0.97 (.91-1.0)	0.35 (.12-.57)
Body shifting	0.62 (.44-.79)	0.81 (.56-1.0)	0.91 (.76-1.0)	0.41 (.15-.68)
Hyperventilation/cough/sigh	0.54 (.39-.71)	0.89 (.74-.96)	0.94 (.84-1.0)	0.39 (.15-.63)
ELECTROGRAPHIC				
Seizure duration ⩾ 56 seconds	0.71 (.57-.85)	0.78 (.53-1.0)	0.93 (.79-1.0)	0.48 (.18-.78)
Temporal LRA*	0.89 (.78-1.0)	0.42 (.23-.60)	0.88 (.77-.98)	0.47 (.10-.84)
LRA frequency ⩾ 6.5 Hz	0.76 (.63-.92)	0.79 (.62-.97)	0.94 (.87-1.0)	0.46 (.18-.75)

* Lateralized rhythmic activity on ictal EEG.

onset, mean seizure duration, frequency of LRA during the ictal EEG, manual automatisms, and historical risk factors for epilepsy. For example, the estimated probabilities that a patient with MTLE has age of seizure onset of 13 years or less, seizure duration of at least 56 seconds, or seizures with maximal LRA frequency of at least 6.5 Hz was 0.80, 0.71, and 0.76, respectively. With one exception, the estimates for positive predictive value exceeded 90% for all the variables listed. However, the negative predictive value estimates were low in comparison. Therefore, if one were to use these variables to classify patients as MTLE or NTLE, the presence of an attribute would be a good indicator of MTLE, but a large number of patients without the attribute would likely be misclassified. Thus, when examined individually, the presence of a particular variable is a good predictor of MTLE, but its absence does not reliably predict NTLE. In addition, because of the small sample size, these values may not reflect true values.

In a larger study, patients were classified as NTLE or MTLE based on history of febrile seizures, presence of abdominal auras and contralateral dystonic posturing, and ipsilateral mesial temporal spike predominance (Pfänder, 2002). Based on the combination of these variables, the likelihood of correctly identifying MTLE was 73%. However, using this model, 19% of NTLE and 30% of MTLE cases were misclassified.

■ Conclusions

A growing body of literature supports the contention that, in many cases, it may be possible to differentiate between NTLE and MTLE on the basis of clinical features, seizure semiology, and ictal surface EEG recordings during presurgical evaluation. While seizure semiology and surface EEG features may be indistinguishable in some cases, most studies suggest that NTLE seizures lack features commonly exhibited in MTLE, including abdominal auras, oral and manual automatisms, and contralateral dystonia. Similarly, surface ictal EEG recordings show a higher rate of early bilateral changes and hemispheric, rather than temporal, maximum rhythms. The ability to distinguish between NTLE and MTLE during non-invasive evaluation would be advantageous, particularly in non-lesional NTLE cases which generally require intracranial EEG monitoring and more extensive or tailored resections.

References

- Cendes F, Li LM, Watson C, et al. Is ictal recording mandatory in temporal lobe epilepsy? Not when the interictal electroencephalogram and hippocampal atrophy coincide. *Arch Neurol* 2000; 57: 497-500.
- Duchowny M, Jayakar P, Resnick T, Levin B, Alvarez L. Posterior temporal epilepsy: electroclinical features. *Ann Neurol* 1994; 35: 427-31.
- Ebersole JS. *Neocortical Epilepsies: Advances in Neurology*, Vol. 84. Philadelphia: Lippincott Williams & Wilkins, 2000, pp. 353-63.
- Ebersole JS, Pacia SV. Localization of temporal lobe foci by ictal EEG patterns. *Epilepsia* 1996; 37: 386-99.
- Ebner A. *Epileptic seizures and syndromes*. London: John Libbey & Company Ltd., 1994, pp. 375-82.

- Foldvary N, Lee N, Thwaites G, Mascha E, Hammel J, Kim H, *et al.* Clinical and electrographic manifestations of lesional neocortical temporal lobe epilepsy. *Neurology* 1997; 49: 757-63.
- Gil-Nagel A, Risinger MW. Ictal semiology in hippocampal *versus* extrahippocampal temporal lobe epilepsy. *Brain* 1997; 120: 183-92.
- Maillard L, Vignal JP, Gavaret M, Guye M, Biraben A, McGonigal A, *et al.* Semiologic and electrophysiologic correlations in temporal lobe seizure subtypes. *Epilepsia* 2004; 45: 1590-9.
- Mihara T, Inoue Y, Hiyoshi T, Watanabe Y, Kubota Y, Tottori, *et al.* Localizing value of seizure manifestations of temporal lobe epilepsies and the consequence of analyzing their sequential appearance. *Jpn J Psychiatry Neurol* 1993; 47: 175-82.
- O'Brien TJ, Kilpatrick C, Murrie V, Vogrin S, Morris K, Cook MJ. Temporal lobe epilepsy caused by mesial temporal sclerosis and temporal neocortical lesions. A clinical and electroencephalographic study of 46 pathologically proven cases. *Brain* 1996; 119: 2133-41.
- Pacia SV, Ebersole JS. Intracranial EEG substrates of scalp ictal patterns from temporal lobe foci. *Epilepsia* 1997; 38: 642-54.
- Pacia SV, Devinsky O, Perrine K, Ravdin, Luciano D, Vazquea B, *et al.* Clinical features of neocortical temporal lobe epilepsy. *Ann Neurol* 1996; 40: 724-30.
- Phänder M, Arnold S, Henkel A, Weil S, Werhahn KJ, Eisensehr I, *et al.* Clinical features and EEG findings differentiating mesial from neocortical temporal lobe epilepsy. *Epileptic Disord* 2002; 4: 189-95.

Section III:
Clinical and experimental neurophysiology of mesial temporal lobe epilepsies

Non-invasive and invasive EEG in mesial temporal epilepsy

Hajo M. Hamer[1], Philippe Kahane[2,3], Hans O. Lüders[4]

[1] Epilepsy Center Hessen, Department of Neurology, University Hospitals Giessen and Marburg GmbH & Philipps-University Marburg, Marburg, Germany
[2] Department of Neurology & GIN Inserm U836-UJF-CEA, Grenoble University Hospital, France
[3] CTRS-Inserm IDEE, Lyon University Hospital, France
[4] Epilepsy Center, University Hospitals, Case Medical Center, Cleveland, USA

Non-invasive EEG

Scalp EEG and sphenoidal electrodes

Scalp electrodes only detect brain activity which is synchronized within at least 6 cm^2 of cortex (Cooper *et al.*, 1965; Fernandez Torre *et al.*, 1999b; Barkley & Baumgartner, 2003; Tao *et al.*, 2005). This is because cerebral activity is attenuated by the impedance of the cerebrospinal fluid, meninges, skull and scalp. Therefore, scalp EEG only reveals a small percentage of interictal epileptiform discharges (IEDs) which can be recorded by depth or subdural electrodes from mesial temporal structures (Carreno & Lüders, 2001; So, 2001) *(Figure 1)*. Closely spaced scalp electrodes and scalp electrodes placed caudally to the standard international 10-20 system (essentially in the face area and immediately anterior to the ear lobe) can improve the yield of spike detection and also assist in better localization of the source of the spikes (Morris III, *et al.*, 1986; Hamer *et al.*, 1999). Surface electrodes, placed 1 cm above a point, which is one third the distance between the external auditory meatus and the external canthus (T1 and T2 which correspond approximately to FT9 and FT10 electrode placement of the 10-10 system, respectively), are intended to cover the temporal pole and are frequently used in patients with suspected mesial temporal lobe epilepsy (MTLE).

Sphenoidal electrodes are placed beneath the zygomatic arch, approximately 2.0 cm anterior to the incisura intertragica, 3 to 4 cm under the skin, and record close to the foramen ovale (FO). Sphenoidal electrodes can record epileptiform activity which does not appear at anterior temporal electrodes for only a minority of patients with MTLE *(Figure 2)* (Marks *et al.*, 1992; Tuunainen *et al.*, 1994; Kanner & Jones, 1997; Pacia *et al.*, 1998; Provini *et al.*, 1999). Some studies even concluded that sphenoidal electrodes are of little

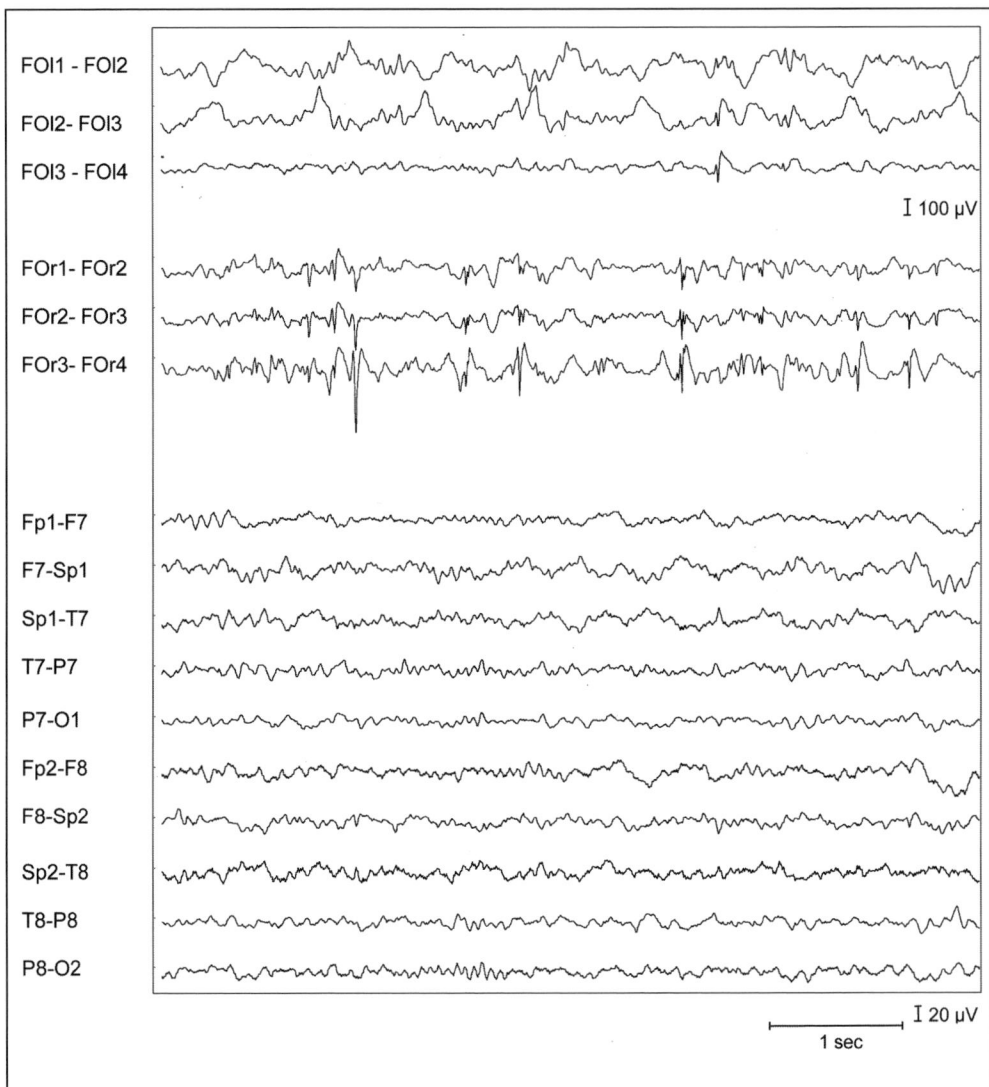

Figure 1. Invasive video-EEG monitoring with bilateral FO electrodes in a 38-year-old patient with bitemporal epilepsy.
In addition, scalp electrodes were attached according to the International 10-20 system and sphenoidal electrodes were bilaterally inserted. Note the IEDs recorded maximally at the fourth contact of the right FO electrode while the scalp and sphenoidal electrodes failed to detect these IEDs. FOr1, FOr2, FOr3, FOr4: four contacts of the right FO electrode; FOl1, FOl2, FOl3, FOl4: four contacts of the left FO electrode; Sp1: left sphenoidal electrode; Sp2: right sphenoidal electrode.

use because spikes detected at sphenoidal electrodes can also be seen consistently in other 10-10 system electrodes (Fernandez Torre et al., 1999a; Kissani et al., 2001; Mintzer et al., 2002). The real value of sphenoidal electrodes, like other 10-10 system electrodes, is the analysis of the field distribution of spikes recorded with additional electrodes. Additional electrodes significantly improve our ability to resolve the inverse solution and, therefore, predict the most likely source of a given spike. Spikes with the maximal amplitude at the sphenoidal electrodes can arise from the mesial or lateral temporal lobe or from an orbitofrontal focus (Marks et al., 1992). In patients with MTLE, sphenoidal electrodes usually register higher amplitudes of IED compared to scalp electrodes (Morris, III et al., 1989; Kanner et al., 1995; Foldvary 2000). However, sphenoidal electrodes still fail to detect a large proportion of IED recorded with FO electrodes or other invasive electrodes (Fernandez Torre et al., 1999a) *(Figure 1)*.

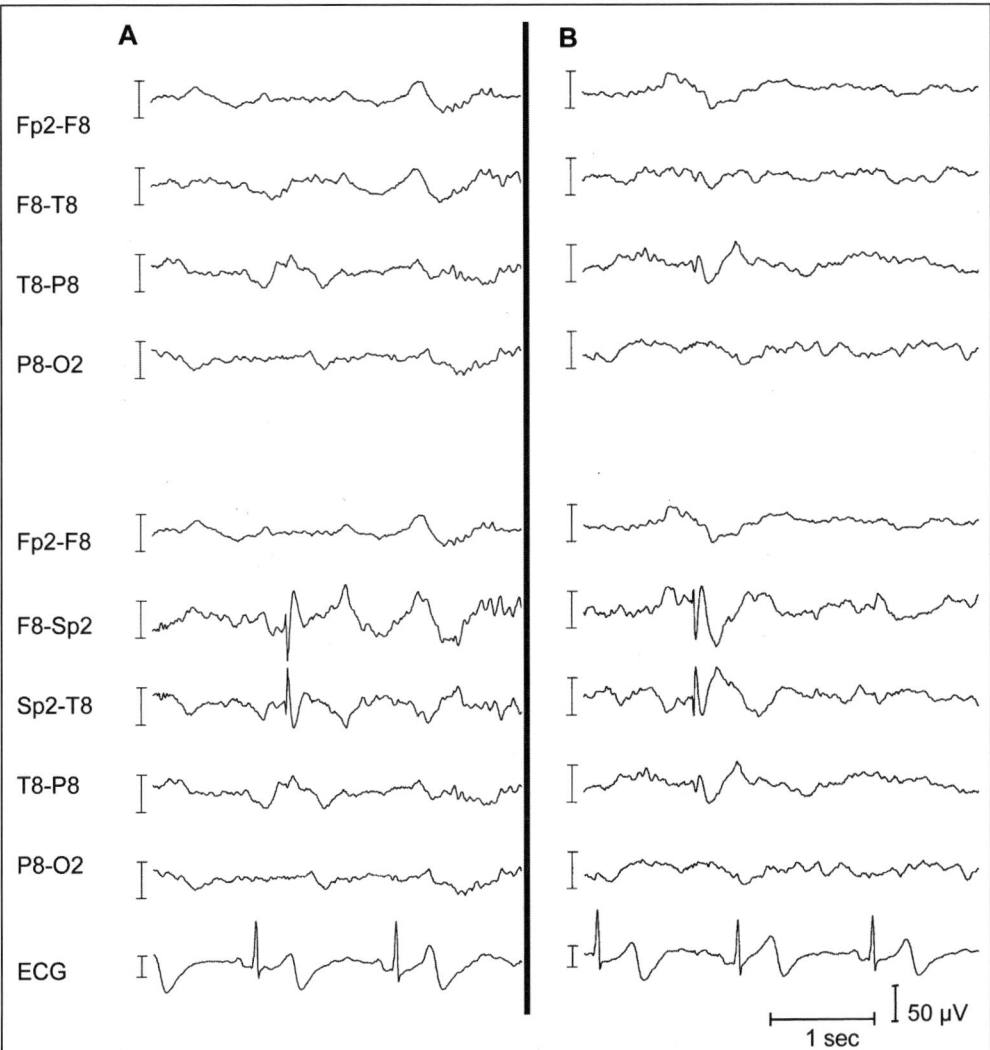

Figure 2. Two examples of IEDs of a 39-year-old patient with right mesial temporal epilepsy due to hippocampal sclerosis.
Scalp electrodes were attached according to the International 10-20 system and additional sphenoidal electrodes were bilaterally inserted (Sp2: right sphenoidal electrode). Note the sharp waves recorded by the sphenoidal electrode but not by the scalp electrodes. ECG: electrocardiogram.

Sensitivity and specificity of interictal scalp EEG

Overall, 10% of patients with epilepsy are expected not to show any IED on scalp EEG during wakefulness or sleep, in spite of prolonged or repeated recordings (Chung et al., 1991; Adachi et al., 1998; Binnie & Stefan, 1999). The yield from a single EEG is substantially increased in patients investigated within one or two days after a seizure, and is greater in patients with monthly seizures than in those who had been seizure-free for a year (Marsan & Zivin, 1970; Sundaram et al., 1990; King et al., 1998). The frequency of IEDs is higher in NREM sleep than during wakefulness which makes it advisable to include sleep recordings (Malow et al., 1999; Klein et al., 2003). In addition, IED in NREM sleep provides more accurate information for lateralization of epileptogenesis than during wakefulness (Adachi et al., 1998). The duration of recording may also affect the detection rate of interictal spiking (Gotman & Koffler, 1989). However, spikes and sharp waves must be differentiated from benign variants which are frequently recorded in the temporal area and may resemble IED (Binnie & Stefan, 1999; Foldvary, 2000).

In general, the frequency, morphological characteristics and sleep state dependence of interictal epileptiform activity cannot be used to predict the aetiology or severity of MTLE (Foldvary, 2000). However, there are reports that rhythmic spiking on a slow background activity (not associated with behavioural changes) is relatively characteristic of focal cortical dysplastic lesions (Palmini et al., 1995; Gambardella et al., 1996; Rosenow et al., 1998). As mentioned above, several studies have shown that the majority of mesial and neocortical temporal IEDs fail to be recorded by surface electrodes. However, IEDs which are recorded by extracranial EEG tend to show a better correlation with the seizure origin compared to IEDs recorded by invasive electrodes (Blume et al., 1993). This suggests that widely synchronous interictal spikes more likely arise from the epileptogenic area than spikes with relatively smaller fields.

In addition to IED, there is evidence that temporal intermittent rhythmic delta activity (TIRDA) strongly correlates with the clinical diagnosis of temporal lobe epilepsy (TLE) (Reiher et al., 1989; Blume et al., 1993; Gambardella et al., 1995) *(Figure 3)*. TIRDA was seen in 0.3% of all recordings obtained in a general EEG laboratory (Normand et al., 1995), but in as many as 28% of patients evaluated for temporal lobe resections (Geyer et al., 1999). A significant association was also found between MTLE and TIRDA (Di Gennaro et al., 2003). Focal intermittent delta activity is reported to identify the side of MTLE with a sensitivity and specificity of > 90% (Gambardella et al., 1995).

Distribution of interictal epileptiform discharges

In MTLE, IEDs tend to produce a stereotyped pattern on the scalp and usually are highly restricted to anterior temporal electrodes (Williamson et al., 1993; Ebner & Hoppe, 1995; Hamer et al., 1999). This may be due to the location of the neuronal generators within the temporal lobe and anatomical characteristics of the brain surface, such as skull discontinuities (Fernandez Torre et al., 1999b). Using three-dimensional multiple dipole modelling, two possible sources of interictal spikes in patients suffering from hippocampal sclerosis (HS) were identified (Baumgartner et al., 1995). The first source involved the mesio-basal aspect of the temporal lobe (hippocampus and parahippocampal gyrus) and was followed within 40 milliseconds by activation of the anterior temporal lobe neocortex. Extracranially recorded IED in mesial and not in lateral TLE frequently show a negative pole in the anterior temporal region or at the sphenoidal electrode and a widespread positive pole over the vertex (Ebersole & Wade 1991). As a rule, patients with HS have more than 90% IEDs in the anterior temporal region. The rare occurrence of lateral temporal and frontal spikes/sharp waves in adult patients with HS may be due to spread of epileptic discharges to the temporal neocortex or to the orbito-frontal cortex via the limbic system (Ebersole & Wade 1991). Frequent posterior temporal or extratemporal sharp waves decrease the likelihood of HS (Hamer et al., 1999). Bilateral independent spikes and/or slow waves, as well as precentral spike-and-wave complexes, suggest an epileptogenic area extending outside the limits of the temporal lobe (Barba et al., 2007). Most (Bengzon et al., 1968; Dodrill et al., 1986; Keogan et al., 1992; Barry et al., 1992; Salanova et al., 1996; McIntosh et al., 2001), but not all studies (Chung et al., 1991; Cascino et al., 1996) confirmed the finding that IEDs confined to the anterior temporal region are predictive of good postoperative outcome after TLE surgery.

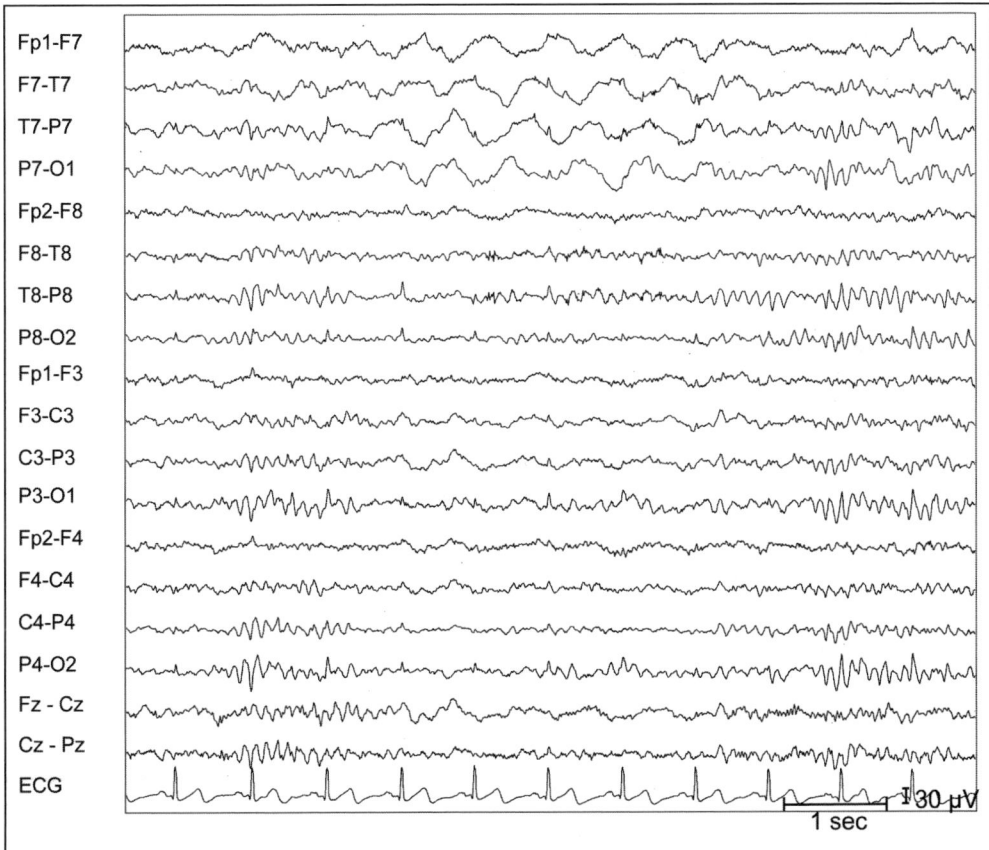

Figure 3. Interictal EEG of a 21-year-old patient with left temporal lobe epilepsy due to hippocampal sclerosis. Scalp electrodes were attached according to the International 10-20 system. Note the temporal intermittent rhythmic delta activity (TIRDA) in the left temporal region. ECG: electrocardiogram.

Children with MTLE tend to have a more widespread irritative zone showing mid, posterior or bilateral temporal, extratemporal, or even generalised IED (Mohamed et al., 2001). Tumours in the mesial temporal region tend to cause wider distributed IEDs compared to HS or developmental abnormalities (Aykut-Bingol et al., 1998; Hamer et al., 1999; Kameyama et al., 2001). This is also true for seizure patterns in patients with mesial temporal tumours (Bösebeck et al., 2002). This may be caused by local neuronal injury, oedema, ischaemia or other electrical and/or biochemical effects of the structural lesion on susceptible neighbouring brain tissue or homologous contralateral areas (Spencer et al., 1984; Awad et al., 1991b).

Lateralizing value of interictal discharges

In extracranial EEG recordings, interictal discharges can have a more reliable lateralizing value than ictal changes in MTLE (Sammaritano et al., 1987). In a series of patients with TLE, the presence of a single interictal spike focus in the antero-temporal region accurately predicted temporal lobe onset whether the surface ictal EEG was focal, regional or lateralized to the same hemisphere (Kanner et al., 1993). If IEDs were exclusive or clearly preponderant on the side of surgery, they almost always predicted good postoperative outcome (Chee et al., 1993; Blume et al., 1993; 2001; Salanova et al., 1994; 1996; Hufnagel et al., 1994; Steinhoff et al., 1995; Holmes et al., 1996; Pataraia et al., 1998; Radhakrishnan et al., 1998; Serles et al., 1998; Malow et al., 1999; McIntosh et al., 2001; So, 2001; Janszky et al., 2005; Kelemen et al., 2006). In a study of 59 patients who had temporal lobectomy, 92% of patients with > 90% lateralization of interictal spikes had a good surgical outcome, whereas only 50% with < 90% had a favourable outcome (Chung et al., 1991). It remains controversial whether preoperative IED frequency is associated with postoperative outcome (Janszky et al., 2003b; Di Gennaro et al., 2004; Krendl et al., 2008). Concordance between structural MRI and interictal EEG was more closely associated with good surgical outcome than concordance between MRI and ictal EEG findings with non-lateralizing interictal EEG (Cascino et al., 1996; Gilliam et al., 1997; Pataraia et al., 1998; Serles et al., 1998; Cendes et al., 2000). These findings may not fully be applicable to tumour patients who can show a wide irritative zone (Hamer et al., 1999) and whose postoperative seizure outcome is not affected by bilateral IEDs (Morris et al., 1998).

The incidence of bilateral IEDs in TLE is estimated to lie between 20% and 44% and may be more when investigated with invasive EEG (So, 2001). The probability of bilateral IEDs was positively correlated with the duration of EEG monitoring (Cascino et al., 1996; Ergene et al., 2000). Bilateral IEDs were associated with higher seizure frequency in unilateral disease suggesting that "mirror foci" are produced by seizures and not epileptiform discharges (Janszky et al., 2003a). Hence, bitemporal IEDs can reflect bilateral damage, dysfunction at a distance, or secondary epileptogenesis (Margerison & Corsellis 1966; Sammaritano et al., 1987; Aykut-Bingol et al., 1998). Bitemporal IEDs increase the likelihood that seizures arise independently from both sides (Steinhoff et al., 1995) and substantially decrease the chance of a favourable postoperative outcome (Schulz et al., 2000). However, subjects with bitemporal IEDs, but MRI hippocampal abnormalities concordant with the ictal onset region, may still have a good to excellent surgical outcome (Barry et al., 1992; Williamson et al., 1993; Holmes et al., 1997; Hamer et al., 1999; Malow et al., 1999).

Prognostic relevance of postoperative IEDs

In both temporal and extratemporal epilepsy, absence of IEDs in the six-month or one-year postoperative scalp EEG monitoring period was associated with good postoperative outcome (Godoy et al., 1992; Lüders et al., 1994; Patrick et al., 1995; Morris et al., 1998; Aronica et al., 2001; Hildebrandt et al., 2005). The prognostic value of a three-month postoperative EEG monitoring period remains controversial (Cascino et al., 1992; Kirkpatrick et al., 1993; Tuunainen et al., 1994; Radhakrishnan et al., 1998). The presence of IEDs on the early extracranial postoperative EEG (within one or two weeks after surgery) were not found to be of prognostic value in most studies (So et al., 1989; Salanova et al., 1992; Radhakrishnan et al., 1998; Ficker et al., 1999; Mintzer et al., 2005). There are conflicting results on the prognostic value of IEDs on post-resection electrocorticography (ECoG) and several studies found an association between post-resection IEDs and less favourable outcome (So et al., 1989; Fiol et al., 1991; McBride et al., 1991; Salanova et al., 1996; Wennberg et al., 1998) while others did not (Godoy et al., 1992; Shih et al., 1994; Tuunainen et al., 1994; Tran et al., 1995; Radhakrishnan et al., 1998; Ficker et al., 1999; McIntosh et al., 2001; Chen et al., 2006). The lack of agreement of these studies may be due to differences in the patient populations (e.g. lesional *versus* non-lesional cases), the recording techniques and the anaesthetic agents used during surgery. Even in the studies confirming the association of post-resection IEDs and seizure continuation, the percentage of patients with post-resection persistence of IEDs, but still favourable outcome, varied from 18% to 47% (So et al., 1989; Fiol et al., 1991; Salanova et al., 1996; Hildebrandt et al., 2005; Kipervasser et al., 2007) which can make it difficult to estimate the prognosis in individual cases.

Ictal EEG

Non-invasive ictal EEG manifestations of seizures arising from the temporal lobe have been studied extensively. As for the recording of IEDs, it is preferable to record seizures during sleep. Buechler et al. reported that sleep seizure recordings were less disturbed by artefacts, were 2.5 times more likely to have a focal EEG onset, were four times more likely to lateralize the seizure correctly and preceded the clinical seizure for a longer time compared to seizure recordings during wakefulness (Buechler et al., 2008).

Rhythmic 5-9 Hz activity, lateralized or localized to the temporal region, appearing within the first 30 seconds of the electrographic or clinical seizure onset, is observed in 65-90% of patients with MTLE *(Figure 4)* (Risinger et al., 1989; Williamson et al., 1993; Ebner & Hoppe 1995; Ebersole & Pacia, 1996; Pataraia et al., 1998; Vossler et al., 1998; Foldvary et al., 2001; Caboclo et al., 2007). In addition, however, several other ictal surface EEG patterns may also occur in MTLE such as attenuation of EEG activity, cessation of IED, repetitive spiking and rhythmic delta or beta activity (Steinhoff et al., 1995). Rhythmic theta activity at ictal onset was significantly more common in patients with moderate to marked hippocampal atrophy (79%) than those with mild or no hippocampal atrophy (19%), and a positive correlation between the median frequency of the initial ictal discharges and the severity of HS has been reported (Vossler et al., 1998).

Patients with 5-9 Hz ictal patterns at seizure onset with a limited antero-temporal distribution were significantly more likely to be seizure-free after anterior temporal lobectomy than those with irregular, slow rhythms (< 5 Hz) with a widespread temporal distribution (Assaf & Ebersole, 1999). A seizure-free outcome was observed in 83% of patients with

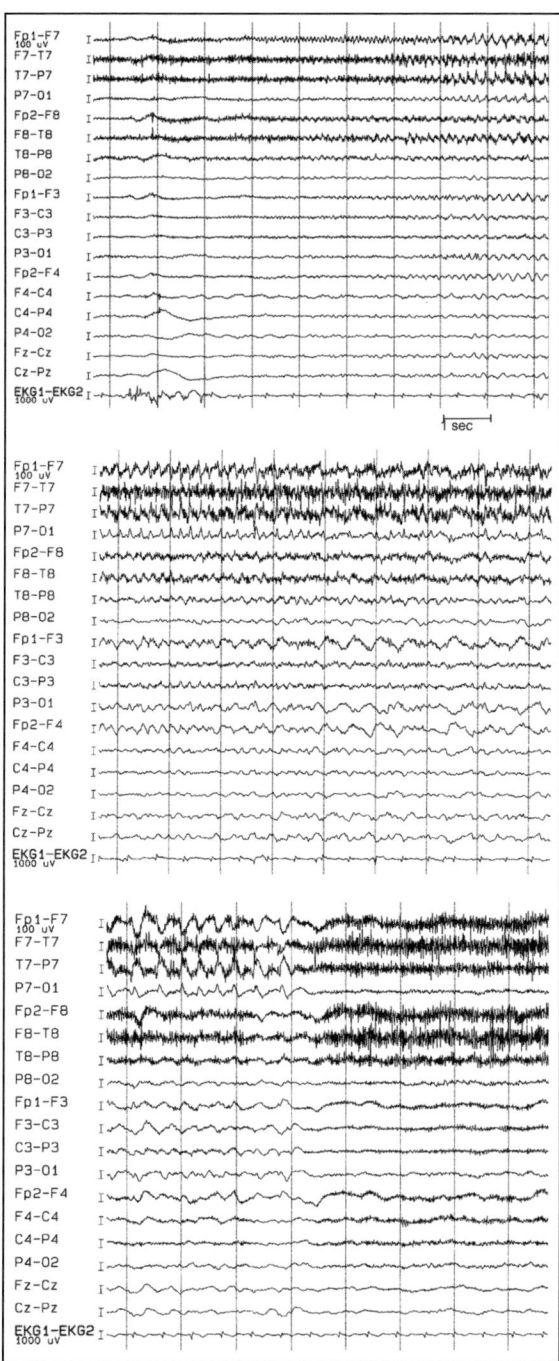

Figure 4. Ictal EEG of a 35-year-old patient with left temporal lobe epilepsy due to hippocampal sclerosis. Scalp electrodes were attached according to the International 10-20 system. Note the evolving left temporal seizure, maximum at the left anterior temporal electrodes. EKG: electrocardiogram.

ictal recordings localized to the lesioned temporal lobe, compared to 63% with non-lateralized seizure patterns or 46% with seizures which propagated to the contralateral hemisphere (Schulz et al., 2000; Lee et al., 2006; Kelemen et al., 2006). The ictal onset was rarely incorrectly lateralized to the contralateral temporal lobe due to a severely sclerotic hippocampus (the so called "burned-out hippocampus"). This was observed in five of 109 cases with suspected TLE who underwent depth electrode evaluation at two epilepsy centres (Mintzer et al., 2004). Bilateral independent seizure onsets, asynchrony of ictal activity over the two temporal lobes and switch of ictal activity from one hemisphere to the other are all strongly correlated with bitemporal epileptogenicity (Steinhoff et al., 1995).

The post-ictal EEG can also be valuable in lateralizing seizures in MTLE. Regional or lateralized delta activity or EEG attenuation are reliable predictors of the side of seizure origin (Kaibara & Blume 1988; Walczak et al., 1992; Hufnagel et al., 1995). In a series of 29 patients with TLE, lateralized post-ictal delta activity predicted the side of seizure origin in 96% of cases (Jan et al., 2001).

The results of several studies suggest that non-invasive ictal recordings do not improve the localization of epilepsy in patients with suspected TLE in whom MRI and interictal EEG are concordant (Gilliam et al., 1997; Pataraia et al., 1998; Cendes et al., 2000). In 84 patients with unilateral hippocampal atrophy and concordant interictal EEG, over 90% of patients had an excellent postoperative outcome regardless of whether ictal EEG was concordant or discordant (Cambier et al., 2001).

▪ Invasive EEG

The number of patients with epilepsy and HS requiring intracranial EEG studies has been markedly reduced over the last decades due to growing experience with this syndrome and better neuroimaging. There is general agreement that non-invasive evaluation is sufficient in unilateral MTLE with concordant non-invasive testing. Even in the case of bilateral IEDs, surgery is usually indicated without preceding invasive monitoring if the scalp ictal EEG, neuroimaging and neuropsychology all point to the same side. However, bilateral independent ictal patterns on surface EEG should lead us to suspect bilateral disease. In this situation, invasive recordings should be performed if the MRI and other neuroimaging studies indicate unilateral or predominantly unilateral disease (Diehl & Lüders, 2000). Invasive studies may also be indicated in non-lesional cases (no clear lesion on MRI), or cases with widespread lesions on MRI. Moreover, invasive monitoring can be of great value when presurgical non-invasive studies cannot differentiate between MTLE, neocortical temporal lobe epilepsy or extratemporal lobe epilepsy ("pseudotemporal" epilepsy) or suggest that the epileptogenic zone extends outside the boundaries of a standard temporal lobectomy (temporal *versus* temporal "plus" epilepsy).

Foramen ovale electrodes

The "semi-invasive" technique of recording with FO electrodes was designed to evaluate patients with suspected MTLE when non-invasive work-up could not rule out bilateral disease (Wieser et al., 1985; Gloor 1991; Williamson et al., 1993; Gil-Nagel & Risinger 1997; Carter et al., 1998). The main aim of recording with FO electrodes is to verify seizure origin at the mesio-basal temporal lobe structures and to prove constant lateralization or propagation times from one hippocampus to the other, mostly in non-lesional patients (Wieser & Siegel, 1991; Alarcon et al., 2001; Zumsteg et al., 2006).

Compared to intracerebral depth and subdural electrodes, FO electrodes are less invasive and have a rate of serious complications which is low but not negligible (Wieser et al., 1985; Schuler et al., 1993; Steude et al., 1993; Sperling, 1997). Most complications are transitory such as haematoma, facial pain or hypoesthesia, but also subarachnoid haemorrhage or meningitis have been described (Velasco et al., 2006).

The most reliable seizure onset patterns recorded with FO electrodes are low-amplitude fast discharges, frequently preceded by a localized electrodecrement (Wieser & Siegel, 1991). In the absence of these patterns, the localization of the seizure onset zone should be questioned. The findings obtained by FO recordings were very similar to those seen with depth electrodes in a group of five patients who underwent simultaneous recording with both types of electrodes (Velasco et al., 2006). However, there is a risk of falsely lateralizing or localizing the ictal onset zone by overlooking the spread of a seizure from outside the mesial temporal structures into the mesio-basal structures (Binnie et al., 1994). In addition, discharges confined to the amygdala may not be detected (Wieser & Siegel, 1991). Due to these limitations, FO electrodes are now only used infrequently.

Subdural strip and grid electrodes

In MTLE, as in other focal epilepsies, intracranial electrodes are specifically useful in the design of an appropriate invasive EEG study. The use of invasive recordings with bitemporal subdural recordings enable the assessment of the side of temporal epileptogenesis in many patients whose scalp data have been inconclusive in this respect (Blume et al., 2001). Subdural electrodes can be placed over the temporal and frontal lobes to differentiate between a temporal and frontal epileptogenic zone. Subdural electrodes may be applied to patients when it is not clear whether the ictal onset zone involves the mesial or lateral aspect of the temporal lobe, and the exact extent of the epileptogenic zone is of concern especially in non-lesional cases. Basal temporal subdural strip electrode placement and lateral temporal grid coverage is recommended in these patients (Lüders et al., 1989; Cohen-Gadol & Spencer, 2003; Zijlmans et al., 2008). Patients who are not rendered seizure-free postoperatively may be candidates for a second surgical procedure which also requires frequently invasive recordings to identify the exact location and extent of the residual epileptogenic zone in relation to remaining tissue (Awad et al., 1991a). About 50% of these patients become seizure-free after second surgery and 30% have a reduction of greater than 90% in seizure frequency (Awad et al., 1991a).

The advantages of subdural strip electrodes over depth electrodes include: easier implantation with no stereotactic equipment, coverage of larger cortical areas, definition of the exact extent and distribution of the epileptogenic zone within one temporal lobe and possibly a lower risk of haemorrhage (Lüders et al., 1989; Diehl & Lüders, 2000). Disadvantages include: the relatively inaccurate placement by virtue of the insertion technique and the inability to record from buried structures. In MTLE, the concordance between subdural and depth electrodes is high as long as the mesial electrodes of the subtemporal subdural strips record the mesial to collateral sulcus from the parahippocampal region (Eisenschenk et al., 2001).

The ictal patterns seen in subdural electrodes covering the mesial temporal cortex are similar to those recorded by FO electrodes. High-frequency, low-voltage activity is most common at seizure onset, although rhythmic discharges greater than 2 Hz in the beginning of the seizure and periodic spiking prior to seizure onset have also been described (Spencer et al., 1992). A widespread ictal pattern at onset should raise the suspicion that the intracranial electrodes are inserted at a distance from the seizure onset zone. A long latency of typical ictal patterns prior to interhemispheric spread is associated with good postoperative prognosis in MTLE (Lieb et al., 1986).

Monitoring with subdural grids is associated with transient complications in 10-25% of patients and with more severe complications, such as osteomyelitis or infarction, in 2% (Hamer et al., 2002; Burneo et al., 2006). Transient complications are reported in 0-3% of cases during recordings with strip electrodes (Cohen-Gadol & Spencer, 2003; Burneo et al., 2006).

Depth electrodes

The main advantage of using chronically implanted "depth" electrodes is that they penetrate brain tissue directly, thus allowing access without any theoretical restriction to almost any cortical (and even subcortical) area involved in the epileptic process. This is of special interest in temporal lobe epilepsies, since it provides recordings from deep, buried structures such as the amygdala, hippocampus, planum temporalis, or insula, as well as from the sulcal cortex. Such a technique carries some risks, predominantly haemorrhage, which are relatively low and vary from 1 to 4% (Van Buren, 1987). Depth electrodes should be placed stereotactically, and their positioning strategy varies according to the results of the non-invasive presurgical testing. The stereo-electroencephalography (SEEG) method of Talairach and Bancaud evaluates all areas potentially involved in the onset, propagation, and clinical expression of seizures (Kahane & Francoine, 2008). In such cases, spatial sampling needs to be generous, to generate information which permits adequate definition of the region for resection (Munari et al., 1994a). The implantation strategy in suspected MTLE cases usually includes the amygdalo-hippocampal complex (and therefore the second temporal convolution), the temporo-polar cortex, the first temporal gyrus and, when relevant, the baso-temporal region (see also the chapter by Bartlomei). Additionally, the investigation of extratemporal areas must be wide enough to provide information not only to customize a more extensive cortectomy (if necessary), but also to identify a possible extratemporal origin of seizures which could not have been anticipated with certainty from scalp EEG and clinical findings. Proceeding this way, it has been shown that although MRI evidence of HS is correlated with the side of epileptogenesis, it is not always predictive of the site of seizure onset within the temporal lobe (King et al., 1997). Indeed, seizures may arise from the amygdala (Munari et al., 1994b; Spanedda et al., 1997), entorhinal cortex (Bartolomei et al., 2005), temporal pole (Chabardès et al., 2005), and even the temporal neocortex (Munari et al., 1994b; Arzimanoglou & Kahane, 2008). Accordingly, depth EEG patterns may differ from one region to another. A characteristic pattern of slow (1-2 Hz) periodic spike activity, referred to as hypersynchronous seizure onset (Velasco et al., 2000), is seen almost exclusively in the hippocampus. In contrast, a rhythmic polyspike activity of > 13 Hz (Wennberg et al., 2002) or a low-voltage fast onset (Velasco et al., 2000) is more common in regional onsets, as well as in temporal lobe seizures which involve the temporo-polar region from onset (Chabardès et al., 2005) or the entorhinal cortex (Bartolomei et al., 2005). Also, the classic distinction between medial and lateral temporal lobe discharges is an oversimplification, and other types of temporal lobe seizures exist which include the classic medial and lateral subtypes as well as the medial-lateral or lateral-medial subtype (Bartolomei et al., 1999; Maillard et al., 2004). MTL epileptogenic zones may even incorporate a participating network that extends beyond these traditional medial and lateral TL areas, including the orbito-frontal cortex, the insula, the frontal and parietal operculum, or the temporo-parieto-occipital junction, a finding described using the term of temporal "plus" epilepsy (Munari et al., 1989; Kahane et al., 2001; Ryvlin & Kahane, 2005; Barba et al., 2007). However, the precise evaluation of the ictal onset zone depends on the spatial sampling of the intracerebral investigation. Therefore, caution is required to ascertain that the fast discharge, which is supposed to mark the ictal onset, is really localized to the place where it has been recorded from (i.e. a volume of brain tissue of approximating 1 cm^3).

ECoG

A major disadvantage of intraoperative electrocorticography is the usual absence of ictal activity (Stefan et al., 2008). Moreover, successful localization of the irritative zone may rely heavily on the selection of the site for electrocorticography which only allows recording with a limited number of electrodes. Intraoperative recording with many electrodes (64 electrodes and more) is difficult to perform because of the long set-up time that such recordings require. This may lead to the conclusion that chronic evaluation techniques may often be preferable to acute intraoperative testing in MTLE, in spite of higher risks of chronic monitoring *versus* acute electrocorticography (Rosenbaum et al., 1986; McBride et al., 1991; Cascino et al., 1995; Schwartz et al., 1997; Hamer et al., 2002; Burneo et al., 2006).

Studies which included only patients with confirmed TLE due to HS reported contradictory findings regarding the possible association of spikes outside the area of the planned resection and surgical outcome in pre-resection ECoG (Schwartz et al., 1997; Chen et al., 2006). Both studies similarly did not find post-resection ECoG to be helpful. In patients with lesions, such as tumours invading the mesial structures, there is evidence suggesting that the persistence of spikes beyond the lateral margins of the resection does not impact on the final outcome (Tran et al., 1995). Therefore, in many epilepsy surgery centres no ECoG is used in cases with MTLE.

■ Conclusions

The great value of scalp recorded IEDs in lateralizing and localizing temporal epileptogenesis and predicting postoperative outcome in MTLE has been increasingly recognized in recent years, in spite of scalp EEG failing to detect most of the epileptiform activity recorded by intracranial electrodes. In the vast majority of patients with MTLE, interictal epileptiform activity is highly restricted to anterior temporal electrodes including sphenoidal electrodes. Bilateral IEDs can be generated by unilateral TLE but decrease the chance of postoperative seizure freedom. In general, the absence of IEDs in the six-month or one-year postoperative scalp EEG monitoring period is associated with good postoperative outcome.

Non-invasive EEG remains also extremely useful for the recording of seizures in MTLE. However, ictal recordings cannot precisely delineate the seizure onset zone and have a lower diagnostic yield compared to IEDs.

The need for invasive electrodes in patients with MTLE has declined over the last decades. Appropriate invasive electrodes (depth electrodes, subdural electrodes or a combination of depth and subdural electrodes) should be used in those cases in which the non-invasive evaluation cannot define the precise localization and extent of the epileptogenic zone. Electrocorticography and FO electrodes do not appear to be contributory in most cases of MTLE.

References

- Adachi N, Alarcon G, Binnie CD, Elwes RD, Polkey CE, Reynolds EH. Predictive value of interictal epileptiform discharges during non-REM sleep on scalp EEG recordings for the lateralization of epileptogenesis. *Epilepsia* 1998; 39: 628-32.
- Alarcon G, Kissani N, Dad M, Elwes RD, Ekanayake J, Hennessy MJ, *et al.* Lateralizing and localizing values of ictal onset recorded on the scalp: evidence from simultaneous recordings with intracranial foramen ovale electrodes. *Epilepsia* 2001; 42: 1426-37.
- Aronica E, Leenstra S, van Veelen CW, van Rijen PC, Hulsebos TJ, Tersmette AC, *et al.* Glioneuronal tumors and medically intractable epilepsy: a clinical study with long-term follow-up of seizure outcome after surgery. *Epilepsy Res* 2001; 43: 179-91.
- Arzimanoglou A, Kahane P. The ictal onset zone: general principles, pitfalls and caveats. In: Lüder HO, ed. *Textbook of Epilepsy Surgery*. London: Informa Healthcare, 2008, pp. 597-602.
- Assaf BA, Ebersole JS. Visual and quantitative ictal EEG predictors of outcome after temporal lobectomy. *Epilepsia* 1999; 40: 52-61.
- Awad IA, Nayel MH, Lüders H. Second operation after the failure of previous resection for epilepsy. *Neurosurgery* 1991a; 28: 510-8.
- Awad IA, Rosenfeld J, Ahl J, Hahn JF, Lüders H. Intractable epilepsy and structural lesions of the brain: mapping, resection strategies, and seizure outcome. *Epilepsia* 1991b; 32: 179-86.
- Aykut-Bingol C, Bronen RA, Kim JH, Spencer DD, Spencer SS. Surgical outcome in occipital lobe epilepsy: implications for pathophysiology. *Ann Neurol* 1998; 44: 60-9.
- Barba C, Barbati G, Minotti L, Hoffmann D, Kahane P. Ictal clinical and scalp-EEG findings differentiating temporal lobe epilepsies from temporal "plus" epilepsies. *Brain* 2007; 130: 1957-67.
- Barkley GL, Baumgartner C. MEG and EEG in epilepsy. *J Clin Neurophysiol* 2003; 20: 163-78.
- Barry E, Sussman NM, O'Connor MJ, Harner RN. Presurgical electroencephalographic patterns and outcome from anterior temporal lobectomy. *Arch Neurol* 1992; 49: 21-7.
- Bartolomei F, Khalil M, Wendling F, Sontheimer A, Regis J, Ranjeva JP, *et al.* Entorhinal cortex involvement in human mesial temporal lobe epilepsy: an electrophysiologic and volumetric study. *Epilepsia* 2005; 46: 677-87.
- Bartolomei F, Wendling F, Vignal JP, Kochen S, Bellanger JJ, Badier JM, *et al.* Seizures of temporal lobe epilepsy: identification of subtypes by coherence analysis using stereo-electro-encephalography. *Clin Neurophysiol* 1999; 110: 1741-54.
- Baumgartner C, Lindinger G, Ebner A, Aull S, Serles W, Olbrich A, *et al.* Propagation of interictal epileptic activity in temporal lobe epilepsy. *Neurology* 1995; 45: 118-22.
- Bengzon AR, Rasmussen T, Gloor P, Dussault J, Stephens M. Prognostic factors in the surgical treatment of temporal lobe epileptics. *Neurology* 1968; 18: 717-31.
- Binnie CD, Elwes RD, Polkey CE, Volans A. Utility of stereoelectroencephalography in preoperative assessment of temporal lobe epilepsy. *J Neurol Neurosurg Psychiatry* 1994; 57: 58-65.
- Binnie CD, Stefan H. Modern electroencephalography: its role in epilepsy management. *Clin Neurophysiol* 1999; 110: 1671-97.
- Blume WT. Current trends in electroencephalography. *Curr Opin Neurol* 2001; 14: 193-7.
- Blume WT, Borghesi JL, Lemieux JF. Interictal indices of temporal seizure origin. *Ann Neurol* 1993; 34: 703-9.
- Blume WT, Holloway GM, Wiebe S. Temporal epileptogenesis: localizing value of scalp and subdural interictal and ictal EEG data. *Epilepsia* 2001; 42: 508-14.
- Bösebeck F, Schulz R, May T, Ebner A. Lateralizing semiology predicts the seizure outcome after epilepsy surgery in the posterior cortex. *Brain* 2002; 125: 2320-31.
- Buechler RD, Rodriguez AJ, Lahr BD, So EL. Ictal scalp EEG recording during sleep and wakefulness: diagnostic implications for seizure localization and lateralization. *Epilepsia* 2008; 49: 340-2.

- Burneo JG, Steven DA, McLachlan RS, Parrent AG. Morbidity associated with the use of intracranial electrodes for epilepsy surgery. Can J Neurol Sci 2006; 33: 223-7.
- Caboclo LO, Garzon E, Oliveira PA, Carrete H, Jr., Centeno RS, Bianchin MM, et al. Correlation between temporal pole MRI abnormalities and surface ictal EEG patterns in patients with unilateral mesial temporal lobe epilepsy. Seizure 2007; 16: 8-16.
- Cambier DM, Cascino GD, So EL, Marsh WR. Video-EEG monitoring in patients with hippocampal atrophy. Acta Neurol Scand 2001; 103: 231-7.
- Carreno M, Lüders HO. General principles of presurgical evaluation. In: Lüders HO, Comair YG (eds). Epilepsy Surgery. Philadelphia: Lippincott Williams & Wilkins, 2001, pp. 185-99.
- Carter DA, Lassiter AT, Brown JA. Cost-efficient localization of seizures of mesiotemporal onset with foramen-ovale electrodes. Neurol Res 1998; 20: 153-60.
- Cascino GD, Kelly PJ, Sharbrough FW, Hulihan JF, Hirschorn KA, Trenery MR. Long-term follow-up of stereotactic lesionectomy in partial epilepsy: predictive factors and electroencephalographic results. Epilepsia 1992; 33: 639-44.
- Cascino GD, Trenery MR, Jack CR, Jr., Dodick D, Sharbrough FW, So EL, et al. Electrocorticography and temporal lobe epilepsy: relationship to quantitative MRI and operative outcome. Epilepsia 1995; 36: 692-6.
- Cascino GD, Trenery MR, So EL, Sharbrough FW, Shin C, Lagerlund TD, et al. Routine EEG and temporal lobe epilepsy: relation to long-term EEG monitoring, quantitative MRI, and operative outcome. Epilepsia 1996; 37: 651-6.
- Cendes F, Li LM, Watson C, Andermann F, Dubeau F, Arnold DL. Is ictal recording mandatory in temporal lobe epilepsy? Not when the interictal electroencephalogram and hippocampal atrophy coincide. Arch Neurol 2000; 57: 497-500.
- Chabardès S, Kahane P, Minotti L, Tassi L, Grand S, Hoffmann D, Benabid AL. The temporopolar cortex plays a pivotal role in temporal lobe seizures. Brain 2005; 128: 1818-31.
- Chee MW, Morris HH, III, Antar MA, Van Ness PC, Dinner DS, Rehm P, Salanova V. Presurgical evaluation of temporal lobe epilepsy using interictal temporal spikes and positron emission tomography. Arch Neurol 1993; 50: 45-8.
- Chen X, Sure U, Haag A, Knake S, Fritsch B, Muller HH, et al. Predictive value of electrocorticography in epilepsy patients with unilateral hippocampal sclerosis undergoing selective amygdalohippocampectomy. Neurosurg Rev 2006; 29: 108-13.
- Chung MY, Walczak TS, Lewis DV, Dawson DV, Radtke R. Temporal lobectomy and independent bitemporal interictal activity: what degree of lateralization is sufficient? Epilepsia 1991; 32: 195-201.
- Cohen-Gadol AA, Spencer DD. Use of an anteromedial subdural strip electrode in the evaluation of medial temporal lobe epilepsy. Technical note. J Neurosurg 2003; 99: 921-3.
- Cooper R, Winter AL, Crow HJ. Comparison fo subcortical, cortical and scalp activity using chronically indwelling electrodes in man. Electroencephalogr Clin Neurophysiol 1965; 18: 217-28.
- Di Gennaro G, Quarato PP, Onorati P, Colazza GB, Mari F, Grammaldo LG, et al. Localizing significance of temporal intermittent rhythmic delta activity (TIRDA) in drug-resistant focal epilepsy. Clin Neurophysiol 2003; 114: 70-8.
- Di Gennaro G, Quarato PP, Sebastiano F, Esposito V, Onorati P, Mascia A, et al. Postoperative EEG and seizure outcome in temporal lobe epilepsy surgery. Clin Neurophysiol 2004; 115: 1212-9.
- Diehl B, Lüders HO. Temporal lobe epilepsy: when are invasive recordings needed? Epilepsia 2000; 41 (Suppl 3): S61-S74.
- Dodrill CB, Wilkus RJ, Ojemann GA, Ward AA, Wyler AR, van Belle G, Tamas L. Multidisciplinary prediction of seizure relief from cortical resection surgery. Ann Neurol 1986; 20: 2-12.
- Ebersole JS, Pacia SV. Localization of temporal lobe foci by ictal EEG patterns. Epilepsia 1996; 37: 386-99.

- Ebersole JS, Wade PB. Spike voltage topography identifies two types of frontotemporal epileptic foci. *Neurology* 1991; 41: 1425-33.
- Ebner A, Hoppe M. Noninvasive electroencephalography and mesial temporal sclerosis. *J Clin Neurophysiol* 1995; 12: 23-31.
- Eisenschenk S, Gilmore RL, Cibula JE, Roper SN. Lateralization of temporal lobe foci: depth *versus* subdural electrodes. *Clin Neurophysiol* 2001; 112: 836-844.
- Ergene E, Shih JJ, Blum DE, So NK. Frequency of bitemporal independent interictal epileptiform discharges in temporal lobe epilepsy. *Epilepsia* 2000; 41: 213-8.
- Fernandez Torre JL, Alarcon G, Binnie CD, Polkey CE. Comparison of sphenoidal, foramen ovale and anterior temporal placements for detecting interictal epileptiform discharges in presurgical assessment for temporal lobe epilepsy. *Clin Neurophysiol* 1999a; 110: 895-904.
- Fernandez Torre JL, Alarcon G, Binnie CD, Seoane JJ, Juler J, Guy CN, Polkey CE. Generation of scalp discharges in temporal lobe epilepsy as suggested by intraoperative electrocorticographic recordings. *J Neurol Neurosurg Psychiatry* 1999b; 67: 51-8.
- Ficker DM, So EL, Mosewich RK, Radhakrishnan K, Cascino GD, Sharbrough FW. Improvement and deterioration of seizure control during the postsurgical course of epilepsy surgery patients. *Epilepsia* 1999; 40: 62-7.
- Fiol ME, Gates JR, Torres F, Maxwell RE. The prognostic value of residual spikes in the postexcision electrocorticogram after temporal lobectomy. *Neurology* 1991; 41: 512-6.
- Foldvary N. Focal epilepsy and surgical evaluation. In: Levin KH, Lüders HO (eds). *Comprehensive Clinical Neurphysiology*. Philadelphia: Saunders Company, 2000, pp. 481-96.
- Foldvary N, Klem G, Hammel J, Bingaman W, Najm I, Lüders H. The localizing value of ictal EEG in focal epilepsy. *Neurology* 2001; 57: 2022-8.
- Gambardella A, Gotman J, Cendes F, Andermann F. Focal intermittent delta activity in patients with mesiotemporal atrophy: a reliable marker of the epileptogenic focus. *Epilepsia* 1995; 36: 122-9.
- Gambardella A, Palmini A, Andermann F, Dubeau F, Da Costa JC, Quesney LF, *et al*. Usefulness of focal rhythmic discharges on scalp EEG of patients with focal cortical dysplasia and intractable epilepsy. *Electroencephalogr Clin Neurophysiol* 1996; 98: 243-9.
- Geyer JD, Bilir E, Faught RE, Kuzniecky R, Gilliam F. Significance of interictal temporal lobe delta activity for localization of the primary epileptogenic region. *Neurology* 1999; 52: 202-5.
- Gil-Nagel A, Risinger MW. Ictal semiology in hippocampal *versus* extrahippocampal temporal lobe epilepsy. *Brain* 1997; 120 (Pt 1): 183-92.
- Gilliam F, Bowling S, Bilir E, Thomas J, Faught E, Morawetz R, *et al*. Association of combined MRI, interictal EEG, and ictal EEG results with outcome and pathology after temporal lobectomy. *Epilepsia* 1997; 38: 1315-20.
- Gloor P. Preoperative electroencephalographic investigation in temporal lobe epilepsy: extracranial and intracranial recordings. *Can J Neurol Sci* 1991; 18: 554-8.
- Godoy J, Lüders H, Dinner DS, Morris HH, Wyllie E, Murphy D. Significance of sharp waves in routine EEGs after epilepsy surgery. *Epilepsia* 1992; 33: 285-8.
- Gotman J, Koffler DJ. Interictal spiking increases after seizures but does not after decrease in medication. *Electroencephalogr Clin Neurophysiol* 1989; 72: 7-15.
- Hamer HM, Morris HH, Mascha EJ, Karafa MT, Bingaman WE, Bej MD, *et al*. Complications of invasive video-EEG monitoring with subdural grid electrodes. *Neurology* 2002; 58: 97-103.
- Hamer HM, Najm I, Mohamed A, Wyllie E. Interictal epileptiform discharges in temporal lobe epilepsy due to hippocampal sclerosis *versus* medial temporal lobe tumors. *Epilepsia* 1999; 40: 1261-8.
- Hildebrandt M, Schulz R, Hoppe M, May T, Ebner A. Postoperative routine EEG correlates with long-term seizure outcome after epilepsy surgery. *Seizure* 2005; 14: 446-51.

- Holmes MD, Dodrill CB, Ojemann GA, Wilensky AJ, Ojemann LM. Outcome following surgery in patients with bitemporal interictal epileptiform patterns. *Neurology* 1997; 48: 1037-40.
- Holmes MD, Dodrill CB, Wilensky AJ, Ojemann LM, Ojemann GA. Unilateral focal preponderance of interictal epileptiform discharges as a predictor of seizure origin. *Arch Neurol* 1996; 53: 228-32.
- Hufnagel A, Elger CE, Pels H, Zentner J, Wolf HK, Schramm J, Wiestler OD. Prognostic significance of ictal and interictal epileptiform activity in temporal lobe epilepsy. *Epilepsia* 1994; 35: 1146-53.
- Hufnagel A, Poersch M, Elger CE, Zentner J, Wolf HK, Schramm J. The clinical and prognostic relevance of the postictal slow focus in the electrocorticogram. *Electroencephalogr Clin Neurophysiol* 1995; 94: 12-8.
- Jan MM, Sadler M, Rahey SR. Lateralized postictal EEG delta predicts the side of seizure surgery in temporal lobe epilepsy. *Epilepsia* 2001; 42: 402-5.
- Janszky J, Pannek HW, Janszky I, Schulz R, Behne F, Hoppe M, Ebner A. Failed surgery for temporal lobe epilepsy: predictors of long-term seizure-free course. *Epilepsy Res* 2005; 64: 35-44.
- Janszky J, Rasonyi G, Clemens Z, Schulz R, Hoppe M, Barsi P, et al. Clinical differences in patients with unilateral hippocampal sclerosis and unitemporal or bitemporal epileptiform discharges. *Seizure* 2003a; 12: 550-4.
- Janszky J, Schulz R, Hoppe M, Ebner A. Spikes on the postoperative EEG are related to preoperative spike frequency and postoperative seizures. *Epilepsy Res* 2003b; 57: 153-8.
- Kahane P, Francoine S. Stereoelectroencephalography. In: Lüders HO (ed). *Textbook of Epilepsy Surgery* London: Informa Healthcare, 2008, pp. 649-58.
- Kahane P, Huot JC, Hoffmann D. Perisylvian cortex involvement in seizures affecting the temporal lobe. In: Avanzini G, Beaumanoir A, Miral L, (eds). *Limbic Seizures in Children.* London: John Libbey, 2001, pp. 115-27.
- Kaibara M, Blume WT. The postictal electroencephalogram. *Electroencephalogr Clin Neurophysiol* 1988; 70: 99-104.
- Kameyama S, Fukuda M, Tomikawa M, Morota N, Oishi M, Wachi M, et al. Surgical strategy and outcomes for epileptic patients with focal cortical dysplasia or dysembryoplastic neuroepithelial tumor. *Epilepsia* 2001; 42 (Suppl 6): 37-41.
- Kanner AM, Jones JC. When do sphenoidal electrodes yield additional data to that obtained with antero-temporal electrodes? *Electroencephalogr Clin Neurophysiol* 1997; 102: 12-9.
- Kanner AM, Morris HH, Lüders H, Dinner DS, Van Ness P, Wyllie E. Usefulness of unilateral interictal sharp waves of temporal lobe origin in prolonged video-EEG monitoring studies. *Epilepsia* 1993; 34: 884-9.
- Kanner AM, Ramirez L, Jones JC. The utility of placing sphenoidal electrodes under the foramen ovale with fluoroscopic guidance. *J Clin Neurophysiol* 1995; 12: 72-81.
- Kelemen A, Barsi P, Eross L, Vajda J, Czirjak S, Borbely C, et al. Long-term outcome after temporal lobe surgery-prediction of late worsening of seizure control. *Seizure* 2006; 15: 49-55.
- Keogan M, McMackin D, Peng S, Phillips J, Burke T, Murphy S, et al. Temporal neocorticectomy in management of intractable epilepsy: long-term outcome and predictive factors. *Epilepsia* 1992; 33: 852-61.
- King D, Bronen RA, Spencer DD, Spencer SS. Topographic distribution of seizure onset and hippocampal atrophy: relationship between MRI and depth EEG. *Electroencephalogr Clin Neurophysiol* 1997; 103: 692-7.
- King MA, Newton MR, Jackson GD, Fitt GJ, Mitchell LA, Silvapulle MJ, Berkovic SF. Epileptology of the first-seizure presentation: a clinical, electroencephalographic, and magnetic resonance imaging study of 300 consecutive patients. *Lancet* 1998; 352: 1007-11.

- Kipervasser S, Nagar S, Chistik V, Kramer U, Fried I, Neufeld MY. The prognostic significance of interictal epileptiform activity in postoperative EEGs of patients with mesial temporal lobe epilepsy. *Clin EEG Neurosci* 2007; 38: 137-42.
- Kirkpatrick PJ, Honavar M, Janota I, Polkey CE. Control of temporal lobe epilepsy following en bloc resection of low-grade tumors. *J Neurosurg* 1993; 78: 19-25.
- Kissani N, Alarcon G, Dad M, Binnie CD, Polkey CE. Sensitivity of recordings at sphenoidal electrode site for detecting seizure onset: evidence from scalp, superficial and deep foramen ovale recordings. *Clin Neurophysiol* 2001; 112: 232-40.
- Klein KM, Knake S, Hamer HM, Ziegler A, Oertel WH, Rosenow F. Sleep but not hyperventilation increases the sensitivity of the EEG in patients with temporal lobe epilepsy. *Epilepsy Res* 2003; 56: 43-9.
- Krendl R, Lurger S, Baumgartner C. Absolute spike frequency predicts surgical outcome in TLE with unilateral hippocampal atrophy. *Neurology* 2008; 71: 413-8.
- Lee SA, Yim SB, Lim YM, Kang JK, Lee JK. Factors predicting seizure outcome of anterior temporal lobectomy for patients with mesial temporal sclerosis. *Seizure* 2006; 15: 397-404.
- Lieb JP, Engel J, Jr., Babb TL. Interhemispheric propagation time of human hippocampal seizures. I. Relationship to surgical outcome. *Epilepsia* 1986; 27: 286-93.
- Lüders H, Hahn J, Lesser RP, Dinner DS, Morris HH 3rd, Wyllie E, et al. Basal temporal subdural electrodes in the evaluation of patients with intractable epilepsy. *Epilepsia* 1989; 30: 131-42.
- Lüders H, Murphy D, Awad I, Wyllie E, Dinner DS, Morris HH 3rd, Rothner AD. Quantitative analysis of seizure frequency 1 week and 6, 12, and 24 months after surgery of epilepsy. *Epilepsia* 1994; 35: 1174-8.
- Maillard L, Vignal JP, Gavaret M, Guye M, Biraben A, McGonigal A, et al. Semiologic and electrophysiologic correlations in temporal lobe seizure subtypes. *Epilepsia* 2004; 45: 1590-9.
- Malow BA, Selwa LM, Ross D, Aldrich MS. Lateralizing value of interictal spikes on overnight sleep-EEG studies in temporal lobe epilepsy. *Epilepsia* 1999; 40: 1587-92.
- Margerison JH, Corsellis JA. Epilepsy and the temporal lobes. A clinical, electroencephalographic and neuropathological study of the brain in epilepsy, with particular reference to the temporal lobes. *Brain* 1966; 89: 499-530.
- Marks DA, Katz A, Booke J, Spencer DD, Spencer SS. Comparison and correlation of surface and sphenoidal electrodes with simultaneous intracranial recording: an interictal study. *Electroencephalogr Clin Neurophysiol* 1992; 82: 23-9.
- Marsan CA, Zivin LS. Factors related to the occurrence of typical paroxysmal abnormalities in the EEG records of epileptic patients. *Epilepsia* 1970; 11: 361-81.
- McBride MC, Binnie CD, Janota I, Polkey CE. Predictive value of intraoperative electrocorticograms in resective epilepsy surgery. *Ann Neurol* 1991; 30: 526-32.
- McIntosh AM, Wilson SJ, Berkovic SF. Seizure outcome after temporal lobectomy: current research practice and findings. *Epilepsia* 2001; 42: 1288-1307.
- Mintzer S, Cendes F, Soss J, Andermann F, Engel J, Jr., Dubeau F, et al. Unilateral hippocampal sclerosis with contralateral temporal scalp ictal onset. *Epilepsia* 2004; 45: 792-802.
- Mintzer S, Nasreddine W, Passaro E, Beydoun A. Predictive value of early EEG after epilepsy surgery. *J Clin Neurophysiol* 2005; 22: 410-4.
- Mintzer S, Nicholl JS, Stern JM, Engel J. Relative utility of sphenoidal and temporal surface electrodes for localization of ictal onset in temporal lobe epilepsy. *Clin Neurophysiol* 2002; 113: 911-6.
- Mohamed A, Wyllie E, Ruggieri P, Kotagal P, Babb T, Hilbig A, et al. Temporal lobe epilepsy due to hippocampal sclerosis in pediatric candidates for epilepsy surgery. *Neurology* 2001; 56: 1643-9.

- Morris HH 3rd, Kanner A, Lüders H, Murphy D, Dinner DS, Wyllie E, Kotagal P. Can sharp waves localized at the sphenoidal electrode accurately identify a mesiotemporal epileptogenic focus? *Epilepsia* 1989; 30: 532-9.
- Morris HH 3rd, Lüders H, Lesser RP, Dinner DS, Klem GH. The value of closely spaced scalp electrodes in the localization of epileptiform foci: a study of 26 patients with complex partial seizures. *Electroencephalogr Clin Neurophysiol* 1986; 63: 107-11.
- Morris HH, Matkovic Z, Estes ML, Prayson RA, Comair YG, Turnbull J, et al. Ganglioglioma and intractable epilepsy: clinical and neurophysiologic features and predictors of outcome after surgery. *Epilepsia* 1998; 39: 307-13.
- Munari C, Hoffmann D, Francione S, Kahane P, Tassi L, Lo RG, Benabid AL. Stereo-electroencephalography methodology: advantages and limits. *Acta Neurol Scand* 1994a; 152 (Suppl): 56-67.
- Munari C, Rosler J, Jr., Musolino A, Betti OO, Daumas-Duport C, Missir O, Chodkiewiez JP. Differential diagnosis between tumoural and non-tumoural intracranial lesions in children: a stereotactic approach. *Acta Neurochir Suppl (Wien)* 1989; 46: 75-8.
- Munari C, Tassi L, Kahane P, Francione S, di Leo M, Quarato PP. Analysis of clinical symptomatology during stereo-EEG recorded mesiotemporal seizures. In: Wolf P (ed). *Epileptic Seizures and Syndromes*. London: John Libbey, 1994b, pp. 335-57.
- Normand MM, Wszolek ZK, Klass DW. Temporal intermittent rhythmic delta activity in electroencephalograms. *J Clin Neurophysiol* 1995; 12: 280-284.
- Pacia SV, Jung WJ, Devinsky O. Localization of mesial temporal lobe seizures with sphenoidal electrodes. *J Clin Neurophysiol* 1998; 15: 256-61.
- Palmini A, Gambardella A, Andermann F, Dubeau F, Da Costa JC, Olivier A, et al. Intrinsic epileptogenicity of human dysplastic cortex as suggested by corticography and surgical results. *Ann Neurol* 1995; 37: 476-487.
- Pataraia E, Lurger S, Serles W, Lindinger G, Aull S, Leutmezer F, Bacher J, et al. Ictal scalp EEG in unilateral mesial temporal lobe epilepsy. *Epilepsia* 1998; 39: 608-14.
- Patrick S, Berg A, Spencer SS. EEG and seizure outcome after epilepsy surgery. *Epilepsia* 1995; 36: 236-40.
- Provini F, Plazzi G, Tinuper P, Vandi S, Lugaresi E, Montagna P. Nocturnal frontal lobe epilepsy. A clinical and polygraphic overview of 100 consecutive cases. *Brain* 1999; 122 (Pt 6): 1017-31.
- Radhakrishnan K, So EL, Silbert PL, Jack CR, Jr., Cascino GD, Sharbrough FW, O'Brien PC. Predictors of outcome of anterior temporal lobectomy for intractable epilepsy: a multivariate study. *Neurology* 1998; 51: 465-71.
- Reiher J, Beaudry M, Leduc CP. Temporal intermittent rhythmic delta activity (TIRDA) in the diagnosis of complex partial epilepsy: sensitivity, specificity and predictive value. *Can J Neurol Sci* 1989; 16: 398-401.
- Risinger MW, Engel J, Jr., Van Ness PC, Henry TR, Crandall PH. Ictal localization of temporal lobe seizures with scalp/sphenoidal recordings. *Neurology* 1989; 39: 1288-93.
- Rosenbaum TJ, Laxer KD, Vessely M, Smith WB. Subdural electrodes for seizure focus localization. *Neurosurgery* 1986; 19: 73-81.
- Rosenow F, Lüders HO, Dinner DS, Prayson RA, Mascha E, Wolgamuth BR, et al. Histopathological correlates of epileptogenicity as expressed by electrocorticographic spiking and seizure frequency. *Epilepsia* 1998; 39: 850-6.
- Ryvlin P, Kahane P. The hidden causes of surgery-resistant temporal lobe epilepsy: extratemporal or temporal plus? *Curr Opin Neurol* 2005; 18: 125-7.
- Salanova V, Andermann F, Olivier A, Rasmussen T, Quesney LF. Occipital lobe epilepsy: electroclinical manifestations, electrocorticography, cortical stimulation and outcome in 42 patients treated between 1930 and 1991. Surgery of occipital lobe epilepsy. *Brain* 1992; 115 (Pt 6): 1655-80.

- Salanova V, Andermann F, Rasmussen T, Olivier A, Quesney L. The running down phenomenon in temporal lobe epilepsy. *Brain* 1996; 119 (Pt 3): 989-96.
- Salanova V, Markand ON, Worth R. Clinical characteristics and predictive factors in 98 patients with complex partial seizures treated with temporal resection. *Arch Neurol* 1994; 51: 1008-13.
- Sammaritano M, de Lotbiniere A, Andermann F, Olivier A, Gloor P, Quesney LF. False lateralization by surface EEG of seizure onset in patients with temporal lobe epilepsy and gross focal cerebral lesions. *Ann Neurol* 1987; 21: 361-9.
- Schuler P, Neubauer U, Schulemann H, Stefan H. Brain-stem lesions in the course of a presurgical re-evaluation by foramen-ovale electrodes in temporal lobe epilepsy. *Electroencephalogr Clin Neurophysiol* 1993; 86: 301-2.
- Schulz R, Lüders HO, Hoppe M, Tuxhorn I, May T, Ebner A. Interictal EEG and ictal scalp EEG propagation are highly predictive of surgical outcome in mesial temporal lobe epilepsy. *Epilepsia* 2000; 41: 564-70.
- Schwartz TH, Bazil CW, Walczak TS, Chan S, Pedley TA, Goodman RR. The predictive value of intraoperative electrocorticography in resections for limbic epilepsy associated with mesial temporal sclerosis. *Neurosurgery* 1997; 40: 302-9.
- Serles W, Pataraia E, Bacher J, Olbrich A, Aull S, Lehrner J, et al. Clinical seizure lateralization in mesial temporal lobe epilepsy: differences between patients with unitemporal and bitemporal interictal spikes. *Neurology* 1998; 50: 742-7.
- Shih YH, Yiu CH, Su MS, Yen DJ, Ho DM, Liu RS, Chen CC. Temporal lobectomy in adults with intractable epilepsy. *J Formos Med Assoc* 1994; 93: 307-13.
- So N, Olivier A, Andermann F, Gloor P, Quesney LF. Results of surgical treatment in patients with bitemporal epileptiform abnormalities. *Ann Neurol* 1989; 25: 432-9.
- So NK. Interictal electroencephalography in temporal lobe epilepsy. In: Lüders HO, Comair YG (eds). *Epilepsy Surgery*. Philadelphia: Lippincott Williams & Wilkins, 2001, pp. 393-402.
- Spanedda F, Cendes F, Gotman J. Relations between EEG seizure morphology, interhemispheric spread, and mesial temporal atrophy in bitemporal epilepsy. *Epilepsia* 1997; 38: 1300-14.
- Spencer DD, Spencer SS, Mattson RH, Williamson PD. Intracerebral masses in patients with intractable partial epilepsy. *Neurology* 1984; 34: 432-6.
- Spencer SS, Guimaraes P, Katz A, Kim J, Spencer D. Morphological patterns of seizures recorded intracranially. *Epilepsia* 1992; 33: 537-45.
- Sperling MR. Clinical challenges in invasive monitoring in epilepsy surgery. *Epilepsia* 1997; 38 (Suppl 4): S6-12.
- Stefan H, Hopfengartner R, Kreiselmeyer G, Weigel D, Rampp S, Kerling F, et al. Interictal triple ECoG characteristics of temporal lobe epilepsies: An intraoperative ECoG analysis correlated with surgical outcome. *Clin Neurophysiol* 2008; 119: 642-52.
- Steinhoff BJ, So NK, Lim S, Lüders HO. Ictal scalp EEG in temporal lobe epilepsy with unitemporal *versus* bitemporal interictal epileptiform discharges. *Neurology* 1995; 45: 889-96.
- Steude U, Stodieck S, Schmiedek P. Multiple contact foramen ovale electrode in the presurgical evaluation of epileptic patients for selective amygdala-hippocampectomy. *Acta Neurochir (Wien)* 1993; 58 (Suppl): 193-4.
- Sundaram M, Hogan T, Hiscock M, Pillay N. Factors affecting interictal spike discharges in adults with epilepsy. *Electroencephalogr Clin Neurophysiol* 1990; 75: 358-60.
- Tao JX, Ray A, Hawes-Ebersole S, Ebersole JS. Intracranial EEG substrates of scalp EEG interictal spikes. *Epilepsia* 2005; 46: 669-76.
- Tran TA, Spencer SS, Marks D, Javidan M, Pacia S, Spencer DD. Significance of spikes recorded on electrocorticography in nonlesional medial temporal lobe epilepsy. *Ann Neurol* 1995; 38: 763-70.

- Tuunainen A, Nousiainen U, Mervaala E, Pilke A, Vapalahti M, Leinonen E, et al. Postoperative EEG and electrocorticography: relation to clinical outcome in patients with temporal lobe surgery. *Epilepsia* 1994; 35: 1165-73.
- Van Buren JM. Complications of surgical procedures in the diagnosis and treatment of epilepsy. In: Engel J (ed). *Surgical Treatment of the Epilepsies*. New York: Raven Press, 1987, pp. 465-75.
- Velasco AL, Wilson CL, Babb TL, Engel J, Jr. Functional and anatomic correlates of two frequently observed temporal lobe seizure-onset patterns. *Neural Plast* 2000; 7: 49-63.
- Velasco TR, Sakamoto AC, Alexandre V, Jr., Walz R, Dalmagro CL, Bianchin MM, et al. Foramen ovale electrodes can identify a focal seizure onset when surface EEG fails in mesial temporal lobe epilepsy. *Epilepsia* 2006; 47: 1300-7.
- Vossler DG, Kraemer DL, Knowlton RC, Kjos BO, Rostad SW, Wyler AR, et al. Temporal ictal electroencephalographic frequency correlates with hippocampal atrophy and sclerosis. *Ann Neurol* 1998; 43: 756-62.
- Walczak TS, Radtke RA, Lewis DV. Accuracy and interobserver reliability of scalp ictal EEG. *Neurology* 1992; 42: 2279-85.
- Wennberg R, Arruda F, Quesney LF, Olivier A. Preeminence of extrahippocampal structures in the generation of mesial temporal seizures: evidence from human depth electrode recordings. *Epilepsia* 2002; 43: 716-26.
- Wennberg R, Quesney F, Olivier A, Rasmussen T. Electrocorticography and outcome in frontal lobe epilepsy. *Electroencephalogr Clin Neurophysiol* 1998; 106: 357-68.
- Wieser HG, Elger CE, Stodieck SR. The "foramen ovale electrode": a new recording method for the preoperative evaluation of patients suffering from mesio-basal temporal lobe epilepsy. *Electroencephalogr Clin Neurophysiol* 1985; 61: 314-22.
- Wieser HG, Siegel AM. Analysis of foramen ovale electrode-recorded seizures and correlation with outcome following amygdalohippocampectomy. *Epilepsia* 1991; 32: 838-50.
- Williamson PD, French JA, Thadani VM, Kim JH, Novelly RA, Spencer SS, et al. Characteristics of medial temporal lobe epilepsy: II. Interictal and ictal scalp electroencephalography, neuropsychological testing, neuroimaging, surgical results, and pathology. *Ann Neurol* 1993; 34: 781-7.
- Zijlmans M, Huiskamp GM, van Huffelen AC, Spetgens WP, Leijten FS. Detection of temporal lobe spikes: comparing nasopharyngeal, cheek and anterior temporal electrodes to simultaneous subdural recordings. *Clin Neurophysiol* 2008; 119: 1771-7.
- Zumsteg D, Friedman A, Wieser HG, Wennberg RA. Propagation of interictal discharges in temporal lobe epilepsy: correlation of spatiotemporal mapping with intracranial foramen ovale electrode recordings. *Clin Neurophysiol* 2006; 117: 2615-26.

Magnetoencephalograhpy findings in medial temporal lobe epilepsy

Hideaki Shiraishi

Department of Pediatrics, Hokkaido University School of Medicine, Japan

Magnetoencephalography (MEG) is a technique that arose from the superconductivity theory and is now applied to clinical investigations (Cohen *et al.*, 1968; Hämäläinen *et al.*, 1993). Studies of epileptic patients are a particularly useful application of MEG, because MEG provides better spatial and temporal resolution than electroencephalography (EEG).

Many reports have described the application of MEG for clinical investigations of epileptic patients (Knake *et al.*, 2004; Grondin *et al.*, 2006; Cappel *et al.*, 2006; Mäkelä *et al.*, 2006; Shibazaki *et al.*, 2007; Rampp *et al.*, 2007; Schwartz *et al.*, 2008). MEG currently plays an important role in the definition of the epileptogenic lesion in epileptic surgery candidates, especially those with neocortical epileptic lesions (Nakasato *et al.*, 1994; Sutherling *et al.*, 1987; Shiraishi *et al.*, 2001; Oishi *et al.*, 2006; Otsubo *et al.*, 2001; 2005). By comparison, MEG analysis is more difficult when used to investigate medial temporal lobe epilepsy (MTLE), because the medial temporal structure is hidden anatomically in the depth of the temporal lobe (Shigeto *et al.*, 2002; Pataraia *et al.*, 2005). For this reason, the MEG current is not always detected because of the inherently low signal-to-noise ratio. In general, MEG can detect magnetic activity to a depth of less than 2 cm (Shigeto *et al.*, 2002). In this chapter, we describe the application of MEG for the diagnosis of MTLE in patients using specific analysis paradigms.

■ MEG source analysis

The MEG data are digitally filtered with a pass band of 3 to 30 Hz for offline analysis. Segments containing abnormal paroxysms are selected manually. Individual spikes aligned on the basis of the peak latency are analyzed. The distribution of brain activity generating the spikes is determined using two source estimation approaches: the equivalent current dipole (ECD) model and dynamic statistical parametric mapping (dSPM). The ECD model is appropriate when the underlying brain activity is focal, *i.e.* restricted to a relatively small region of the brain. For non-focal brain activity, the distributed source models, including dSPM, are expected to be better suited than the ECD model for determining the distribution of brain activity generating the spikes.

Equivalent current dipoles

Equivalent current dipoles (ECDs) are calculated with the "xfit" software (Elekta-Neuromag Ltd.) using the single-dipole model. The conductivity geometry of the head is assumed to be spherically symmetrical. Dipoles are calculated for each time point measurement (every 2.5 ms) within a period of 100 ms at the vicinity of each MEG spike. All sensors are included in the analyses, with no selection of regions of interest. The initial location for the iterative fit of the ECD is chosen to be under the sensor with the largest signal. The ECD with the best goodness of fit (GOF) is selected as the representative ECD of that particular MEG spike. The GOF is a measure of how well the ECD model explains the measured signals. A dipole fit is accepted when the GOF is greater than 70%. To visualize anatomical locations, the ECDs are superimposed on the MRI from each patient.

Dynamic statistical parametric mapping

The dynamic statistical parametric mapping (dSPM) method (Dale et al., 2000) is based on a noise-normalized minimum L2-norm estimate. For dSPM analysis, we use an anatomically constrained, distributed source model, which assumes the sources are located in the cerebral cortex. The cortical surface is segmented from high-resolution MRI using the FreeSurfer software (Dale et al., 1999; Fischl et al., 1999) and subsampled to approximately 2,500 elements per hemisphere. The source model consists of current dipole vectors located at each element. The forward solution is calculated using a boundary element method (BEM) model.

The dSPM approach used to estimate the time course of activity at each cortical location is based on the generalised least-squares or weighted minimum-norm solution (Hämäläinen, 1994; Dale, 1993); in this case, the estimate is normalized for noise sensitivity, thus providing a statistical parametric map (Dale et al., 2000). The noise normalization reduces the variation in the point-spread function between locations (Liu et al., 2002). Simulations have suggested that the spatial resolution is 15 mm or better (Dale et al., 2000; Liu et al., 2002). Maps are calculated at 2.5-ms intervals. The significance of modulation at each site is calculated using an F-test (Dale et al., 2000; Dhond et al., 2001). These statistical maps differ from maps of estimated source strengths, since the estimated noise variance is not constant across different cortical locations. However, since the same noise covariance estimates are used at all time points for given cortical locations, source strength at a given location over time is directly proportional to the statistical maps. The current approach provides dynamic statistical parametric maps of cortical activity, similar to the statistical maps typically generated using fMRI or PET data, but with a millisecond temporal resolution.

Short-time Fourier transform analysis

Short-time Fourier transform (STFT) analysis is used to reveal the distributions of MEG polyspikes (Oppenheim et al., 1999). The MATLAB (MathWorks, Natick, MA, USA) program is used to execute the STFT for the MEG signals. Each signal is divided into small sequential frames, and fast Fourier transformation (FFT) is applied to each frame.

In the present study, the STFT was implemented using a 256-point window. The time of each window was 426.7 ms (*i.e.* 256 points × 1,000 ms/600 Hz). The window was shifted every four points, which corresponded to 6.7 ms (*i.e.* 1,000 ms/600 Hz × 4 points). FFT was applied to each window. This process was repeated for all selected signals. The time-frequency distributions are displayed as graphs.

Fourier transform is performed with frequencies in the ranges of 3-30 Hz, 30-50 Hz, and 50-100 Hz. A spectrum is considered to be aberrant when it is observed to be isolated from the background frequency spectrum in the graph. An aberrant frequency spectrum on the graph is superimposed onto the reconstructed 3D-MRI.

Electrocortigogram

An electrocorticogram (ECoG) study is performed during surgery. The ECoG data are collected using the Ceegraph system (Bio-Logic, Mundelein, IL, USA), with a sampling rate of 512 Hz. A 4 × 5 grid electrode array was used in the second case report. The recording is performed for at least one minute at each electrode location.

Case report 1

We report the case of a 17-year-old girl. Her epilepsy started when she was 11 years old with simple partial seizures described as cephalic sensation, and complex partial seizures described as motion arrest, oral automatism, and bilateral manual automatisms lasting for 2-3 minutes without dystonic posturing or secondary generalised tonic-clonic seizures (GTCs). Over time, her seizures had become more frequent and occurred more than once per week.

She had a selective amygdala-hippocampectomy at 15 years of age and has been seizure-free for three years (Engel class I).

EEG, MEG, MRI, SPECT, and PET findings are shown in *Figure 1*. Her spike sources were localized by ECDs at the pole and base of the left temporal lobe. The location and distribution of her ECDs were consistent with the typical location and distribution of the horizontal ECD described in MTLE (Stefan *et al.*, 2003). ECDs are not always located at the hippocampus, but may be located at other areas of the temporal lobe. It is not always possible to detect MEG activity because of the low signal-to-noise ratio.

Case report 2

We report the case of a nine-year-old girl. Her epilepsy started at one month of age with complex partial seizures with motion arrest and cyanosis. Her seizures evolved to daily simple partial seizures, described as ictal fear and cephalic sensations, and complex partial seizures with motion arrest and autonomic change (cyanotic face) for three to four minutes without dystonic posturing.

At the age of nine years she underwent resection of focal cortical dysplasia at the medial aspect of the left temporal lobe and the head of the hippocampus. She has now been seizure-free for one year and eight months. Initial EEG and MEG measurements showed no epileptiform discharges *(Figure 2A)*. Sequential EEG and MEG measurements demonstrated activity in the right occipital and left frontal areas, but not to the same level of activity recorded from the left temporal area, where the focal cortical dysplasia was located *(Figure 2B)*. Furthermore, EEG and MEG measurements showed intermittent, but prolonged rhythmic activity in the left frontal and temporal region *(Figure 2B)*. This rhythmic activity was no longer observed after her operation *(Figure 2C)*.

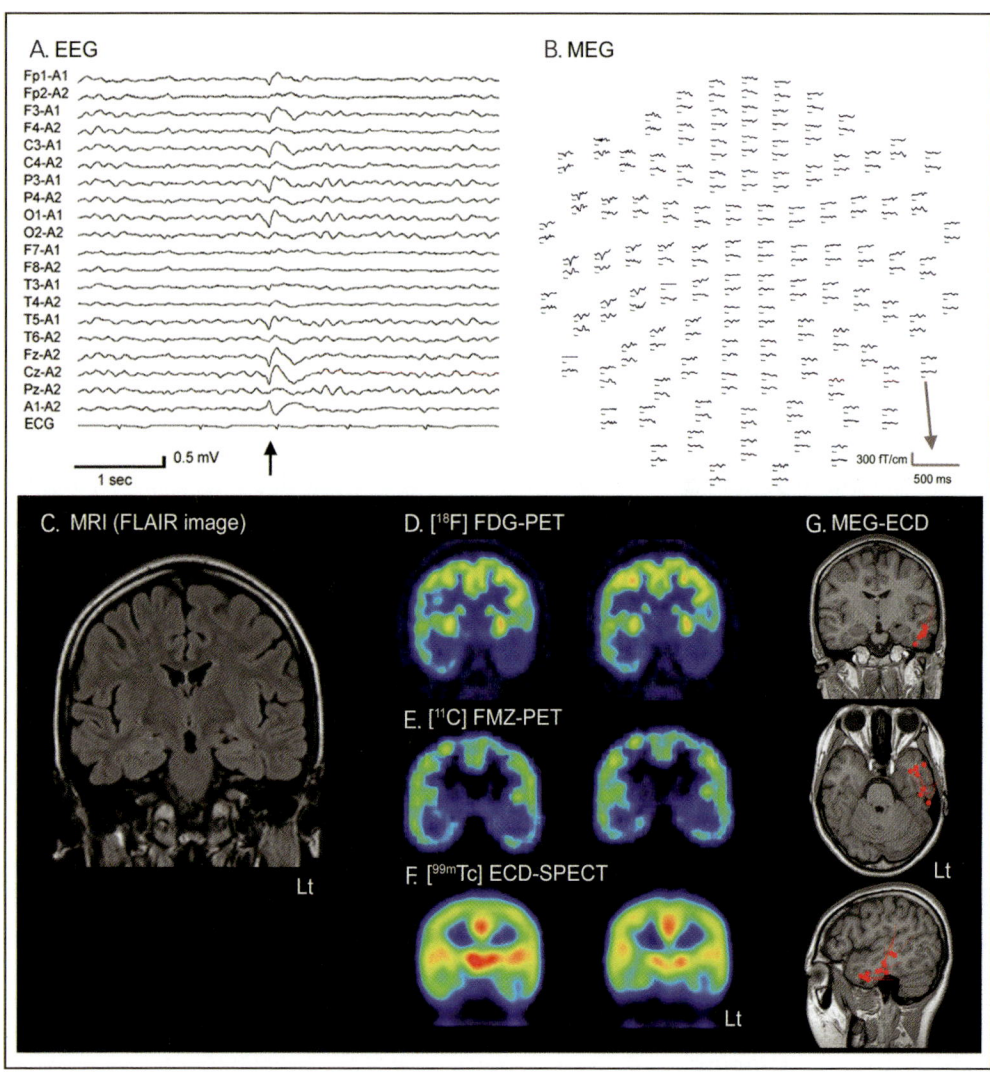

Figure 1. Case 1: EEG, MEG, MRI, PET and interictal SPECT.
A. EEG showing left hemispheric positive spikes which were reflected by the epileptic current at reference electrode A1. **B.** MEG showing spikes in the left temporal region. **C.** MRI showing atrophy and sclerosis of the left hippocampus of the patient. **D.** [^{18}F] Fluorodeoxyglucose (FDG) positron emission CT (PET) showing hypometabolism in the left medial temporal lobe. **E.** [^{11}C] Flumazenil (FMZ) PET showing low benzodiazepine receptor binding in the left medial temporal lobe. **F.** Interictal [^{99m}Tc] ethylcysteinate dimer (ECD) single photon emission CT (SPECT) showing low perfusion in left medial temporal structures. **G.** The location of MEG ECDs of epileptiform activity were located at the pole and base of the left temporal lobe in a horizontal direction.

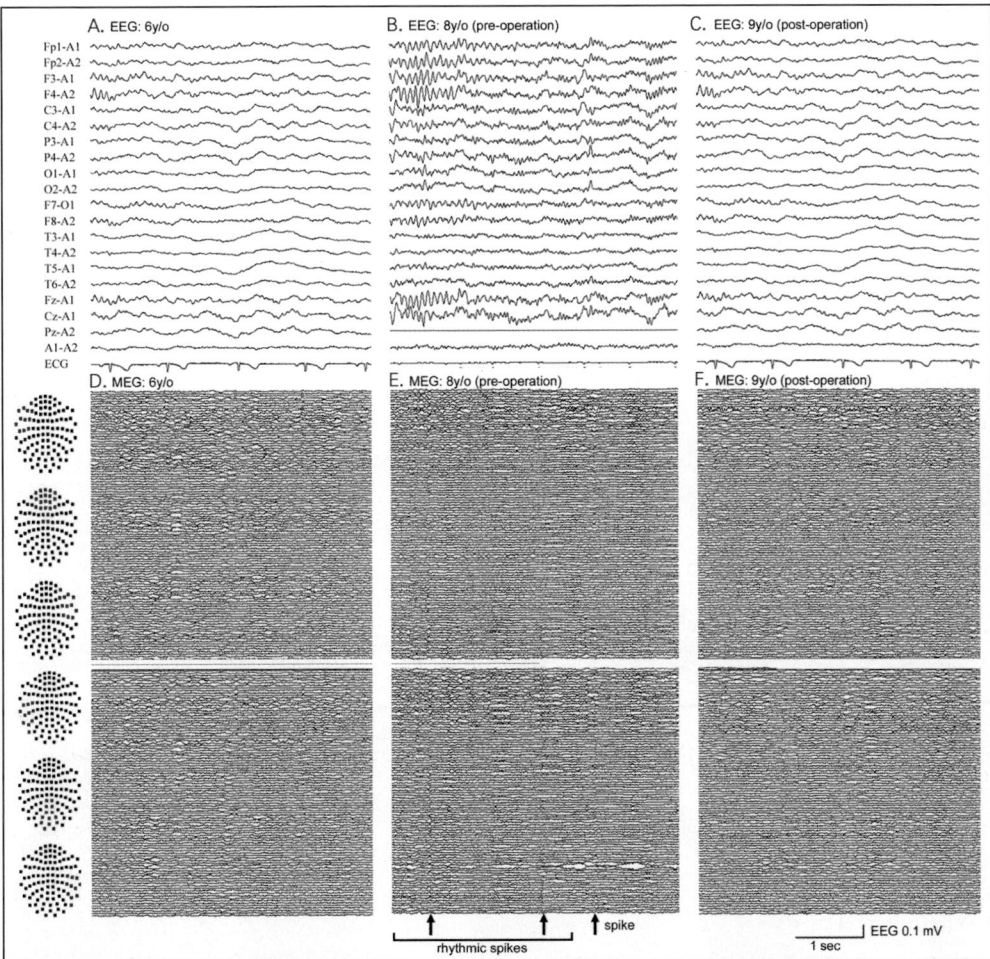

Figure 2. Case 2: EEG and MEG.
A. EEG at six years of age on her first visit showing no epileptiform discharges. **B.** EEG at eight years of age just before her operation showing prolonged rhythmic spiking with 10 Hz oscillation at Fp1, Fp2, F3, F4, F7, F8 and Fz. Independent spikes were detected at Fp1, Fp2, F3, C3, P3, P4, O1, O2 and Cz. **C.** EEG at nine years of age after her operation showing fragmental rhythmic activities at F3, F4 F7, F8 and Fz. **D.** MEG at six years of age on her first visit showing no epileptiform discharge. **E.** MEG at eight years of age just before her operation showing continuous aberrant oscillation at approximately 20 Hz at the left frontal area and the occipito-parietal area (quoted). MEG shows the frequent occurrence of an independent spike at the right occipital area and the left frontal area (arrow). **F.** MEG at nine years of age after her operation showing a spatially restricted oscillation band at the left frontal area at approximately 16 Hz.

To investigate the widespread spikes in MEG just before the operation, ECDs were located at the left superior frontal gyrus and the right supra-marginal gyrus (*Figure 3B*). dSPM analysis revealed genesis of the spikes at the right supra-marginal gyrus and propagation to left superior frontal gyrus and medial aspect (*Figure 3C*). In this situation, the ECD measurements only represented propagation of activity from a distinct epileptogenic area.

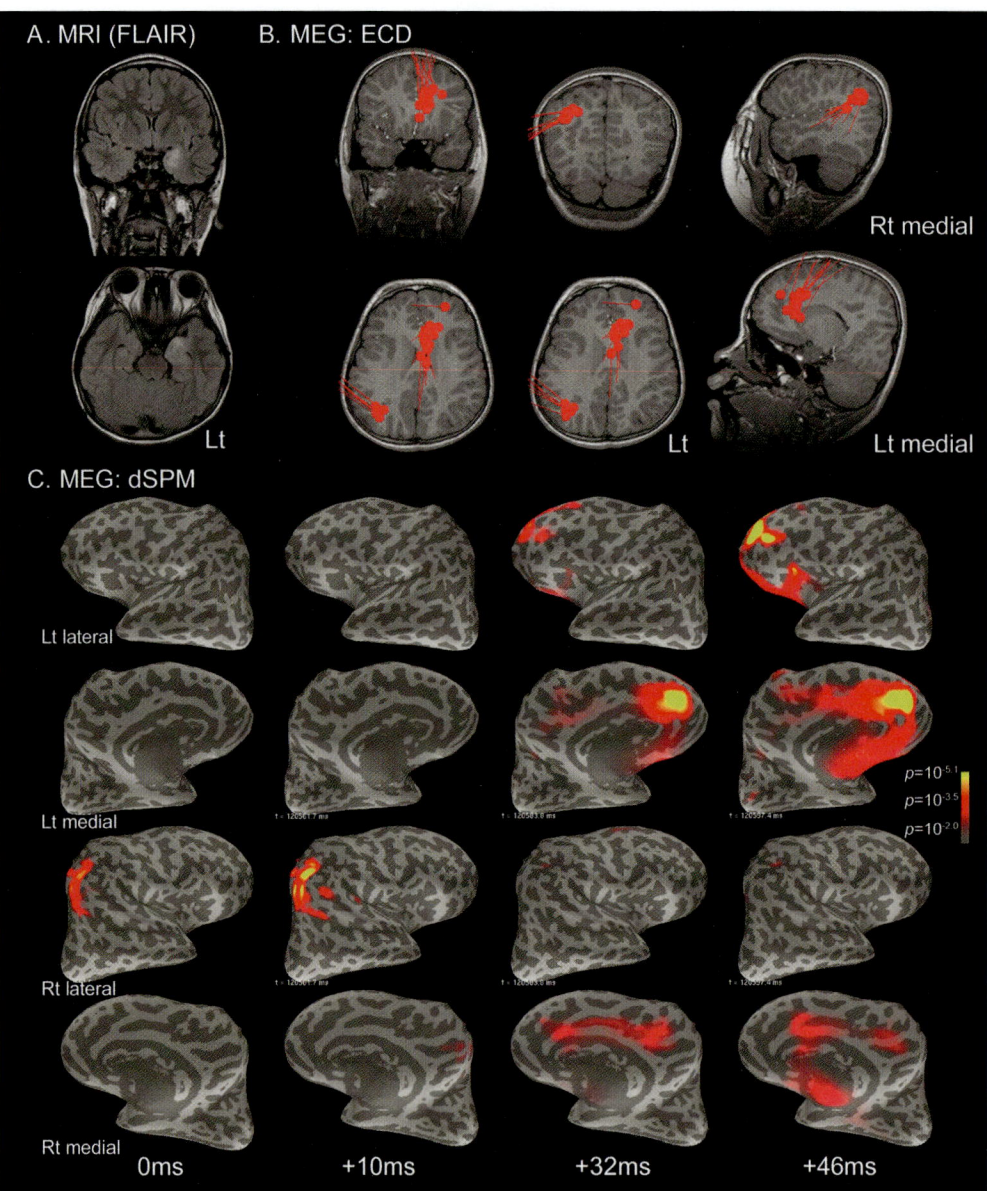

Figure 3. Case 2: MRI and MEG.
A. MRI FLAIR images showing focal cortical dysplasia at the left temporal para-hippocampal gyrus, uncus and hippocampus. **B.** ECDs were located at the left superior frontal gyrus and the right supra-marginal gyrus. **C.** dSPM snapshots demonstrated epileptiform activity generated in the right supra-marginal gyrus, which propagated to the left superior frontal gyrus and the corresponding medial aspect. In inflated MRI, dark and light grey areas revealed the sulcus and gyrus, respectively. The area in yellow, the point of transition from red to yellow, and the point of transition from grey to red, represent statistical values with $p = 10^{-5.1}$, $10^{-3.5}$, and $10^{-2.0}$, respectively.

She underwent SFT analysis for preoperative and postoperative rhythmic activity (*Figure 4A, 4C*). SFT analyses demonstrated rhythmic activity in the ipsilateral frontal lobe and within a broad region of the lateral aspect of the temporal lobe (*Figure 4B*). After the operation these rhythmic activities disappeared and became localized to the left pre- and post-central gyrus (*Figure 4D*).

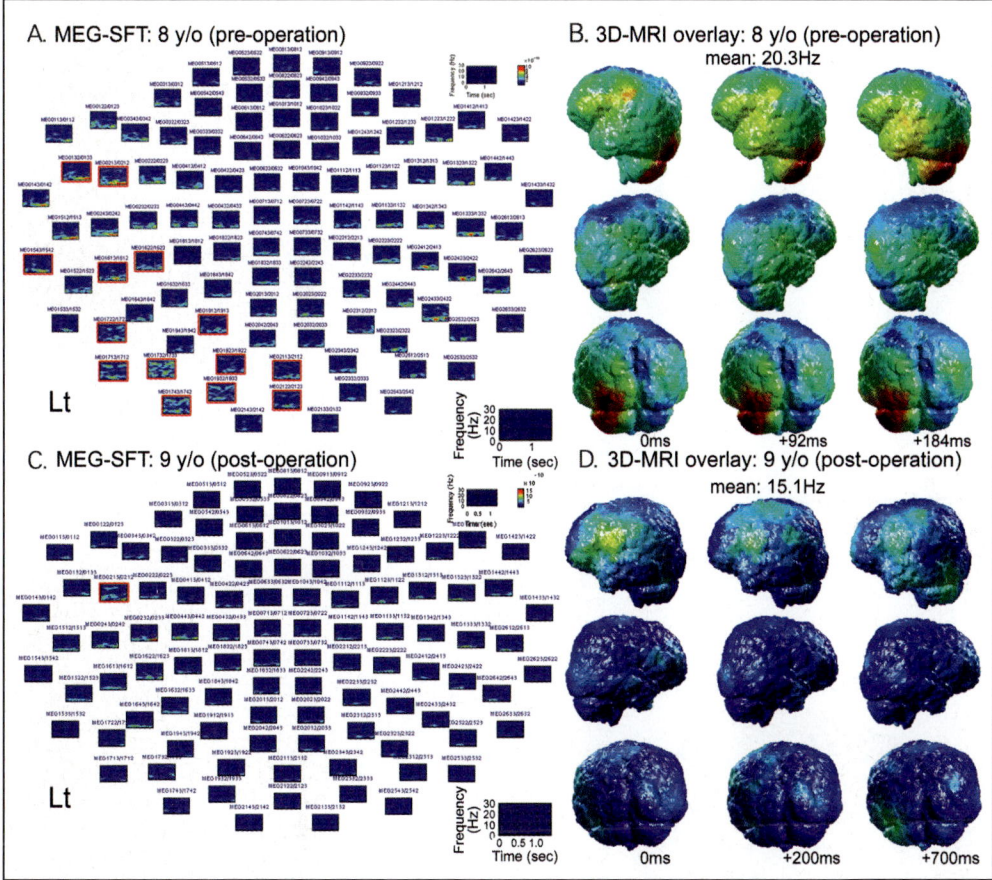

Figure 4. Case 2: STFT analysis.
A. STFT at eight years of age just before her operation showed aberrant magnetological oscillation at the left occipital and temporal and frontal areas at approximately 20 Hz (surrounded by red lines). **B.** EG signal from (A), superimposed on the 3D MRI image showing broad aberrant oscillation in the left lateral occipital lobe, the inferior, middle, and superior temporal gyrus, the angular gyrus, the supra-marginal gyrus and the inferior frontal gyrus (red and yellow areas). **C.** STFT at nine years of age after her operation showing aberrant magnetic field oscillation in the left frontal region at approximately 20 Hz (surrounded by red lines). **D.** MEG signal from (C), superimposed on the 3D MRI image showing broad aberrant oscillation in the left angular gyrus and the inferior frontal gyrus (red and yellow area).

She underwent ECoG during the operation. Just before the dysplasia resection, continuous rhythmic spikes at approximately 20 Hz were detected at the lower area of the left pre- and post-central gyrus and supra-marginal gyrus (*Figure 5A*). This activity disappeared and the irritative zone became more restricted to the left pre-frontal gyrus and supra-marginal gyrus from where epileptiform activity with lower amplitude was now recorded (*Figure 5B*). These findings provide clear evidence of the power reduction of the irritative zone after surgery.

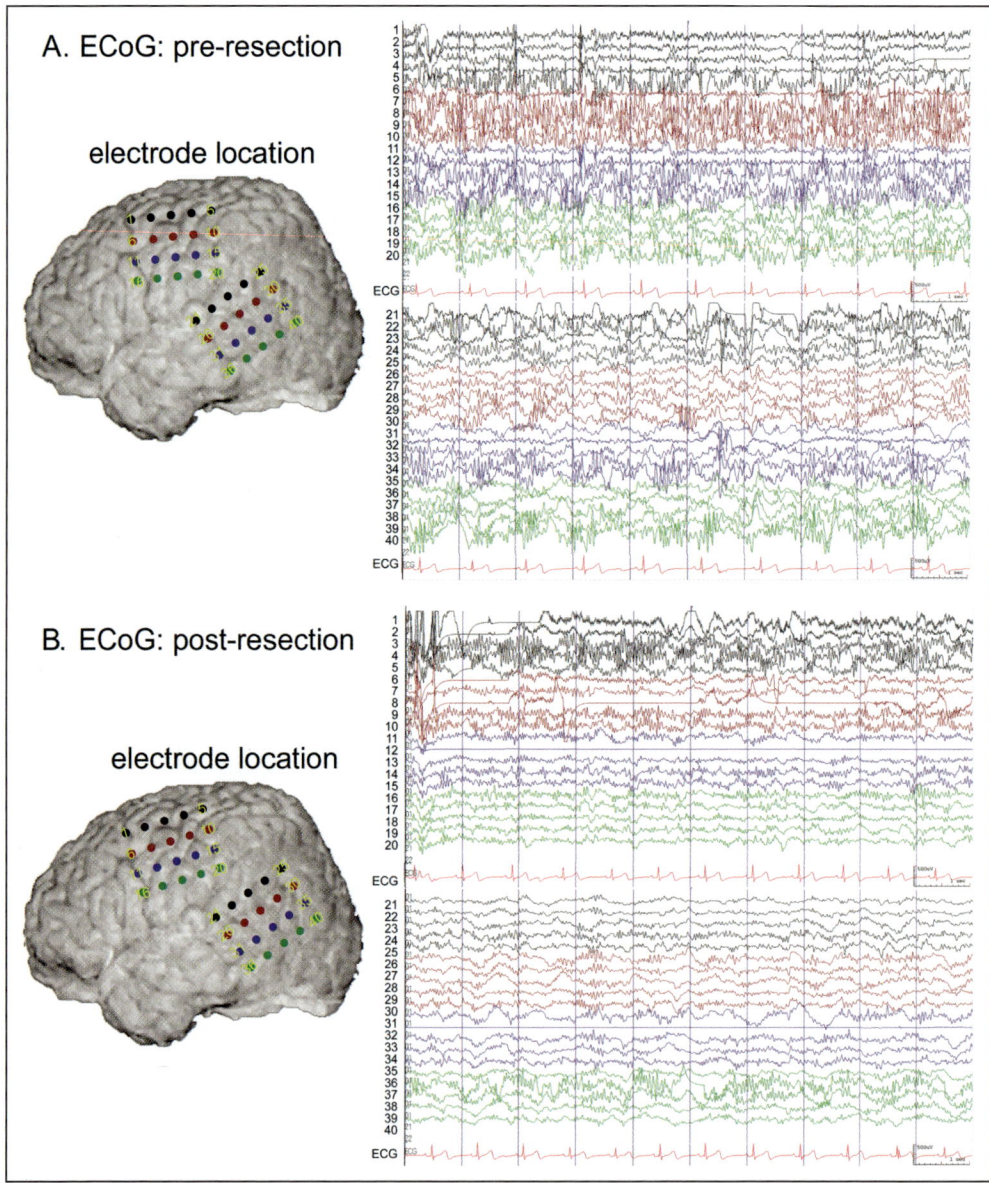

Figure 5. Case 2: ECoG.
A. ECoG during the operation before resection of the lesion demonstrating continuous aberrant rhythmic discharges at 20 Hz in electrode 5, 6, 7, 8, 9, 10, 13, 14, 15, 28, 19, 33, 34, 39 and 10 at approximately 500 µV. **B.** ECoG during the operation after resection of the lesion demonstrating an aberrant oscillation area at electrode 3, 4, 9, 10, 37 and 38 at approximately 250 µV.

Discussion and conclusion

MEG analysis is not the optimal tool for the identification of the epileptogenic area in patients with MTLE. MEG is reported to detect only about 50% of the ECoG spikes generated from medial temporal structures (Shigeto et al., 2002; Pataraia et al., 2005). However, a seizure-free (Engel class I) outcome was achieved in more than 90% of the patients after epilepsy surgery when the results using the ECD model showed horizontal currents from the ipsilateral medial temporal lobe (Assafa et al., 2004). Furthermore, in patients with medial temporal sclerosis (MTS) on MRI and a definite history of complex partial seizures (CPS), negative MEG findings provide further evidence that MTLE patients are good surgical candidates.

In this chapter, the investigation of epileptic rhythmic activity by MEG, which may reveal the presence of widespread aberrant epileptic discharges from medial temporal structures, was discussed. For follow-up evaluation in MTLE patients who have undergone surgery, MEG holds the potential to non-invasively grade the propensity for seizure recurrence. At this stage, the evidence highlights the potential of MEG as a valuable non-invasive tool before and after surgery for sequential evaluation, especially in paediatric patients.

References

- Assafa BA, Karkarb KM, Laxerc KD, Garciab PA, Austin EJ, Nicholas M, et al. Magnetoencephalography source localization and surgical outcome in temporal lobe epilepsy. *Clin Neurophysiol* 2004; 115: 2066-76.
- Cappell J, Schevon C, Emerson RG. Magnetoencephalography in epilepsy: tailoring interpretation and making inferences. *Curr Neurol Neurosci Rep* 2006; 6: 327-31.
- Cohen D. Magnetoencephalography: evidence of magnetic fields produced by alpha-rhythm currents. *Science* 1968; 161: 784-6.
- Dale AM, Fischl B, Sereno MI. Cortical surface-based analysis. I. Segmentation and surface reconstruction. *Neuroimage* 1999; 9: 179-94.
- Dale AM, Liu AK, Fischl BR, Buckner RL, Belliveau JW, Lewine JD, et al. Dynamic statistical parametric mapping: combining fMRI and MEG for high-resolution imaging of cortical activity. *Neuron* 2000; 26: 55-67.
- Dale AM, Sereno MI. Improved localization of cortical activity by combining EEG and MEG with MRI cortical surface reconstruction: A linear approach. *J Cogn Neurosci* 1993; 5: 162-76.
- Dhond RP, Buckner RL, Dale AM, Marinkovic KM, Halgren E. Spatiotemporal maps of brain activity underlying word generation and their modification during repetition priming. *J Neurosci* 2001; 21: 3564-71.
- Fischl B, Sereno MI, Tootell RB, Dale AM. High-resolution intersubject averaging and a coordinate system for the cortical surface, *Hum Brain Mapp* 1999; 8: 272-84.
- Grondin R, Chuang S, Otsubo H, Holowka S, Snead OC 3rd, Raybaud C, et al. The role of magnetoencephalography in pediatric epilepsy surgery. *Childs Nerv Syst* 2006; 22: 779-85.
- Hämäläinen M, Hari R, Ilmoniemi RJ, Knuutila J, Lounasmaa OV. Magnetoencephalography: theory, instrumentation, and application to noninvasive studies of the working human brain. *Rev Mod Phys* 1993; 65: 413-97.
- Hämäläinen MS, Ilmoniemi RJ. Interpreting magnetic fields of the brain: minimum norm estimates. *Med Biol Eng Compu* 1994; 32: 35-42.

- Knake S, Grant PE, Stufflebeam SM, Wald LL, Shiraishi H, Rosenow F, et al. Aids to telemetry in the presurgical evaluation of epilepsy patients: MRI, MEG and other non-invasive imaging techniques. *Suppl Clin Neurophysiol* 2004; 57: 494-502.
- Liu AK, Dale AM, Belliveau JW. Monte Carlo simulation studies of EEG and MEG localization accuracy. *Hum Brain Mapp* 2002; 16: 47-62.
- Mäkelä JP, Forss N, Jääskeläinen J, Kirveskari E, Korvenoja A, Paetau R. Magnetoencephalography in neurosurgery. *Neurosurgery* 2006; 59: 493-510; 510-1.
- Nakasato N, Levesque MF, Barth DS, Baumgartner C, Rogers RL, Sutherling WW. Comparisons of MEG, EEG, and ECoG source localization in neocortical partial epilepsy in humans. *Electroencephalogr Clin Neurophysiol* 1994; 91: 171-8.
- Oishi M, Kameyama S, Masuda H, Tohyama J, Kanazawa O, Sasagawa M, et al. Single and multiple clusters of magnetoencephalographic dipoles in neocortical epilepsy: Significance in characterizing the epileptogenic zone. *Epilepsia* 2006; 47: 355-64.
- Oppenheim A, Schafer RW. *Discrete-Time Signal Processing*. Englewood Cliffs: Prentice Hall, 1999.
- Otsubo H, Ochi A, Elliott I, Chuang SH, Rutka JT, Jay V, et al. MEG predicts epileptic zone in lesional extrahippocampal epilepsy: 12 pediatric surgery cases. *Epilepsia* 2001; 42: 1523-30.
- Otsubo H, Iida K, Okuda C, Ochi A, Pang E, Weiss SK, et al. Neurophysiological findings of neuronal migration disorders: intrinsic epileptogenicity of focal cortical dysplasia on EEG, ECoG, and MEG. *J Child Neurol* 2005; 20: 357-63.
- Pataraia E, Lindinger G, Deecke L, Mayer D, Baumgartner C. Combined MEG/EEG analysis of the interictal spike complex in mesial temporal lobe epilepsy. *Neuroimage* 2005; 24: 607-14.
- Rampp S, Stefan H. Magnetoencephalography in presurgical epilepsy diagnosis. *Expert Rev Med Devices* 2007; 4: 335-47.
- Schwartz ES, Dlugos DJ, Storm PB, Dell J, Magee R, Flynn TP, et al. Magnetoencephalography for pediatric epilepsy: how we do it. *AJNR Am J Neuroradiol* 2008; 29: 832-7.
- Shibasaki H, Ikeda A, Nagamine T. Use of magnetoencephalography in the presurgical evaluation of epilepsy patients. *Clin Neurophysiol* 2007; 118: 1438-48.
- Shigeto H, Morioka T, Hisada K, Nishio S, Ishibashi H, Kira D, et al. Feasibility and limitations of magnetoencephalographic detection of epileptic discharges: simultaneous recording of magnetic fields and electrocorticography. *Neurol Res* 2002; 24: 531-6.
- Shiraishi H, Watanabe Y, Watanabe M, Inoue Y, Fujiwara T, Yagi K. Interictal and ictal magnetoencephalographic study in patients with medial frontal lobe epilepsy. *Epilepsia* 2001; 42: 875-82.
- Stefan H, Hummel C, Scheler G, Genow A, Druschky K, Tilz C, et al. Magnetic brain source imaging of focal epileptic activity: a synopsis of 455 cases. *Brain* 2003; 126: 2396-405.
- Sutherling WW, Crandall PH, Engel J Jr, Darcey TM, Cahan LD, Barth DS. The magnetic field of complex partial seizure agrees with intracranial localizations. *Ann Neurol* 1987; 21: 548-58.

The relevance of high frequency oscillations in the pathophysiology and diagnosis of mesial temporal lobe epilepsy

Julia Jacobs

Department of Neuropediatrics, University of Freiburg, Germany

High frequency oscillations (HFOs) are generally considered to be distinct oscillatory events with frequencies above the gamma band (Urrestarazu et al. 2007; Staba et al. 2004). In recent years, they have attracted increasing interest as they mainly occur in epileptic tissue. Band frequencies in the higher range are not as well defined as the commonly used lower frequency bands (alpha, beta, theta, and delta) and, thus, definitions of HFOs vary. Most groups distinguish between lower frequency oscillations, referred to as "ripple" (~ 100 to ~ 250 Hz) and faster oscillations referred to as "fast ripples" (FR) (~ 250 to ~ 500 Hz) (Staba et al., 2002; Jacobs et al., 2008). HFOs are believed to be generated over very small surface areas. In animal models, FR-generating sites are suggested to be as small as 1 mm^3. As a result of these small generating sites, reports of HFOs, as they are described below, are exclusively derived from intracranial EEG recordings.

HFOs are found in the mesial temporal as well as neocortical areas (Bragin et al., 2002a; Worrell et al., 2004). HFOs generated in the mesial temporal areas are more common and prominent than those in neocortex *(Figure 1)*. Mesial HFOs occur with rates of around 22/min and 20/min for ripples and fast ripples, respectively, while neocortical HFOs only occur with rates of around 5/min and 2/min for ripples and fast ripples, respectively (Jacobs et al., 2008; 2009d). Within the mesial temporal structures, rates are lower in the amygdala than in hippocampus and parahippocampus *(Table 1)*.

Moreover, mesial temporal HFOs have greater amplitude and longer duration. In the hippocampus, the duration for ripples is around 97 ms and 43 ms for fast ripples, while those in the neocortex are considerably shorter with a duration of 77 ms for ripples and 22 ms for fast ripples (Jacobs et al., 2008). Reasons for the frequent occurrence and length of HFOs in the mesial temporal structures are unclear but may reflect a higher level of epileptogenicity and result from their unique anatomical structure.

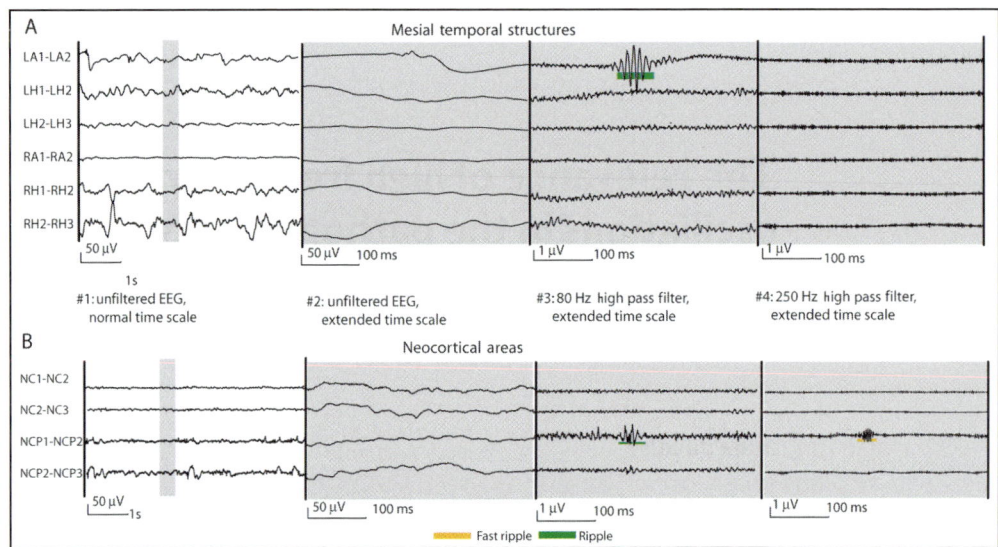

Figure 1. Example of a ripple in the **(A)** mesial temporal structures (hippocampus) and **(B)** neocortex. Neocortical ripples and fast ripples are usually much smaller than mesiotemporal ones. In the present example this difference is shown for ripples, while only a neocortical fast ripple can be seen. The thin grey section #1 is expanded in time and amplitude in sections #2, #3, and #4. Note that sections #3 and #4 have a much higher gain that #1 and #2. Figure is modified with permission from Jacobs et al., 2009d.

Table I. Rates (per minute) of ripples and fast ripples in the different anatomical regions marked in 12 consecutive patients
HFOs were much more frequent in the mesial temporal structures. Within each structure, HFOs were always significantly more frequent in the SOZ than outside the SOZ. ns: non-significant.
Reproduced with permission from Jacobs et al., 2009d

	Ripples rates		Significance	Fast ripples rates		Significance
	SOZ	Non-SOZ		SOZ	Non-SOZ	
Mesial temporal structures	29.2	14.2	< 0.001	21.8	3.0	< 0.001
Neocortex	9.7	4.9	< 0.001	5.1	2.1	0.05
Amygdala	24.2	14.2	0.003	12.5	7.6	ns
Hippocampus	34.5	15.6	< 0.001	27.1	1.2	< 0.001
Parahippocampus	18	14.2	n.s.	22.7	1.9	< 0.001

While it is a commonly accepted fact that ripples can occur in the hippocampus under physiological as well as pathological conditions, this matter is still under discussion for fast ripples. Some groups consider all fast ripples to be pathological while others distinguish a third type of oscillation referred to as "pathological HFO" (pHFO) (Engel, Jr. et al., 2009).

The first association between epilepsy and HFOs was described by microwire recordings in the mesial temporal structures of rodents which developed seizures after kainic acid injection (Bragin et al., 1999a). This was followed by studies in humans with bitemporal refractory epilepsy (Bragin et al., 1999b). Prior to this discovery, the relevance of ripple oscillations as physiological oscillations during memory formation was discovered in healthy rodents (Buzsaki et al., 1992; Chrobak & Buzsaki, 1996). Thus, consideration of the co-occurrence of physiological and pathological HFOs in mesial temporal structures has remained necessary when using HFOs as a diagnostic tool in mesial temporal lobe epilepsy. Over time, however, it became more and more clear that a simple frequency analysis cannot distinguish between physiological and pathological oscillations (Engel Jr. et al., 2009). For ethical reasons, it is not possible to implant intracranial electrodes in healthy patients or healthy tissue from epileptic patients. Reliable reports of physiological HFO activity thus derive only from animal studies. To what extent this knowledge can be translated to humans remains uncertain, especially as relevant frequency bands may be different between different species. Data of physiological HFOs in humans should be examined in the context of limitations; most studies have used the "healthier side" of two affected hippocampi as a reference (Bragin et al., 2002a; Axmacher et al., 2008a). In humans, even the separation between ripples and fast ripples, a concept originating from rodent experiments, may be arbitrary (Zelmann et al., 2009a). Consequently, a division between pHFO and physiological HFO now remains a theoretical concept and the recording of physiological HFOs cannot be disregarded when analysing pHFOs for diagnostic purposes. This is especially true in the mesial temporal regions for several reasons: 1) spontaneous non-event-related physiological HFOs have only been described in these structures; 2) the related physiological mechanisms such as memory are active during sleep when pHFOs are usually analysed and cannot be willingly suppressed; 3) methods to record and understand physiological HFOs in volunteers, such as MEG and high-resolution surface EEG, are unlikely to be effective in these deeply located structures.

■ Physiological high frequency oscillations

Description of HFOs in the mesial temporal structures therefore requires basic insight of physiological HFOs. Ripple oscillations are network oscillations most likely involved in memory consolidation processes mainly during sleep. They are associated with the synchronization of neuronal activity over large distances and thus facilitate the process of transferring memory information from temporary storage within hippocampal tissue to more permanent memory information in neocortical areas (Sirota et al., 2003). During this process, ripple oscillations occur at the same time as sharp wave complexes and are therefore termed "sharp-wave-ripple complexes" (Siapas & Wilson, 1998; Clemens et al., 2007). The sharp-wave-ripple complexes were shown to be increased during sleep after combined, spatial, visual and emotional memory tasks in rodents as well as humans (Axmacher et al., 2008a, Moelle et al., 2009; Girardeau et al., 2009).

Ripple activity, however, does not always occur in combination with sharp waves and can be observed as rather localized oscillatory events. Bragin and co-workers described large numbers of ripple oscillations in healthy rats as well as in the "healthier" hippocampus opposite to the seizure onset zone (SOZ) in patients with refractory epilepsy (Bragin et al., 1999b; Staba et al., 2002). The presentation of a combined visual and spatial memory task led to an increase of ripple activity in both mesial temporal structures and the extent of the increase was correlated with the recall performance after memory consolidation (Axmacher et al., 2008a). However, the conclusion that ripple oscillations of up to 200 Hz are physiological events, while only fast ripples above 200 Hz are pathological within the mesial temporal structures, would seem to be incorrect (Engel, Jr. et al., 2009). Evidence acquired with standard clinical macro-electrodes suggests that ripples are largely increased in the SOZ and linked to epileptogenesis not only in neocortical but also in mesial temporal structures (Jacobs et al., 2008; 2009a). The number of ripples is relevant for predicting the SOZ, as well as the postsurgical outcome (Jacobs et al., 2008; 2010). It is therefore hypothesized that ripples measured in mesial temporal structures are a mixture of physiological and pathological events, thus physiological HFOs may interfere with the analysis of epileptic HFOs. As shown by Axmacher et al., they may, however, also be a future tool for memory evaluation in epilepsy patients. To achieve this goal, a better analysis of verbal and non-verbal memory consolidation and understanding of their association with ripple activity seems necessary (Axmacher et al., 2008a; 2008b).

One variable that may help to distinguish between physiological and pathological HFOs is spatial distribution. Pathological HFOs are not involved in the synchronization of neurological information over long distances, rather, they are believed to be the result of pathologically synchronized bursts of neurons (Foffani et al., 2007). In the future, this difference in generating mechanisms may allow us to differentiate between both events by looking at features such as propagation and co-occurrence with sleep patterns.

Pathological high frequency oscillations

Pathological HFOs may provide an additional marker for epileptogenic tissue in patients with refractory MTLE. As already mentioned, for now this evaluation remains an invasive option in patients who have already been implanted with intracranial electrodes and therefore provides only additional information to intracranial investigation. Nevertheless, additional investigation of epileptogenic tissue in patients with MTLE can provide several advantages: first, a better prediction of surgical outcome and a better delineation of epileptogenic areas in patients in whom the outcome or the complete seizure onset zone is still uncertain after intracranial recording; second, a better identification of areas of propagation which may be interpreted as areas of SOZ due to limited sampling of intracranial electrodes; third, a reduction of recording time as HFOs, can usually be recorded reliably with only 10 minutes of slow-wave sleep.

However, HFOs can only serve as additional reliable markers of epileptogenicity if they meet the following basic requirements: 1) they have to be independent of other well established markers, such as spikes; 2) their generation has to be stable, reliable and as independent as possible from environmental changes; 3) they have to have a clear pathophysiological link with epilepsy and epileptogenesis.

The relationship between spikes and high frequency oscillations

In studies with micro-electrodes, it was first noticed that HFOs occurred often in the same channels and even at the same time point as interictal epileptic discharges/spikes. This raised the question as to whether both events are related to the same pathomechanism and are dependent on each other, or whether they are actually independent features. This question is not as intuitive to answer as it may appear, as spikes are not visible at the extended time scale or with filtering used to observe HFOs. Moreover, some events resembling HFOs may result from the high-pass filtering of the fast transient nature of a spike. The assessment of macro-electrode recordings has facilitated the evaluation of the spike-HFO relationship, as a large number of electrode contacts have been evaluated covering large brain regions, prompting the observation of spike propagation patterns. In an initial study, three different HFO-spike associations were described (Urrestarazu et al., 2007). First, spikes and ripples could co-occur at the same point in time and HFOs were seen to "ride" on the spike on the unfiltered EEG. Second, both events could co-occur, but without visible HFOs on the unfiltered EEG. In this case, HFOs may have resulted from filtering the fast transient nature of the spike. Third, HFOs could occur at completely independent time points to spikes (Urrestarazu et al., 2007). Approximately 63% of ripples and 48% of fast ripples were reported to occur with spikes, while 44% of spikes co-occurred with ripples and 27% with FRs (Jacobs et al., 2008) *(Figure 2)*. In the mesial temporal structures, an even larger percentage of co-occurrence was reported (Crepon et al., 2010). However, HFOs could also occur in channels that did not show any spiking activity during the recordings. Thus, when considering timing and location, the occurrence of HFOs was not obligatorily linked to the occurrence of spikes, and *vice versa*.

Moreover, patterns of HFOs and spikes are different during intracranial recordings. A reduction of antiepileptic medication was shown to have opposite effects on HFOs and spikes (Zijlmans et al., 2009a). In a study that analysed rates of spikes and HFOs over several nights during an intracranial investigation, the rate of HFOs increased after the reduction of antiepileptic medication and remained stable after recurrent seizures. On the contrary, the rate of spikes remained stable following medication withdrawal and increased after recurrent seizures. Stability or even decrease of spike rates after medication reduction has also been described in previous studies (Gotman 1991; Spencer et al., 2008). Thus, HFOs behave differently to spikes since they increase when medication is lowered.

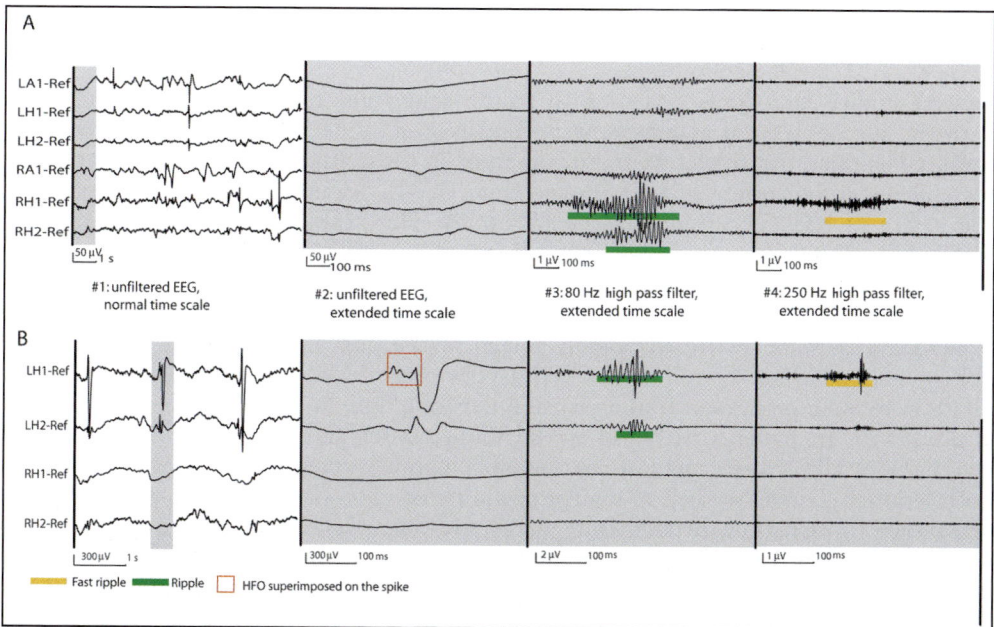

Figure 2. Example of HFOs without spikes **(A)** and "riding on the spike" **(B)**.
They were both recorded from a hippocampal electrode. Figure modified with permission from Jacobs et al., 2008.

Differences were also observed when HFO rates during the transition from the interictal to pre-ictal and ictal period were examined. While HFO rates already increased during the 5 seconds prior to seizures, relative to the interictal period, spikes only increased in the ictal period. For HFOs, the increase and spread during the ictal period was also more focal and limited to the SOZ, relative to spikes (Zijlmans et al., 2011).

In conclusion, HFOs seem to have different pathophysiological mechanisms to spikes and better reflect epileptic activity (Zijlmans et al., 2009a). The relationship between the two is, however, not yet well understood and both events often occur together.

Stability and location

In rodents, fast ripples have previously been described to be spatially stable and the tissue generating fast ripples was not shown to change or vary over time during several weeks of recordings (Bragin et al., 2003). In humans, the time of observation is naturally limited by the time of intracranial recording. Nevertheless, during the limited time of the recording, several studies have indirectly shown that while the actual rates of HFOs may vary over time, the areas that generate HFOs remain stable. For example, HFOs are influenced by vigilance state: they are most frequent in slow-wave sleep and rare in wakefulness and REM sleep (Staba et al., 2004; Bagshaw et al., 2009). However, this does not change the fact that, independent of sleep stage, the channels within the epileptogenic tissue usually have the highest rates (Bagshaw et al., 2009). The same finding was observed in the study of Zijlmans et al (2009a) who described the effect of AED reduction and seizures; even if the actual rates varied between the night-time periods investigated, their localisation and relative differences between areas remained the same (Zijlmans et al., 2009a).

High frequency oscillations and epileptogenicity

Several studies in rodents treated with kainic acid point towards a close relationship between fast ripples and epileptogenesis (Bragin et al., 1999a; 2003; 2005). After acute status epilepticus, fast ripples were only observed in those animals which developed chronic epilepsy and recurrent seizures (Bragin et al., 2004). Seizure frequency correlated with the extent of HFO occurrence in the rat brains. Thus, HFOs appear to represent epileptogenic changes in rat mesial temporal structures. In humans, the development of epilepsy cannot be observed and for this reason, good correlation with the SOZ is used as a variable. In micro as well as macro-electrode recordings from the human hippocampus, HFOs were interictally clearly linked to the side of predominant seizure onset (Bragin et al., 2002b; Worrell et al., 2008; Jacobs et al., 2008) (Figure 3). During seizures, HFOs were more prominent in the seizure onset zone than in areas of propagation (Jirsch et al., 2006). In patients with widespread seizure onset and an indication of recorded propagation, HFOs were rare. In the mesial temporal structures, HFOs were linked to both lesional changes as well as epileptogenic tissue. The ratio of fast ripples to ripples was shown to increase with increasing atrophy (Staba et al., 2007). Moreover, increased HFO rates within the hippocampus were directly linked to areas of hippocampal atrophy and therefore may reflect neuron loss and synaptic reorganisation (Ogren et al., 2009). When comparing lesional areas inside and outside the SOZ, as well as areas of SOZ outside the lesion, HFOs however, were more closely linked to the actual site of SOZ than to the lesion (Jacobs et al., 2009a). An increase of HFOs was also not limited to

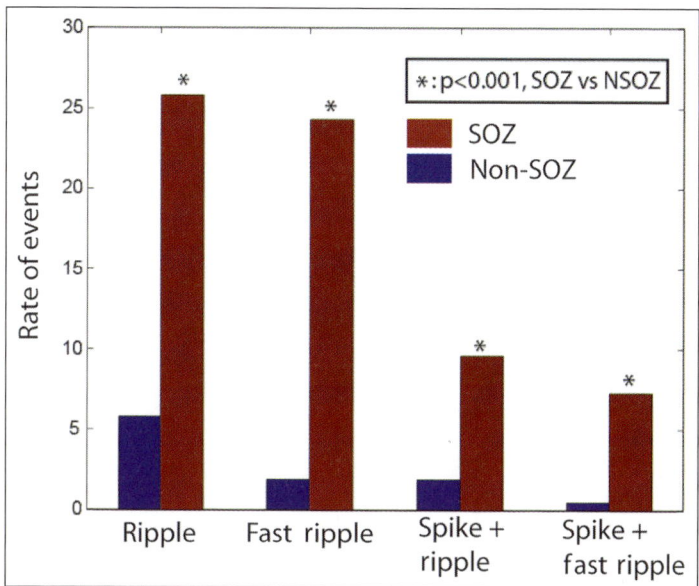

Figure 3. Differences in rates of HFOs between SOZ channels and non-SOZ channels taken from 20 patients recorded with depth macro-electrodes at the Montreal Neurological Institute.
Note that not only rates of ripples or fast ripples, but also rates of spikes with ripples and spikes with fast ripples are significantly higher in the SOZ than outside the SOZ ($p < 0.001$); the same is not true for spikes alone.

patients with atrophy and sclerosis but could also be seen in non-lesional mesial temporal lobe epilepsy and patients with developmental malformation in the mesial temporal structures (Jacobs et al., 2010).

In bitemporal epilepsy, the seizures actually recorded during the monitoring period may not always reflect the actual seizure distribution between left and right hippocampus. In some centres, electrical stimulation is used to further delineate the seizure onset, however, results are contradictory with regards to whether stimulation responses, in the form of after-discharges, auras and seizures, can actually indicate the hippocampus which is mostly involved. One study indicated that, independent of the delineated SOZ, the same areas which responded to stimulation correlated with those generating HFOs. In detail, rates of HFOs were greatest in those areas which needed the lowest current to evoke a stimulation response, which could be either after discharges with propagation, auras or seizures (Jacobs et al., 2010).

The most important evidence for HFOs as markers of epileptogenicity, however, is the correlation between their surgical removal and postsurgical outcome. In a study of 20 patients, 10 of whom had mesial temporal lobe epilepsy, all patients with minimal removal of HFO-generating tissue had a poor surgical outcome (Jacobs et al., 2010) (*Figure 4*). Thus, such an outcome could have been predicted in this study. However, in three patients the majority of HFO-generating tissue was removed but the patients continued to have seizures nevertheless. This finding may be explained by the limited electrode coverage which cannot record HFOs in other brain areas and therefore reflects a true limitation of the technique for neocortical epilepsies, since postsurgical outcome may not be predictable. This limitation, however, is less an issue in mesial temporal epilepsy as the affected structures are better defined and easier to cover with electrodes. For now, the usefulness of HFOs in planning the extent of a resection is still questionable due to the many limitations of the technique.

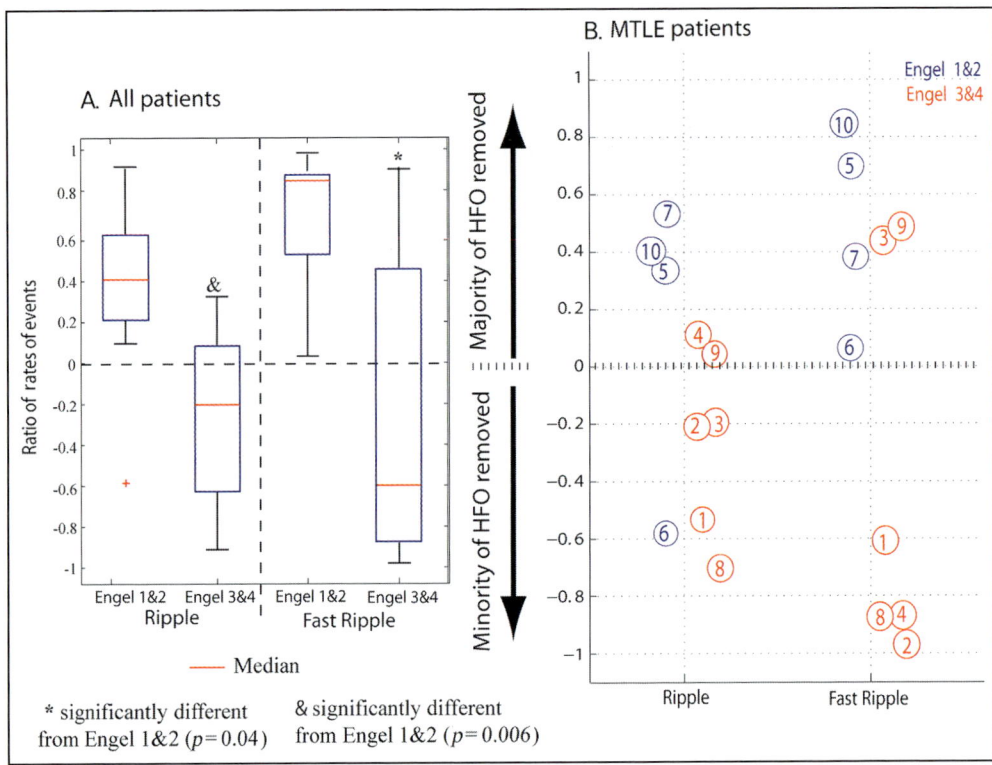

Figure 4. Correlation between the removal of HFOs and postsurgical outcome.
Normalized ratios were recorded for HFO rates in areas which were surgically removed and areas which remained. Ratios between 0 and 1 reflect patients for whom the majority of HFOs was removed and ratios between 0 and – 1 reflect those for whom minimal areas were taken out. In patients with a good outcome, significantly more HFO-generating areas were removed relative to those with a bad outcome. **A.** All patients (20 patients) and **B.** individual ratios of patients with MTLE. Figure modified with permission from Jacobs et al., 2010.

■ Practical aspects

Currently, the analysis of HFOs is performed using two different approaches; several groups have worked with automatic detection tools, while others have relied on visual marking of the events. At present, both techniques have advantages and disadvantages for research purposes. However, for long-term clinical use, an automatic detection tool is essential. Automatic detection analysis, which is often semi-automatic since data have to be confirmed visually, has the great advantage of being fast and reviewer-independent. Currently, most automatic methods are based on frequency analysis, although there are no standard methods in use among the different research groups (Staba *et al.*, 2002; Gardner *et al.*, 2007). All techniques face problems in detection since areas identified may be strongly dependent on the brain region and the baseline from which they are recorded. They also fail to provide information about the relationship between spikes and HFOs. As for mesial temporal epilepsies, some techniques already seem to be very reliable and HFOs may be easier to detect using a threshold, since the actual events are longer and larger in amplitude (Crepon et al., 2010). For research purposes, visual HFO marking is also used; this allows more detailed analysis, but requires hours of work for each patient, even when only 5 to 10 minutes of interictal EEG is analysed (Staba et al., 2004; Jacobs et al., 2008). Visual approaches are reviewer-dependent and should be validated by a measurement of inter-rater agreement (Zelmann et al., 2009b).

A centre wanting to implement an HFO-directed approach should also consider the size of the electrodes used in their routine. Theoretically, the possibility of recording HFOs should be largely dependent on the size of the effective surface area of the contact; it has been hypothesised that the larger the contact the lower the signal to noise ratio. Even if it cannot be proven that the events recorded with micro-electrodes are the same as those seen with macro-electrodes, their electrophysiological pattern and shapes appear to be comparable. Additionally, simultaneous recordings with micro and macro-contacts using hybrid electrodes did not reveal substantial differences in the amount or characteristics of the recorded HFOs (Worrell et al., 2008; Chatillon et al., 2009). Further investigation is required to establish whether this applies to the various macro-contact types used commercially. Moreover, it remains unclear whether cortical strips and depth contacts implanted in the same patient with MTLE are comparable.

■ Diagnostic value of high frequency oscillations in mesial temporal lobe epilepsies

A measurement which could allow us to clearly identify tissues which generate seizures (SOZ), or even the whole epileptogenic zone including tissue which has the potential to generate seizures, would considerably enhance the diagnostic possibilities in patients with refractory epilepsy. Furthermore, a marker to differentiate between the more and less epileptogenic hippocampus would enable a more precise prediction of postsurgical outcome in patients with MTLE. HFOs may have the potential to provide both types of information, as they seem to mirror the epileptogenic potential of the tissue. They are closely linked to pathogenesis in mesial temporal lobe epilepsy and reflect the degree of atrophy and disease activity (Staba et al., 2007; Ogren et al., 2009). They are more reliable and precise indicators of epileptic areas than spikes, and possibly even the SOZ (Jacobs et al., 2008; 2010). Information on HFOs can be gained during the interictal period and after very short recordings of only 10 minutes (Zelmann et al., 2009b). However, results should be interpreted carefully, as reliable recording and detection tools are still in the process of becoming established.

The occurrence of physiological HFOs has been discussed before, but their practical consequences should again be emphasised here. HFO rates are significantly higher in the mesial temporal structures, as are spikes with HFOs. This seems to be a reflection of epileptogenic potential on the one hand, but also, on the other hand, a result of the sum of physiological and pathological HFOs. As long as physiological and pathological HFOs cannot be distinguished, higher rates of HFOs in a hippocampus may either reflect a lower threshold for seizures or better memory function. Additionally, HFO rates in the mesial temporal structures cannot be easily compared with those in neocortical structures. This is not problematic if patients are only implanted either in the neocortex or in the mesial temporal structures, since HFO rates suitably delineate the SOZ within each of these structures.

Problems occur in those patients with a combination of electrodes in the mesial temporal and neocortical structures and a simple comparison of rates may not be possible. In a patient with a suspected lesion in the frontal lobe and an unclear seizure onset, rates of ripples of 10/minute in the hippocampus, which is a relatively low rate for this structure, may be less relevant than a rate of 5/minute in the frontal lesion, as healthy neocortical structures usually do not show any spontaneous ripples (Jacobs et al., 2008). Thus, physiological HFOs may interfere with our interpretation and methods of differentiating both types have to be established. If this is accomplished, physiological HFOs may be used as a measurement of memory capacity of the affected hippocampus, while pHFOs reflect epileptic potential.

Techniques to record mesial temporal HFOs remain invasive and linked to chronic intracranial investigations, especially in MTLE where structures lie too deep to expect visible HFOs on the surface. Semi-invasive electrodes, such as sphenoidal contacts, may, however, reduce any distress to the patient, as physiological ripples have already been recorded with these techniques (Clemens et al., 2007). Other approaches using shorter intra-operative recordings are also under current evaluation.

In the future, HFOs will most likely represent an additional marker in presurgical diagnostics, supplementing established methods such as structural and functional imaging. Nevertheless, studies with a large number of patients from different centres, as well as with different recording techniques, are necessary before HFOs can be considered a reliable marker of epileptogenicity and used to tailor surgical resection.

References

- Axmacher N, Elger CE, Fell J. Ripples in the medial temporal lobe are relevant for human memory consolidation. *Brain* 2008a; 131: 1806-17.
- Axmacher N, Helmstaedter C, Elger CE, Fell J. Enhancement of neocortical-medial temporal EEG correlations during non-REM sleep. *Neural Plast* 2008b: 563028.
- Bagshaw AP, Jacobs J, LeVan P, Dubeau F, Gotman J. Effect of sleep stage on interictal high-frequency oscillations recorded from depth macroelectrodes in patients with focal epilepsy. *Epilepsia* 2009; 50: 617-28.
- Bragin A, Azizyan A, Almajano J, Wilson CL, Engel J, Jr. Analysis of chronic seizure onsets after intrahippocampal kainic acid injection in freely moving rats. *Epilepsia* 2005; 46: 1592-8.
- Bragin A, Engel J, Jr., Wilson CL, Fried I, Buzsaki G. High-frequency oscillations in human brain. *Hippocampus* 1999b; 9: 137-42.
- Bragin A, Engel J, Jr., Wilson CL, Fried I, Mathern GW. Hippocampal and entorhinal cortex high-frequency oscillations (100-500 Hz) in human epileptic brain and in kainic acid-treated rats with chronic seizures. *Epilepsia* 1999a; 40: 127-37.
- Bragin A, Mody I, Wilson CL, Engel J, Jr. Local generation of fast ripples in epileptic brain. *J Neurosci* 2002b; 22: 2012-21.
- Bragin A, Wilson CL, Almajano J, Mody I, Engel J, Jr. High-frequency oscillations after status epilepticus: epileptogenesis and seizure genesis. *Epilepsia* 2004; 45: 1017-23.
- Bragin A, Wilson CL, Engel J. Spatial stability over time of brain areas generating fast ripples in the epileptic rat. *Epilepsia* 2003; 44: 1233-7.

- Bragin A, Wilson CL, Staba RJ, Reddick M, Fried I, Engel J, Jr. Interictal high-frequency oscillations (80-500 Hz) in the human epileptic brain: entorhinal cortex. *Ann Neurol* 2002a; 52: 407-15.
- Buzsaki G, Horvath Z, Urioste R, Hetke J, Wise K. High-frequency network oscillation in the hippocampus. *Science* 1992; 256: 1025-7.
- Chatillon CE, Zelmann R, Bortel A, Avoli M, Dubeau F, Gotman J. Smaller Size of Macroelectrodes does not improve HFO detection in intracerebral EEG recordings of the chronic epileptic rat. *Epilepsia* 2009; 50 (S11): 18-9.
- Chrobak JJ, Buzsaki G. High-frequency oscillations in the output networks of the hippocampal-entorhinal axis of the freely behaving rat. *J Neurosci* 1996; 16: 3056-66.
- Clemens Z, Molle M, Eross L, Barsi P, Halasz P, Born J. Temporal coupling of parahippocampal ripples, sleep spindles and slow oscillations in humans. *Brain* 2007; 130: 2868-78.
- Crepon B, Navarro V, Hasboun D, Clemenceau S, Martinerie J, Baulac M, et al. Mapping interictal oscillations greater than 200 Hz recorded with intracranial macroelectrodes in human epilepsy. *Brain* 2010; 133 (Pt 1): 33-45.
- Engel J, Jr., Bragin A, Staba R, Mody I. High-frequency oscillations: what is normal and what is not? *Epilepsia* 2009; 50: 598-604.
- Foffani G, Uzcategui YG, Gal B, Menendez dlP. Reduced spike-timing reliability correlates with the emergence of fast ripples in the rat epileptic hippocampus. *Neuron* 2007; 55: 930-41.
- Gardner AB, Worrell GA, Marsh E, Dlugos D, Litt B. Human and automated detection of high-frequency oscillations in clinical intracranial EEG recordings. *Clin Neurophysiol* 2007; 118: 1134-43.
- Girardeau G, Benchenane K, Wiener SI, Buzsaki G, Zugaro MB. Selective suppression of hippocampal ripples impairs spatial memory. *Nat Neurosci* 2009; 12: 1222-3.
- Gotman J. Relationships between interictal spiking and seizures: human and experimental evidence. *Can J Neurol Sci* 1991; 18: 573-6.
- Jacobs J, LeVan P, Chander R, Hall J, Dubeau F, Gotman J. Interictal high-frequency oscillations (80-500 Hz) are an indicator of seizure onset areas independent of spikes in the human epileptic brain. *Epilepsia* 2008; 49: 1893-1907.
- Jacobs J, LeVan P, Chatillon CE, Olivier A, Dubeau F, Gotman J. High frequency oscillations in intracranial EEGs mark epileptogenicity rather than lesion type. *Brain* 2009a; 132: 1022-37.
- Jacobs J, Zijlmans M, Zelmann R, Chatillon CE, Hall J, Olivier A, et al. High-frequency electroencephalographic oscillations correlate with outcome of epilepsy surgery. *Ann Neurol* 2010b; 67: 209-20.
- Jacobs J, Zijlmans M, Zelmann R, Olivier A, Hall J, Gotman J, et al. Value of electrical stimulation and high frequency oscillations (80-500 Hz) in identifying epileptogenic areas during intracranial EEG recordings. *Epilepsia* 2010c; 5: 1573-82.
- Jacobs J, LeVan P, Dubeau F, Gotman J. Generation of high frequency oscillations (80-500 Hz) in different anatomical structures and their relation to the seizure onset zone. *Clin Neurophysiol* 2009d; 120: e29-e30.
- Jirsch JD, Urrestarazu E, LeVan P, Olivier A, Dubeau F, Gotman J. High-frequency oscillations during human focal seizures. *Brain* 2006; 129: 1593-608.
- Moelle M, Eschenko O, Gais S, Sara SJ, Born J. The influence of learning on sleep oscillations and associated spindles and ripples in humans and rats. *Eur J Neurosci* 2009; 29: 1071-81.
- Ogren JA, Wilson CL, Bragin A, Lin JJ, Salamon N, Dutton RA, et al. Three-dimensional surface maps link local atrophy and fast ripples in human epileptic hippocampus. *Ann Neurol* 2009; 66: 783-91.
- Siapas AG, Wilson MA. Coordinated interactions between hippocampal ripples and cortical spindles during slow-wave sleep. *Neuron* 1998; 21: 1123-8.

- Sirota A, Csicsvari J, Buhl D, Buzsaki G. Communication between neocortex and hippocampus during sleep in rodents. *Proc Natl Acad Sci USA* 2003; 100: 2065-9.
- Spencer SS, Goncharova II, Duckrow RB, Novotny EJ, Zaveri HP. Interictal spikes on intracranial recording: behavior, physiology, and implications. *Epilepsia* 2008; 49: 1881-92.
- Staba RJ, Frighetto L, Behnke EJ, Mathern GW, Fields T, Bragin A, et al. Increased fast ripple to ripple ratios correlate with reduced hippocampal volumes and neuron loss in temporal lobe epilepsy patients. *Epilepsia* 2007; 48: 2130-8.
- Staba RJ, Wilson CL, Bragin A, Fried I, Engel J, Jr. Quantitative analysis of high-frequency oscillations (80-500 Hz) recorded in human epileptic hippocampus and entorhinal cortex. *J Neurophysiol* 2002; 88: 1743-52.
- Staba RJ, Wilson CL, Bragin A, Jhung D, Fried I, Engel J, Jr. High-frequency oscillations recorded in human medial temporal lobe during sleep. *Ann Neurol* 2004; 56: 108-15.
- Urrestarazu E, Chander R, Dubeau F, Gotman J. Interictal high-frequency oscillations (100-500 Hz) in the intracerebral EEG of epileptic patients. *Brain* 2007; 130: 2354-66.
- Worrell GA, Gardner AB, Stead SM, Hu S, Goerss S, Cascino GJ, et al. High-frequency oscillations in human temporal lobe: simultaneous microwire and clinical macroelectrode recordings. *Brain* 2008; 131: 928-37.
- Worrell GA, Parish L, Cranstoun SD, Jonas R, Baltuch G, Litt B. High-frequency oscillations and seizure generation in neocortical epilepsy. *Brain* 2004; 127: 1496-506.
- Zelmann R, Jacobs J, Zijlmans M, Chatillon CE, Dubeau F, Gotman J. Is there a natural devision between ripples and fast ripples in humans? *Epilepsia* 2009a; 50 (S11): 32-3.
- Zelmann R, Zijlmans M, Jacobs J, Chatillon CE, Gotman J. Improving the identification of High Frequency Oscillations. *Clin Neurophysiol* 2009b; 120: 1457-64.
- Zijlmans M, Jacobs J, Khan YU, Zelmann R, Dubeau F, Gotman J. Ictal and interictal high frequency oscillations in patients with focal epilepsy. *Clin Neurophysiol* 2011; 122: 664-71.
- Zijlmans M, Jacobs J, Zelmann R, Dubeau F, Gotman J. High-frequency oscillations mirror disease activity in patients with epilepsy. *Neurology* 2009a; 72: 979-86.

Laminar electrodes in patients with temporal lobe epilepsy

Istvan Ulbert

Institute for Psychology, Hungarian Academy of Sciences, Budapest, Hungary
Faculty of Information Technology, Pazmany Peter Catholic University, Budapest, Hungary
National Institute of Neurosciences, Budapest, Hungary

In this chapter we present a new multiple channel laminar microelectrode (laminar multielectrode) system capable of recording local field potential and cellular firing activity in patients with medically intractable focal epilepsy. Microelectrodes offer a more detailed insight into the cortical mechanisms of physiological function (*e.g.* sleep, human cognition) and dysfunction (*e.g.* epilepsy). The results of recordings in patients with mesial temporal lobe epilepsy (MTLE) are presented.

The hippocampus usually plays a central role in the generation and maintenance of paroxysmal activity in MTLE. To monitor elementary neural processes underlying MTLE and understand their function, special microelectrodes were developed and used to elucidate the anatomical sources and network bases of interictal discharges in the mesial temporal lobe and define the functional connections between the closely spaced structures of the human hippocampus. Using microelectrodes, one can record laminar field potentials and single unit activity; laminar field potentials (FP) recorded from the hippocampus yield information about synaptic and cellular properties. Multiple and single unit activity (MUA and SUA) and current source density (CSD) analysis have been developed and used to investigate hippocampal circuitries (Ulbert, 2004a).

■ Technical note on laminar electrodes

All the patients who participated in this research underwent temporal lobectomy (amygdalo-hippocampectomy) as surgical treatment for long-standing medically intractable TLE. Each patient gave fully informed consent and the study was approved by the local IRB. Intraoperative recordings were only performed in the hippocampus and in the middle temporal gyrus (T2) which was later resected (Ulbert, 2004b).

Electrophysiology and surgery

Laminar multicontact microelectrodes (multielectrodes; MEs) were designed with a long shaft to reach deep structures in the brains of animals (Mehta et al., 2000a; Mehta et al., 2000b). In a previous paper (Ulbert et al., 2001a), thumbtack MEs (tMEs) were introduced to sample cortical structures (Ulbert et al., 2001b) in humans. These MEs were not adequate for quick intraoperative hippocampal insertion, and so were redesigned to minimize the additional time needed to mount the device and record during surgery.

The depth ME (dME) is manufactured in the same way as the tME (Ulbert et al., 2001a). The recent design is a 10-cm-long, 350-µm-diameter, sharp tip device with a stainless steel shaft and 24 contacts, formed by the cut end of 25-µm-diameter Pt/Ir wires. Centre-to-centre distance is 100 µm. To mount the dME, it was glued on a precision small sledge with epoxy, which was then attached to a micromanipulator with a screw-lock system, in order to be roughly positioned before the insertion. The micromanipulator was equipped with a precision dial advancing mechanism and a measure, so the depth of the penetration could be controlled with 100 µm accuracy after securing the rough positioning screw. All the equipment, preamplifiers and cables that passed into the surgical field were sterilized in ethylene oxide. The micromanipulator was mounted on a medical instrument holder during surgery, which could be fixed in position and allowed the surgeon to aim towards the hippocampus. Under visual control using an operating microscope, the electrode tip was advanced into the hippocampus after temporal pole resection. The pole resection was performed under general anaesthesia (fentanyl, diprivan and N_2O or isofluran or sevofluran and N_2O) from a small craniotomy (3-5 cm) to reveal the head and the initial part of the body of the hippocampus, which is a routine approach for hippocampectomy. After positioning onto the hippocampal surface, the electrode was advanced into the hippocampus with 2-mm increments. At each 2-mm step, recordings were made for 2-5 min continuously. One or two penetrations were made, usually crossing the CA1, dentate gyrus (DG), hilus, and CA3c. Spatial field potential gradient (PG; first spatial derivative of the laminar field potentials) was collected in the low-frequency band (EEG; 0.1-500 Hz, sampled at 2 kHz/channel, 16 bit) and high-frequency band (MUA: 150-5,000 Hz, sampled at 20 kHz/channel, 12 bit) simultaneously. In two patients, intraoperative electrocorticography (ECoG), and in one patient intracortical tME observations, were performed. Details about the amplifier and acquisition system have been previously published (Ulbert et al., 2001a).

Signal analysis

Our technique for localizing synaptic activity was the current source density analysis. It identifies possible synaptic generators using high-resolution maps of simultaneously recorded field potentials obtained across a laminated neural structure (Freeman et al., 1975). The second spatial derivative of these potentials closely approximates the synaptic current density. Simultaneous multiunit activity and action potential records lend convergent information to the definition of these processes and provide insight into local cellular responses to the field potential being analyzed. The origin of the active synapses and passive current returns are represented by sources and sinks. In cortical structures, current flows in the tangential direction can be assumed to be symmetrical (at least to the first approximation), and thus cancel each other out. Consequently, changes in current in the radial dimension imply local passage of current across the neuronal membrane. Excitatory postsynaptic potentials (EPSP) are due to the passage of positive charge from the extracellular to the intracellular space, termed a sink in CSD. Surrounding the sink are passive sources providing passive current return. In contrast, typical inhibitory postsynaptic potentials (IPSP) are due to active current sources and are surrounded by passive sinks. Active and passive transmembrane current flows can be distinguished using simultaneous MUA. An increase in MUA suggests that simultaneous sinks locate active excitatory synapses, whereas a decrease in MUA suggests that simultaneous sources locate active inhibitory synapses. The origin of these synapses may then be inferred from the known anatomical distribution of different pathways across cortical laminae (Ulbert, 2004b).

In the event of spatial potential gradient recording, the mathematical formulae of computing CSD differ from those used in non-gradient FP recordings, since the first spatial derivation is already performed in an analog fashion by the preamplifier. The CMRR (90 dB) of the preamplifier determines the accuracy of the first derivation, if we do not account for the inter-channel gain differences. Gain mismatches also occur in non-gradient FP recording setups. In our case, gain mismatch was less than 0.1%, corresponding to more than 60 dB ratio, and this is what actually determines CSD accuracy. We used the first spatial derivate formula, with Hamming-window smoothing to calculate CSD, with the correction for upper and lower boundaries. A continuous estimate of MUA was obtained by further filtering (300-3,000 Hz, 24 dB/oct), rectifying, and finally passing the signal through a 50 Hz low pass digital filter, (12 dB/oct) rather than integration (Ulbert, 2004b).

■ Results from neocortical and mesial temporal lobe epilepsy

Several publications have appeared recently in the literature which include the use of the laminar multielectrode technique in the field of human epilepsy research (Fabo et al., 2008; Ulbert et al., 2004a; 2004b) and human cognitive electrophysiology research (Halgren et al., 2006; Knake et al., 2007; Ulbert et al., 2001b; Wang et al., 2005).

We have shown in neocortical epilepsies (Ulbert et al., 2004a) that interictal epileptiform events in humans are initiated by large depolarizations, consistent with the hypothesis that the initial spike part of a spike-wave (SW) complex in humans corresponds to paroxysmal depolarization shifts which were observed previously in animals. Furthermore, the cortical layer where the initial depolarization occurs may differ according to whether the SW is locally generated or propagated from a distant location, and whether the SW is in the direct path of propagation or on the periphery of that path. In cortical regions of the main route of ictal spread, SWs begin with powerful depolarization in layer IV, which spreads to both supra- and infragranular laminae, resembling the normal cortical response to strong feedforward corticocortical or thalamic input. In the periphery of the main route of spread, the depolarization begins and remains supragranular.

Limited data suggests that within the spike initiation zone itself, the SW originates in layer V. Within cortical columns, as well as between cortical areas, the spread of the SW appears to involve the build-up of polysynaptic excitation. The patterns were relatively similar between patients, aetiologies and cortical areas suggesting stereotyped membrane current and firing activity during epileptic events.

In addition to neocortical applications, we have also developed laminar multielectrodes to sample hippocampal activity in humans (Ulbert et al., 2004b) with temporal lobe epilepsy (TLE). We have presented data obtained using a combined approach:

Intraoperative recording of local field potentials and single and multiple unit activity under anaesthesia, accompanied by histology and immunohistochemistry from the same hippocampal region of epileptic patients undergoing temporal lobectomy for drug resistant TLE under anesthesia. The stability of electrophysiology and accuracy of co-registration with histology were tested successfully. We have found large field potential spikes associated with single bursting units in CA1. Intracortical and subdural strip recordings from the lateral temporal cortex showed similar field potential activation patterns. A prominent oscillatory activity was present in the dentate gyrus with a highly localized field potential gradient and multiple unit activity. This pattern could be used as a landmark to define the position of the electrode in the hippocampus. Our findings indicate that some aspects of the local and network epileptiform activity in the hippocampal formation are likely to be preserved under anaesthesia. Electrophysiological identification of the functional state of the hippocampus together with its local structural correlates could further enhance our understanding of this disease.

In order to further investigate whether the subiculum is involved in the epileptic discharge generation in the hippocampal formation and how this is achieved, subicular and lateral temporal lobe electrical activity was recorded under anaesthesia in drug-resistant TLE patients undergoing temporal lobectomy (Fabo et al., 2008). Based on laminar FP, CSD, MUA and spectral analyses, two types of interictal spikes were distinguished in the subiculum. The more frequently occurring spike started with an initial excitatory current in the pyramidal cell layer associated with increased MUA in the same location, followed by later inhibitory currents and decreased MUA. For the other spike type, the initial excitation was confined to the apical dendritic region and was associated with a less prominent MUA increase. Interictal spikes were highly synchronized at spatially distinct locations of the subiculum. Laminar data showed that the peak of the initial excitation occurred within 0-10 ms at subicular sites, separated by 6 mm at the anterior-posterior axis. In addition, initial spike peak amplitudes were highly correlated in most recordings. A subset of subicular and temporal lobe spikes were also highly synchronous, in one case the subicular spikes reliably preceded the temporal lobe discharges. Our results indicate that multiple spike generator mechanisms exist in the human epileptic subiculum suggesting complex network interplay between medial and lateral temporal structures during interictal epileptic activity. The observed widespread intra-subicular synchrony may reflect both intrinsically and extrinsically triggered activity supporting the hypothesis that the subiculum may also play an active role in the distribution of epileptiform activity to other brain regions. Limited data suggest that the subiculum may even play a pacemaker role in the generation of paroxysmal discharges.

References

- Fabo D, Magloczky Z, Wittner L, et al. Properties of in vivo interictal spike generation in the human subiculum. *Brain* 2008; 131 (Pt 2): 485-99.
- Freeman JA, Nicholson C. Experimental optimization of current source-density technique for anuran cerebellum. *J Neurophysiol* 1975; 38: 369-82.
- Halgren E, Wang C, Schomer DL, et al. Processing stages underlying word recognition in the anteroventral temporal lobe. *Neuroimage* 2006; 30: 1401-13.
- Knake S, Wang CM, Ulbert I, et al. Specific increase of human entorhinal population synaptic and neuronal activity during retrieval. *Neuroimage* 2007; 37: 618-22.

- Mehta AD, Ulbert I, Schroeder CE. Intermodal selective attention in monkeys. I: distribution and timing of effects across visual areas. *Cereb Cortex* 2000a; 10: 343-58.
- Mehta AD, Ulbert I, Schroeder CE. Intermodal selective attention in monkeys. II: physiological mechanisms of modulation. *Cereb Cortex* 2000b; 10: 359-70.
- Ulbert I, Halgren E, Heit G, *et al*. Multiple microelectrode-recording system for human intracortical applications. *J Neurosci Methods* 2001a; 106: 69-79.
- Ulbert I, Heit G, Madsen J, *et al*. Laminar analysis of human neocortical interictal spike generation and propagation: current source density and multiunit analysis *in vivo*. *Epilepsia* 2004a; 45 (Suppl 4): 48-56.
- Ulbert I, Karmos G, Heit G, *et al*. Early discrimination of coherent *versus* incoherent motion by multiunit and synaptic activity in human putative MT+. *Hum Brain Mapp* 2001b; 13: 226-38.
- Ulbert I, Magloczky Z, Eross L, *et al*. *In vivo* laminar electrophysiology co-registered with histology in the hippocampus of patients with temporal lobe epilepsy. *Exp Neurol* 2004b; 187: 310-8.
- Wang C, Ulbert I, Schomer DL, *et al*. Responses of human anterior cingulate cortex microdomains to error detection, conflict monitoring, stimulus-response mapping, familiarity, and orienting. *J Neurosci* 2005; 25: 604-13.

Section IV:
Imaging in mesial temporal lobe epilepsies

Structural imaging of mesial temporal lobe epilepsy

Susanne Knake[1], Tim Wehner[1], P. Ellen Grant[2]

[1] *Epilepsy Center Hessen, Department of Neurology, University Hospitals Giessen and Marburg GmbH & Philipps-University Marburg, Marburg, Germany*
[2] *Perinatal and Developmental Science Imaging Center, Children Hospital Boston; Harvard Medical School, Boston, USA*

Magnetic resonance imaging (MRI) has made it possible to evaluate structural alterations in the brains of patients with focal epilepsy. Advances in magnetic field strength as well as new sequences and software developments continue to uncover anatomical substrates of focal epilepsy (Knake, 2005).

A tailored MRI study yields important information with regards to aetiology and prognosis of the patient's epilepsy. It has been shown for both children and adults that the presence of hippocampal sclerosis (HS) or other lesions associated with epilepsy on MRI indicates a reduced chance of achieving seizure freedom with antiepileptic medications alone (Kim, 1999; Cardoso, 2006; Spooner, 2006). On the other hand, the presence of HS on preoperative MRI is a strong predictor of seizure freedom after temporal lobectomy (Berkovic, 1995).

For this reason, every patient with unprovoked seizures should undergo at least one tailored MRI study early in the course of the disease. Key elements of such a study include volumetric 1 mm isotropic T1-weighted sequences (for example MPRAGE or 3D-SPGR) as well as T2-weighted images (T2 TSE or FSE, T2* or SWI, FLAIR). T2 and FLAIR images should be obtained in at least two dimensions, with one plane including coronal 2-3 mm slices angled to the hippocampi (ILAE, 1998). Gradient-echo sequences are used to detect haemosiderin and some calcifications, particularly in the setting of cavernous angiomas. Recently T2* images have been replaced by SWI images as they provide increased conspicuity for subtle foci of haemosiderin and aid differentiation between haemosiderin and calcification based on phase images. The use of gadolinium is not routinely necessary and can be reserved for patients in whom a neoplasm or an inflammatory lesion is suspected. For practical reasons, partiularly to avoid motion artefacts, the scanning time should be limited. A high-quality temporal lobe MRI protocol can be acquired in 30 minutes or less (Knake, 2006). It has been shown repeatedly that such a protocol increases the yield for epileptic lesions two to three-fold compared to "standard" MRI scans (McBride, 1998; von Oertzen, 2002). The advent of 32-channel phased array coils has enabled accelerated image acquisition, and recently, developed prospect motion corrected sequences provide 1 mm isotropic MPRAGE and

FLAIR images with exquisite quality achievable in the same time period. These accelerated prospective motion-corrected protocols are preferred over techniques such as periodically rotated overlapping parallel lines with enhanced reconstruction ("PROPELLER"), as such methods do not remove motion artefacts, but rather make them less obvious and result in images of poorer quality. However, if optimized, PROPELLER sequences can provide good tissue contrast and allow visualization of hippocampal subfields (Ericksson, 2008).

■ Qualitative analysis

HS is the most common histopathological substrate of refractory mesial temporal lobe epilepsy (MTLE). The radiographic features of HS were described shortly after MRI was introduced into practice and have been divided into primary and secondary criteria, with individual primary criteria offering sensitivity and specificity in the range of 75% or more (Kuzniecky, 1997; Oppenheim, 1998), compared to values of 30% or less for secondary criteria (Oikawa, 2001) *(Table I)*.

■ Hallmarks of hippocampal sclerosis

The MRI hallmarks of HS are atrophy of the mesial temporal structures in combination with signal hyperintensity on T2-weighted sequences (Jackson, 1990; Kuzniecky, 1987; Maertens, 1987; Triulzi, 1988). Although mesial temporal atrophy preferentially involves the anterior part of the hippocampus (Bernasconi, 2003), the pattern of hippocampal atrophy is diffuse in most patients (Van Paesschen, 1997).

These findings are most striking in patients with a history of febrile convulsions in childhood (Cendes, 1993; Scott, 2001), but no consistent correlation between severity of imaging findings and other clinical parameters such as age at onset, duration of epilepsy or seizure frequency has been found (Cendes, 1993; Van Paesschen, 1997).

In clinical practice, volume and signal intensity of the hippocampi are typically assessed by side-by-side comparison of the mesial temporal structures. Head rotation has to be taken into account when comparing the size of the hippocampi in individual slices.

Table I. MRI findings of mesial temporal sclerosis

Primary criteria	Reference
Increased hippocampal T2 signal intensity	Kuzniecky, 1987; Jackson, 1994
Hippocampal atrophy	Jackson, 1990; Cascino, 1991
Loss of the internal hippocampal architecture	Oppenheim, 1998; Hanamiya, 2009
Secondary criteria	
Thinning of collateral white matter in adjacent parahippocampal gyrus	Meiners, 1994
Diminished grey white matter demarcation in the ipsilateral temporal lobe	Meiners, 1999; Ryvlin, 2002
Ipsilateral temporal lobe atrophy and enlarged temporal horn	Bronen, 1991
Ipsilateral fornix and mamillary body atrophy	Kim, 1995; Kuzniecky, 1999

Although reformatting techniques allow correction of head rotation in most neuroradiological practices, this technology is often not available to the epileptologist who analyses the patient's MRI.

The radiographic diagnosis of HS depends on both the imaging protocol and the expertise of the reader (McBride, 1998; von Oertzen, 2002a). In one study (von Oertzen, 2002a), HS was diagnosed based on 7% of standard MRI scans read by non-experts, 18% based on the same scans by expert readers and 45% based on the scans by expert readers with the use of a dedicated epilepsy imaging protocol. Although diagnosis of HS is possible using the stated criteria with a sensitivity and specificity of 80-85% or more when validated against histopathology in patients who achieve seizure freedom after hippocampectomy (Kuzniecky, 1997; Cheon, 1998; Koepp, 2005), some important differential diagnoses have to be considered.

Great care should be taken when either primary or secondary criteria are considered alone. Volumetric hippocampal asymmetry up to 8% has been described in healthy control subjects in detailed volumetric studies (Van Paesschen, 1997; Wehner, 2007). Furthermore, the position of the hippocampi has been found to be asymmetric in control subjects (Van Paesschen, 1995). The dominant hippocampus is typically larger compared to the nondominant one. On the other hand, it has been estimated that 5-10% of patients with HS may have T2 signal hyperintensity or loss of the internal hippocampal architecture, but no volumetric atrophy (Jackson, 1994; Van Paesschen, 1997). Hippocampal atrophy is also seen in neurodegenerative diseases, in particular Alzheimer's dementia.

■ Differential diagnosis

If increased hippocampal volume is associated with increased T2 signal, the differential diagnosis includes acute swelling due to recent severe seizure activity (Scott, 2002), recent ischaemic injury or recent inflammation (*e.g.* limbic encephalitis) or more chronic swelling due to infiltrating gliomas, other low grade neoplasms (ganglioglioma and dysembryoplastic neuroepithelial tumours), or cortical dysplasia. Although acute swelling due to acute status epilepticus can progress to mesial temporal sclerosis (MTS) (Provenzale, 2008), MTS is a differential diagnosis for an enlarged hippocampus (Sokol, 2003; Van Paesschen, 1998). Normal variants seen in the hippocampal region not associated with seizures are hippocampal sulcal remnants and choroidal fissure cysts (Yoneoka, 2002; Sasaki, 1993). Both are equal to CSF in signal intensity on all sequences. Hippocampal sulcal remnants are normal variants that occur in about 10% of the population and appear as structures, of 1 mm to a maximum of 2 mm, situated between the dentate gyrus and the cornu ammonis. They result from a failure of normal embryogenic involution of the hippocampal sulcus. Choroidal fissure cysts are seen with increasing frequency with age and are located just above the hippocampus in the choroidal fissure.

Although MTS has been reported in patients who were subsequently found to have nonepileptic seizures during video-EEG monitoring (Benbadis, 2000), it is generally accepted that MTS is a feature highly specific to epilepsy. A recent study of 100 healthy controls and 10 patients with MTS could not identify primary signs of HS such as T2 hyperintensity, hippocampal volume loss or loss of the internal architecture in any of the subjects (Menzler, 2010). HS was not detected in any of the healthy subjects (95% confidence interval, 0%-3.6%), but in all patients with known MTLE-HS. Inter-rater agreement was perfect for the presence of HS. Thirty-three subjects had a unilaterally enlarged temporal horn as an isolated secondary criterion for HS with slight inter-rater agreement. However, hippocampal volume loss without increased T2 signal has been described in 34% of asymptomatic first-degree relatives of patients with familiar MTLE (Kobayashi, 2002).

On the other hand, HS is not infrequently associated with another type of epileptogenic lesion ("dual pathology"), most commonly focal cortical dysplasia. Therefore, the extra-temporal brain parenchyma needs to be carefully examined for the presence of additional pathology. Conversely, hippocampal atrophy, though usually of milder degree, has been reported in up to 29% of patients with extratemporal epilepsy (Adam, 1994).

■ Quantitative analysis techniques

The qualitative criteria outlined above rely on intra-subject side-by-side comparison. Consequently, bilateral abnormalities, which are not uncommon in patients with MTLE (Quigg, 1997), may be underappreciated. Quantitative imaging techniques such as hippocampal volumetry (Jack, 1990) and T2 relaxometry have been developed to overcome this problem and to increase the sensitivity of MRI to detect structural abnormalities in the mesial temporal structures in patients with TLE.

Volumetry

Manual or semiautomatic volumetry is a labour-intensive procedure which requires considerable experience. Hippocampal volumes need to be corrected for hemispheric or intracranial volume and compared to a control group matched for age, sex and handedness. A recent comparison of manual and automated volumetry using two automated segmentation tools (FSL and Freesurfer) found that the manually performed volumetry by an expert is more sensitive to small volumetric changes (Pardoe, 2009).

To our knowledge, the most comprehensive quantitative study of hippocampi in patients with intractable TLE to date examined 100 consecutive patients at one centre and compared them to 22 healthy control subjects (Van Paesschen, 1997). Interestingly, only 40% of patients had unilateral hippocampal atrophy in combination with elevated T2 relaxation times when abnormalities in these quantitative parameters were defined as deviations beyond 2 standard deviations from the mean of the control population, whereas 27% of patients had hippocampal volumes and relaxation times within the normal range. Small numbers of patients had either atrophy restricted to the hippocampal head, body or tail; or elevated hippocampal T2 relaxation times without atrophy, or bilateral or discordant abnormalities in hippocampal volume and relaxation time (Van Paesschen, 1997). Although these data illustrate the spectrum of hippocampal MRI features in patients with TLE, it should be noted that the authors did not differentiate between mesial and neocortical TLE.

Careful volumetric studies have also revealed morphological alterations affecting brain structures outside the hippocampus. In patients with MTLE, volume loss affected all temporal lobe gyri ipsilateral and the superior temporal gyrus contralateral to the seizure focus (Moran, 2001). Entorhinal cortex atrophy, ipsilateral to the seizure focus, has been demonstrated in patients with TLE and normal hippocampal volumes, but not in patients with extratemporal or generalised epilepsy (Bernasconi, 2001; 2003b). Interestingly, nine of the 12 patients in this study who underwent epilepsy surgery had histopathological evidence of HS. Thus, the entorhinal cortex may be more prone to injury than the hippocampus in patients with TLE.

Relaxometry

T2 relaxometry is a technique that quantifies the T2 signal intensity in an operator-defined area of interest. Due to the position of the temporal horn of the lateral ventricle, CSF may be included when sampling the mesial temporal structures, thus introducing a source of error. Whereas T2 relaxation times were initially measured in a single axial slice, advances in MRI technology provide measurement of T2 relaxation times of several hippocampal slices in a few minutes (von Oertzen, 2002b). HS is typically associated with marked elevations in the T2 relaxation time, and the sensitivity of this method to detect HS may exceed 90% (Namer, 1998). However, moderate elevations in hippocampal T2 relaxation time have been found in hippocampi without the characteristic imaging findings of HS, as well as in the contralateral hippocampus or hippocampi of patients with extratemporal epilepsy (Namer, 1998; Scott, 2003; Mueller, 2007). T2 relaxometry mapping of the hippocampi using a multislice sequence correctly lateralized the seizure focus in all 14 patients with hippocampal atrophy and in nine of 11 patients with volumetrically normal hippocampi (Bernasconi, 2000). In parallel to the volumetric changes discussed above, increased T2 relaxation times have been demonstrated to extend beyond the hippocampus into the anterior temporal white matter in patients with TLE due to HS (Briellman, 2004).

Automated post-processing techniques

Another approach to increase the sensitivity of MRI is the use of post-acquisition digital processing methods. Statistical parametric mapping (SPM) and voxel-based morphometry (VBM) are used to compare brain scans on a voxel-by-voxel basis (Ashburner, 2000). VBM has been validated against manual volumetric analysis. Patients with TLE and unilateral hippocampal atrophy were found to have structural brain abnormalities extending beyond the hippocampus, involving the cingulum, thalamus, insula, and frontal lobe, as well as ipsilateral temporopolar, entorhinal, and perirhinal white matter areas (Bernasconi, 2004; Keller, 2004; Cormack, 2005; Düzel, 2006). In a group comparison study, patients with left TLE who continued to experience seizures after a left temporal lobectomy had significantly reduced volumes of the ipsilateral posterior medial temporal lobe and contralateral medial temporal lobe, compared to surgically remedied patients (Keller, 2007). Another set of studies confirmed widespread brain abnormalities in patients with TLE and imaging evidence of HS, but failed to demonstrate consistent imaging abnormalities in a group of patients with TLE without HS (Mueller, 2006; 2007). Thus, findings derived from VBM parallel findings based on manual segmentation of individual brain structures (Bernasconi, 2002; 2003; Moran, 2001). Using automated techniques which examine whole brain neocortical thickness, patients with MTLE were found to have regional neocortical thinning in the lateral temporal cortex, as well as in frontal and occipital regions, compared to healthy control subjects (Lin, 2007; McDonald, 2008).

Diffusion tensor imaging

Diffusion imaging is based on the diffusion properties of water molecules in brain tissue; "diffusion" describes the random microscopic translational motion (Brownian motion) of water molecules (Connelly, 2005). Diffusion behaviour in a highly organized system like the human brain is restricted and complex. The magnitude of water molecular translation with diffusion imaging is referred to as the "Apparent Diffusion Coefficient" (ADC). Diffusion tensor imaging (DTI) provides information about the rate, magnitude, and directionality of water apparent diffusion per voxel in the brain. DTI contrast is therefore influenced by multiple microstructural factors such as cell loss, oedema, myelin and axons. A normalized metric of white matter coherence, termed "fractional anisotropy" (FA) is computed from the diffusion properties within a voxel. Specifically, the more tightly packed and coherent a white matter region is, the more likely the diffusion is dominated by few *versus* many directions and the greater will be the FA value. High FA values result in brighter signal intensity on an FA map. The signal abnormality in the DTI scan is presumed to reflect alterations in tissue properties, especially white matter organizational changes which are characterized by a change in FA and ADC, as compared to healthy matched controls. FA changes have been used to detect microstructural white matter pathology in epilepsy and neurodegenerative diseases (Salat *et al.*, 2005; Wieshmann *et al.*, 1999; Thivard *et al.*, 2005; Rugg-Gunn *et al.*, 2001; Eriksson *et al.*, 2001).

Besides detection of microstructural changes, DTI has been used to estimate fibre orientation in the brain and to evaluate the integrity of large fibre bundles such as the pyramidal tract. However, this technique is still investigational and pathological correlation is necessary to prove the accuracy of these results (Connelly, 2005).

In TLE, several studies have shown decreased FA values in the corpus callosum, the ipsilateral and contralateral temporal lobe, as well as in the frontal lobe of patients with MTLE (Arfanakis *et al.*, 2002; Nilsson *et al.*, 2008b; Kim *et al.*, 2008; Diehl *et al.*, 2008; Focke *et al.*, 2008; Gross *et al.*, 2006; Flugel *et al.*, 2006; Knake *et al.*, 2009). Interestingly, a recent study on children with TLE did not find any changes in FA relative to healthy controls. The preserved FA was in contrast to the reduced FA described in the white matter of adult patients with TLE. The authors suggested that this may relate to differences in the duration of epilepsy or in the vulnerability of white matter to seizures. Microstructural white matter changes therefore seem to occur as a consequence of the seizure-induced functional or structural changes in TLE (Nilsson *et al.*, 2008a).

In TLE, DTI may be used to identify more complex cases in the future. Studies correlating the amount of DTI changes with outcome are lacking but could be used to counsel patients preoperatively in the future.

■ Conclusion

In conclusion, dedicated MRI protocols allow the preoperative diagnosis of epileptic lesions in the mesial temporal lobe in the majority of patients with MTLE. Advances in magnetic field strength, imaging techniques and data post-processing increase the sensitivity and continue to uncover structural alterations in the hippocampi and their connected structures in the brains of patients with MTLE. In conjunction with video-EEG, neuropsychology and nuclear imaging, these data contribute to our understanding of the pathogenesis of the MTLE syndromes.

References

- Adam C, Baulac M, Saint-Hilaire JM, Landau J, Granat O, Laplane D. Value of magnetic resonance imaging-based measurements of hippocampal formations in patients with partial epilepsy. *Arch Neurol* 1994; 51: 130-8.
- Arfanakis K, Hermann BP, Rogers BP, Carew JD, Seidenberg M, Meyerand ME. Diffusion tensor MRI in temporal lobe epilepsy. *Magn Reson Imaging* 2002; 20: 511-9.

- Ashburner J, Friston KJ. Voxel-based morphometry-the methods. *Neuroimage* 2000; 11: 805-21.
- Benbadis SR, Tatum WO, Murtagh FR, Vale FL. MRI evidence of mesial temporal sclerosis in patients with psychogenic nonepileptic seizures. *Neurology* 2000; 55: 1061-2.
- Berkovic SF, McIntosh AM, Kalnins RM, Jackson GD, Fabinyi GC, Brazenor GA, et al. Preoperative MRI predicts outcome of temporal lobectomy: An actuarial analysis. *Neurology* 1995; 45: 1358-63.
- Bernasconi A, Bernasconi N, Caramanos Z, Reutens DC, Andermann F, Dubeau F, et al. T2 relaxometry can lateralize mesial temporal lobe epilepsy in patients with normal MRI. *Neuroimage* 2000; 12: 739-46.
- Bernasconi N, Bernasconi A, Caramanos Z, Dubeau F, Richardson J, Andermann F, Arnold DL. Entorhinal cortex atrophy in epilepsy patients exhibiting normal hippocampal volumes. *Neurology* 2001; 56: 1335-9.
- Bernasconi N, Bernasconi A, Caramanos Z, Antel SB, Andermann F, Arnold DL. Mesial temporal damage in temporal lobe epilepsy: A volumetric MRI study of the hippocampus, amygdala and parahippocampal region. *Brain* 2003; 126: 462-9.
- Bernasconi N, Andermann F, Arnold DL, Bernasconi A. Entorhinal cortex MRI assessment in temporal, extratemporal and idiopathic generalized epilepsy. *Epilepsia* 2003; 44: 1070-4.
- Bernasconi N, Duchesne S, Janke A, Lerch J, Collins DL, Bernasconi A. Whole-brain voxel-based statistical analysis of gray matter and white matter in temporal lobe epilepsy. *Neuroimage* 2004; 23: 717-23.
- Briellmann RS, Jackson GD, Pell GS, Mitchell LA, Abbott DF. Structural abnormalities remote from the seizure focus: a study using T2 relaxometry at 3 T. *Neurology* 2004; 63: 2303-8.
- Bronen RA, Cheung G, Charles JT, Kim JH, Spencer DD, Spencer SS, Sze G, McCarthy G. Imaging findings in hippocampal sclerosis: correlation with pathology. *Am J Neuroradiol* 1991; 12: 933-40.
- Cardoso TA, Coan AC, Kobayashi E, Guerreiro CA, Li LM, Cendes F. Hippocampal abnormalities and seizure recurrence after antiepileptic drug withdrawal. *Neurology* 2006; 67: 134-6.
- Cascino GD, Jack CR Jr, Parisi JE, Sharbrough FW, Hirschorn KA, Meyer FB, et al. Magnetic resonance imaging-based volume studies in temporal lobe epilepsy: pathological correlations. *Ann Neurol* 1991; 30: 31-6.
- Cendes F, Andermann F, Gloor P, Lopes-Cendes I, Andermann E, Melanson D, et al. Atrophy of mesial structures in patients with temporal lobe epilepsy: cause or consequence of repeated seizures? *Ann Neurol* 1993; 34: 795-801.
- Cheon JE, Chang KH, Kim HD, Han MH, Hong SH, Seong SO, et al. MR of hippocampal sclerosis: comparison of qualitative and quantitative assessments. *Am J Neuroradiol* 1998; 19: 465-8.
- Connelly A. MR Diffusion and perfusion imaging in epilepsy. In: Kuzniecky R, Jackson GD (eds.). *Magnetic Resonance in Epilepsy*. San Diego: Elsevier Academic Press, 2005, pp. 315-32.
- Cormack F, Gadian DG, Vargha-Khadem F, Cross JH, Connelly A, Baldeweg T. Extra-hippocampal grey matter density abnormalities in paediatric mesial temporal sclerosis. *Neuroimage* 2005; 27: 635-43.
- Diehl B, Busch RM, Duncan JS, Piao Z, Tkach J, Lüders HO. Abnormalities in diffusion tensor imaging of the uncinate fasciculus relate to reduced memory in temporal lobe epilepsy. *Epilepsia* 2008; 49: 1409-18.
- Düzel E, Schiltz K, Solbach T, Peschel T, Baldeweg T, Kaufmann J, et al. *J Neurology* 2006; 253: 294-300.
- Eriksson SH, Thom M, Bartlett PA, Symms MR, McEvoy AW, Sisodiya SM, Duncan JS. PROPELLER MRI visualizes detailed pathology of hippocampal sclerosis. *Epilepsia* 2008; 49: 33-9
- Eriksson SH, Rugg-Gunn FJ, Symms MR, Barker GJ, Duncan JS. Diffusion tensor imaging in patients with epilepsy and malformations of cortical development. *Brain* 2001; 124: 617-26.

- Flugel D, Cercignani M, Symms MR, et al. Diffusion tensor imaging findings and their correlation with neuropsychological deficits in patients with temporal lobe epilepsy and interictal psychosis. *Epilepsia* 2006; 47: 941-4.
- Focke NK, Yogarajah M, Bonelli SB, Bartlett PA, Symms MR, Duncan JS. Voxel-based diffusion tensor imaging in patients with mesial temporal lobe epilepsy and hippocampal sclerosis. *Neuroimage* 2008; 40: 728-37.
- Gross DW, Concha L, Beaulieu C. Extratemporal white matter abnormalities in mesial temporal lobe epilepsy demonstrated with diffusion tensor imaging. *Epilepsia* 2006; 47: 1360-3.
- Hanamiya M, Korogi Y, Kakeda S, Ohnari N, Kamada K, Moriya J, et al. Partial loss of hippocampal striation in medial temporal lobe epilepsy: pilot evaluation with high-spatial-resolution T2-weighted MR imaging at 3.0 T. *Radiology* 2009; 251: 873-81
- ILAE. Guidelines for neuroimaging evaluation of patients with uncontrolled epilepsy considered for surgery. Commission on neuroimaging of the international league against epilepsy. *Epilepsia* 1998; 39: 1375-6.
- Jack CR Jr, Sharbrough FW, Twomey CK, Cascino GD, Hirschorn KA, Marsh WR, et al. Temporal lobe seizures: lateralization with MR volume measurements of the hippocampal formation. *Radiology* 1990; 175: 423-9.
- Jackson GD, Berkovic SF, Tress BM, Kalnins RM, Fabinyi GC, Bladin PF. Hippocampal sclerosis can be reliably detected by magnetic resonance imaging. *Neurology* 1990; 40: 1869-75.
- Jackson GD, Kuzniecky RI, Cascino GD. Hippocampal sclerosis without detectable hippocampal atrophy. *Neurology* 1994; 44: 42-6.
- Keller SS, Wilke M, Wieshmann UC, Sluming VA, Roberts N. Comparison of standard and optimized voxel based morphometry for analysis of brain changes associated with temporal lobe epilepsy. *Neuroimage* 2004; 23: 860-8.
- Keller SS, Cresswell P, Denby C, Wieshmann U, Eldridge P, Baker G, Roberts N. Persistent seizures following left temporal lobe surgery are associated with posterior and bilateral structural and functional brain abnormalities. *Epilepsy Research* 2007; 74: 131-9.
- Kim JH, Tien RD, Felsberg GJ, Osumi AK, Lee N. Clinical significance of asymmetry of the fornix and mamillary body on MR in hippocampal sclerosis. *Am J Neuroradiol* 1995; 16: 509-15.
- Kim WJ, Park SC, Lee SJ, Lee JH, Kim JY, Lee BI, Kim DI. The prognosis for control of seizures with medications in patients with MRI evidence for mesial temporal sclerosis. *Epilepsia* 1999; 40: 290-3.
- Kim H, Piao Z, Liu P, Bingaman W, Diehl B. Secondary white matter degeneration of the corpus callosum in patients with intractable temporal lobe epilepsy: A diffusion tensor imaging study. *Epilepsy Res* 2008; 81: 136-42.
- Knake S, Grant PE. Magnetic resonance imaging techniques in the evaluation for epilepsy surgery. In: Wyllie E (ed.). *The Treatment of Epilepsy*. 4th edition. Philadelphia: Lippincott, Williams & Wilkins 2006, 1247 p.
- Knake S, Triantafyllou C, Wald LL, Wiggins G, Kirk GP, Larsson PG, et al. 3T phased array MRI improves the presurgical evaluation in focal epilepsies: A prospective study. *Neurology* 2005; 65: 1026-31.
- Knake S, Salat DH, Halgren E, Halko M, Greve DN, Grant PE. Changes in white matter microstructure and patients with temporal lobe epilepsy due to hippocampal sclerosis. *Epileptic Disord* 2009; 11: 244-50.
- Kobayashi E, Li LM, Lopes-Cendes I, Cendes F. Magnetic resonance imaging evidence of hippocampal sclerosis in asymptomatic, first-degree relatives of patients with familial mesial temporal lobe epilepsy. *Arch Neurol* 2002; 59: 1891-4.
- Koepp MJ, Woermann FG. Imaging structure and function in refractory focal epilepsy. *Lancet Neurol* 2005; 4: 42-53.

- Kuzniecky R, de la Sayette V, Ethier R, Melanson D, Andermann F, Berkovic S, et al. Magnetic resonance imaging in temporal lobe epilepsy: pathological correlations. Ann Neurol 1987; 22: 341-7.
- Kuzniecky RI, Bilir E, Gilliam F, Faught E, Palmer C, Morawetz R, Jackson G. Multimodality MRI in mesial temporal sclerosis: relative sensitivity and specificity. Neurology 1997; 49: 774-8.
- Kuzniecky R, Bilir E, Gilliam F, Faught E, Martin R, Hugg J. Quantitative MRI in temporal lobe epilepsy: evidence for fornix atrophy. Neurology 1999 11; 53: 496-501.
- Lin JJ, Salamon N, Lee AD, Dutton RA, Geaga JA, Hayashi KM, et al. Reduced neocortical thickness and complexity mapped in mesial temporal lobe epilepsy with hippocampal sclerosis. Cereb Cortex 2007; 17: 2007-18.
- Maertens PM, Machen BC, Williams JP, Evans O, Bebin J, Bassam B, Lum GB. Magnetic resonance imaging of mesial temporal sclerosis: case reports. J Comput Tomogr 1987; 11: 136-9.
- McDonald CR, Hagler DJ, Ahmadi ME, Tecoma E, IraguiV, Gharapetian L, et al. Regional neocortical thinning in mesial temporal lobe epilepsy. Epilepsia 2008; 49: 794-803.
- McBride MC, Bronstein KS, Bennett B, Erba G, Pilcher W, Berg MJ. Failure of standard magnetic resonance imaging in patients with refractory temporal lobe epilepsy. Arch Neurol 1998; 55: 346-8.
- Meiners LC, van Gils A, Jansen GH, de Kort G, Witkamp TD, Ramos LM, et al. Temporal lobe epilepsy: the various MR appearances of histologically proven mesial temporal sclerosis. AJNR Am J Neuroradiol 1994; 15: 1547-55.
- Meiners LC, van Gils AD, De Kort G, Van Der Graaf Y, Jansen GH, Van Veelen CW. Fast fluid-attenuated inversion recovery (FLAIR) compared with T2-weighted spin-echo in the magnetic resonance diagnosis of mesial temporal sclerosis. Invest Radiol 1999; 34: 134-42.
- Menzler K, Iwinska-ZelderJ, Shiratori K, Jaeger RK, Oertel WH, Hamer HM, et al. Evaluation of MRI criteria for the diagnosis of hippocampal sclerosis in healthy subjects. Epilepsy Res 2010, 89: 349-54.
- Moran NF, Lemieux L, Kitchen ND, Fish DR, Shorvon SD. Extrahippocampal temporal lobe atrophy in temporal lobe epilepsy and mesial temporal sclerosis. Brain 2001; 124: 167-75.
- Mueller SG, Laxer KD, Cashdollar N, Buckley S, Paul C, Weiner MW. Voxel-based optimized morphometry (VBM) of gray and white matter in temporal lobe epilepsy (TLE) with and without mesial temporal sclerosis. Epilepsia 2006; 47: 900-7.
- Mueller SG, Laxer KD, Schuff N, Weiner MW. Voxel-based T2 relaxation rate measurements in temporal lobe epilepsy (TLE) with and without mesial temporal sclerosis. Epilepsia 2007; 48: 220-8.
- Namer IJ, Waydelich R, Armspach JP, Hirsch E, Marescaux C, Grucker D. Contribution of T2 relaxation time mapping in the evaluation of cryptogenic temporal lobe epilepsy. Neuroimage 1998; 7: 304-13.
- Nilsson D, Go C, Rutka JT, et al. Bilateral diffusion tensor abnormalities of temporal lobe and cingulate gyrus white matter in children with temporal lobe epilepsy. Epilepsy Res 2008; 81: 128-35.
- Oikawa H, Sasaki M, Tamakawa Y, Kamei A. The circuit of Papez in mesial temporal sclerosis: MRI. Neuroradiology 2001; 43: 205-10.
- Oppenheim C, Dormont D, Biondi A, Lehericy S, Hasboun D, Clemenceau S, et al. Loss of digitations of the hippocampal head on high-resolution fast spinecho MR: A sign of mesial temporal sclerosis. Am J Neuroradiol 1998; 19: 457-63.
- Provenzale JM, Barboriak DP, VanLandingham K, MacFall J, Delong D, Lewis DV. Hippocampal MRI signal hyperintensity after febrile status epilepticus is predictive of subsequent mesial temporal sclerosis. Am J Roentgenol 2008; 190: 976-83.
- Quigg M, Bertram EH, Jackson T, Laws E. Volumetric magnetic resonance imaging evidence of bilateral hippocampal atrophy in mesial temporal lobe epilepsy. Epilepsia 1997; 38: 588-94.

- Quigg M, Bertram EH, Jackson T. Longitudinal distribution of hippocampal atrophy in mesial temporal lobe epilepsy. *Epilepsy Res* 1997b; 27: 101-10.
- Ryvlin P, Coste S, Hermier M, Maquière F. Temporal pole MRI abnormalities in temporal lobe epilepsy. *Epileptic Disord* 2002; 4 (Suppl 1): S33-39.
- Rugg-Gunn FJ, Eriksson SH, Symms MR, Barker GJ, Duncan JS. Diffusion tensor imaging of cryptogenic and acquired partial epilepsies. *Brain* 2001; 124: 627-36.
- Salat DH, Tuch DS, Hevelone ND, et al. Age-related changes in prefrontal white matter measured by diffusion tensor imaging. *Ann NY Acad Sci* 2005; 1064: 37-49.
- Sasaki M, Sone M, Ehara S, Tamakawa Y. Hippocampal sulcus remnant: potential cause of change in signal intensity in the hippocampus. *Radiology* 1993; 188: 743-6.
- Scott RC, Gadian DG, Cross JH, Wood SJ, Neville BG, Connelly A. Quantitative magnetic resonance characterization of mesial temporal sclerosis in childhood. *Neurology* 2001; 56: 1659-65.
- Scott RC, Gadian DG, King MD, Chong WK, Cox TC, Neville BG, Connelly A. Magnetic resonance imaging findings within 5 days of status epilepticus in childhood. *Brain* 2002; 125: 1951-9.
- Scott RC, Cross JH, Gadian DG, Jackson GD, Neville BG, Connelly A. Abnormalities in hippocampi remote from the seizure focus: a T2 relaxometry study. *Brain* 2003; 126: 1968-74.
- Sokol DK, Demyer WE, Edwards-Brown M, Sanders S, Garg B. From swelling to sclerosis: acute change in mesial hippocampus after prolonged febrile seizure. *Seizure* 2003; 12: 237-40.
- Spooner CG, Berkovic SF, Mitchell LA, Wrennall JA, Harvey AS. New-onset temporal lobe epilepsy in children: Lesion on MRI predicts poor seizure outcome. *Neurology* 2006; 67: 2147-53.
- Thivard L, Lehericy S, Krainik A, et al. Diffusion tensor imaging in medial temporal lobe epilepsy with hippocampal sclerosis. *Neuroimage* 2005; 28: 682-90.
- Triulzi F, Franceschi M, Fazio F, Del Maschio A. Nonrefractory temporal lobe epilepsy: 1.5-T MR imaging. *Radiology* 1988; 166: 181-5.
- Van Paesschen W, Duncan JS, Stevens JM, Connelly A. Longitudinal quantitative hippocampal magnetic resonance imaging study of adults with newly diagnosed partial seizures: one-year follow-up results. *Epilepsia* 39; 1998: 633-9.
- Van Paesschen W, Sisodiya S, Connelly A, Duncan JS, Free SL, Raymond AA, et al. Quantitative hippocampal MRI and intractable temporal lobe epilepsy. *Neurology* 1995; 45: 2233-40.
- Van Paesschen W, Connelly A, King MD, Jackson GD, Duncan JS. The spectrum of hippocampal sclerosis. A quantitative magnetic resonance imaging study. *Annal Neurol* 1997; 41: 41-51.
- Von Oertzen J, Urbach H, Jungbluth S, Kurthen M, Reuber M, Fernandez G, Elger CE. Standard magnetic resonance imaging is inadequate for patients with refractory focal epilepsy. *J Neurol Neurosurg Psychiatry* 2002; 73: 643-7.
- Von Oertzen J, Urbach H, Blumcke I, Reuber M, Traber F, Peveling T, et al. Time-efficient T2 relaxometry of the entire hippocampus is feasible in temporal lobe epilepsy. *Neurology* 2002; 58: 257-64.
- Wehner T, Lapresto E, Tkach J, Liu P, Bingaman W, Prayson RA, et al. The value of interictal diffusion weighted imaging in lateralizing temporal lobe epilepsy. *Neurology* 2007; 68: 122-7.
- Wieshmann UC, Clark CA, Symms MR, Franconi F, Barker GJ, Shorvon SD. Reduced anisotropy of water diffusion in structural cerebral abnormalities demonstrated with diffusion tensor imaging. *Magn Reson Imaging* 1999; 17: 1269-74.
- Yoneoka Y, Kwee IL, Fujii Y, and Nakada T. Criteria for normalcy of cavities observed within the adult hippocampus: high-resolution magnetic resonance imaging study on a 3.0-T system. *J Neuroimaging* 2002; 12: 231-5.

The role of cognitive fMRI in mesial temporal lobe epilepsy

Kirsten Labudda, Friedrich G. Woermann

Bethel Epilepsy Center, Mara Hospital, Bielefeld, Germany

In pharmacoresistant mesial temporal lobe epilepsy (TLE), anterior temporal lobectomy (ATL) is an effective treatment. About 38% to 75% of patients with TLE who undergo ATL become seizure-free, even in the long term (Elsharkawy et al., 2009; Wiebe et al., 2001). In chronic TLE, this circumscribed surgical procedure is always elective. A possible adverse side effect of ATL is postsurgical decline of memory functions, and, less frequently, language functions. Therefore, an individual presurgical cost-benefit analysis is necessary. Physicians need to answer patients' questions as to whether the epileptogenic anterior mesial temporal lobe to be resected is essential for cerebral functions which are important in their everyday life (language and memory, but also emotional processing). For lateralization and localization of language or memory-related brain areas, invasive methods such as the Wada test or electrocortical stimulation have been widely used in the past and are still in use in some circumstances. These methods carry an individual risk due to their invasiveness (Hamer et al., 2002; see also the chapter by Hamer, Kahane and Lüders in this book).

Functional magnetic resonance imaging (fMRI) is non-invasive. It is based on measuring cerebrovascular changes associated with neuronal activation to certain stimuli or tasks. These haemodynamic responses result in changing ratios of oxyhaemoglobin and deoxyhaemoglobin, and in MRI contrast differences which can be measured by exploiting the BOLD (blood oxygenation level dependent) effect. In the last decade, BOLD fMRI has contributed considerably to the identification of brain regions involved in sensory, motor, and cognitive functions. fMRI has also gained importance in the diagnosis of patients with epilepsy. Currently, fMRI is increasingly used to delineate eloquent brain areas from epileptogenic lesions in patients with epilepsy.

It is important to note that the clinical application of fMRI differs fundamentally from its use in neuroscientific research. Clinical fMRI is always conducted in single individuals. Therefore, blocked designs consisting of alternating activation and rest conditions are most frequently used due to their superior yield of contrast differences between neuronal activation and rest (Haller & Bartsch, 2009). Rest conditions of clinical fMRI tasks are often not specific enough to create a narrow contrast between activation and rest. Wide contrasts are appropriate because clinicians need to visualize as many components as possible associated with an important function (*i.e.* the neuronal network). The most important clinical aim of statistical fMRI analysis is to reduce false negative results. If a region is falsely judged as non-relevant for a specific function or task by presurgical fMRI, the subsequent decision to surgically remove this region may result in an unexpected postsurgical loss of function. In the current chapter we summarize the application of fMRI for lateralization and localization of memory functions in patients with TLE. We further review recent efforts to predict postsurgical memory outcome on the basis of presurgical fMRI activation. We additionally give an overview of the use and validity of fMRI language tasks in TLE patients.

■ Memory lateralization and localization

The temporal lobe is closely related to memory functions. Encoding and recall of information is particularly associated with mesial temporal lobe regions such as the hippocampus and parahippocampal gyrus (Eichenbaum & Lipton, 2008; Moscovitch *et al.*, 2006; Piolino *et al.*, 2009). Memory deterioration occurs frequently in patients with mesial TLE and such deficits can be observed in some patients prior to epilepsy surgery. However, 30% to 65% of TLE patients with unimpaired presurgical memory who undergo ATL may suffer from postsurgical memory decline (either learning or recall performance or both) (Baxendale *et al.*, 2007; Gleissner *et al.*, 2002; LoGalbo *et al.*, 2005). Patients with left-sided TLE have a higher risk of postsurgical memory loss, particularly in the verbal domain, whereas memory deterioration in patients with right-sided TLE is less frequent and less severe (Doss *et al.*, 2004; Feigenbaum & Morris, 2004). An important aim of the diagnostic process prior to surgery is to assess the extent to which the epileptogenic temporal lobe and associated structures, which are to be resected, are involved in memory functions. Non-invasive fMRI may become increasingly important for the prediction of postsurgical memory decline once the chosen fMRI tasks can be easily and reproducibly applied and evaluated, and once presurgical fMRI has been shown to predict individual postsurgical memory outcome in substantial numbers of patients.

For lateralising memory functions, different fMRI paradigms have been used for relatively small numbers of TLE patients (see overview in *Table I*). In these tasks, patients normally had to learn or recall verbal or visual stimuli during scanning. Although fMRI tasks differed between studies, results consistently showed that TLE patients had asymmetrically stronger fMRI activity in the temporal lobe, contralateral to the side of seizure onset. In left-sided TLE, memory-related activation was stronger in the right temporal lobe, and in right-sided TLE, left-sided activation was predominant. Reliability of memory lateralization by fMRI seems to be high (for concordance between fMRI and Wada test, see Detre *et al.*, 1998; Golby *et al.*, 2002). In patients with early onset epilepsy, fMRI asymmetry is specifically marked, most likely due to functional reorganisation (Griffin & Tranel, 2007). Patients with TLE and bilateral epileptiform activity or patients with extratemporal epilepsy often show bilateral mesiotemporal fMRI activity without lateralization during memory tasks (Janszky *et al.*, 2004). fMRI memory tasks are most helpful when they lead to symmetric bilateral mesiotemporal activity in healthy subjects. In these cases, possible asymmetric memory-related activation in TLE patients can be objectified most clearly and ascribed to models of hippocampal functioning (ipsilateral hippocampal adequacy *vs.* contralateral functional reserve). Tasks that demand the encoding of faces or the recall of visuo-spatial information from long-term memory, as well as combinations of visual and verbal learning tasks, have been reported (Jokeit *et al.*, 2001; Powell *et al.*, 2007). Simple tasks are preferable since children or patients with cognitive decline may also be studied.

Table I. Summary of the fMRI studies on memory lateralization
(lTLE: left-sided temporal lobe epilepsy; rTLE: right-sided temporal lobe epilepsy; HS: hippocampal sclerosis)

Authors	Year	Patients	Presurgical fMRT task	Main results
Detre *et al.*	1998	7 lTLE patients, 3 rTLE patients, 8 healthy subjects	Encoding of complex visual scenes	Symmetric bilateral mesiotemporal activation in healthy subjects. Asymmetric activation in TLE patients (contralateral > ipsilateral). 100% concordance between Wada test (memory) and fMRI lateralisation.
Dupont *et al.*	2000	7 lTLE patients, 10 healthy subjects	Verbal encoding (words)	Healthy subjects with memory associated bilateral activation within the occipital and ventrolateral prefrontal cortex and within the left superior and inferior temporal lobe. TLE patients with less activation mesio- and laterotemporal, occipitotemporal and occipital. TLE patients with frontal activation increase (compared to healthy subject).
Jokeit *et al.*	2001	16 lTLE patients, 14 rTLE patients (17 with HS, 13 with extrahippo-campal temporal lesions), 17 healthy subjects	Recall of an individual walk through the patient's everyday environment (Roland's Hometown Walk)	Healthy subjects with symmetric bilateral mesiotemporal activations. Asymmetric activation in TLE patients (contralateral > ipsilateral) allowing reliable lateralisation of side of seizure onset (> 90% correct lateralization). Number of voxels activated in the left mesial temporal lobe correlated with presurgical verbal memory performance; number of voxels activated in the right mesial temporal lobe correlated with presurgical non-verbal memory performance.
Golby *et al.*	2002	6 lTLE patients, 3 rTLE patients	Incidental encoding of scenes, faces, patterns and words (some stimuli were repeatedly presented)	lTLE patients with greater right-lateralized mesiotemporal activation. rTLE patients with predominant left-lateralized mesiotemporal activation. In 8 of 9 patients concordance between Wada test (memory) and fMRI lateralization.

Richardson et al.	2003	24 ITLE patients with HS, some with additional amygdala sclerosis, 12 healthy subjects	Incidental verbal encoding task (with neutral and affective words)	Healthy subjects with left mesiotemporal activation, primarily. In TLE patients mainly right-sided mesiotemporal activation.
Janszky et al.	2004	60 TLE patients, 20 patients with extratemporal epilepsy	Recall of an individual walk through the patient's everyday environment (Roland's Hometown Walk)	Mesiotemporal activation contralateral > ipsilateral in 75% of the TLE patients but only in 45% of patients with extratemporal epilepsy. Atypical fMRI activation pattern (i.e. bilateral or ipsilateral mesiotemporal) associated with bilateral epileptiform EEG activity.
Schaefer et al.	2006	7 ITLE patients, 7 patients with idiopathic generalized epilepsy	Verbal encoding and recall	Patients with idiopathic epilepsy with bilateral hippocampal activation. ITLE patients without significant memory associated activation. ITLE patients with less hippocampal but greater fusiform activation compared to the patients with idiopathic epilepsy.

■ Prediction of postsurgical memory deterioration

Some retrospective studies have demonstrated the use of presurgical fMRI for the prediction of postsurgical memory impairment. A relationship between ipsilateral mesiotemporal activation (particularly within the hippocampus and parahippocampal gyrus) and changes in postsurgical memory has been suggested *(Table II)*. In right-sided TLE patients, the postsurgical decline of non-verbal memory functions was linked to stronger presurgical fMRI activation in the ipsilateral, *i.e.* right-sided mesial temporal lobe (Janszky *et al.*, 2005). In left-sided TLE, left-sided activity was associated with postsurgical verbal memory decrements (Powell *et al.*, 2007; Richardson *et al.*, 2004). Thus, patients with stronger fMRI activation within the ipsilateral epileptogenic mesial temporal lobe were at a higher risk of postsurgical (material-specific) memory impairment. These results support the so-called "adequacy hypothesis" (Chelune, 1995). This hypothesis claims that the extent of functional ipsilateral epileptogenic mesial temporal lobe, prior to surgery, determines postsurgical memory outcome. The more memory function is supported by the mesial temporal lobe to be resected, the greater is the risk for postsurgical memory loss.

Some findings suggest that verbal memory decline can only be predicted by presurgical fMRI activation from verbal memory tasks (*e.g.* Powell *et al.*, 2007). Non-verbal fMRI tasks may be needed to predict non-verbal memory deterioration. However, other results imply that memory changes can be predicted "across modality". Frings *et al.* (2008) demonstrated an association between left-sided hippocampal activation induced by a visuospatial memory task and verbal memory changes in patients with left-sided TLE.

Table II. Summary of fMRI studies on the prediction of postsurgical memory changes
(lTLE: left-sided temporal lobe epilepsy; rTLE: right-sided temporal lobe epilepsy; HS: hippocampal sclerosis)

Authors	Year	Patients	Presurgical fMRT task	Results
Rabin et al.	2004	15 lTLE patients, 20 rTLE patients, 30 healthy subjects	Encoding of complex scenes	Symmetric bilateral mesiotemporal activation in healthy subjects. Asymmetric activation in TLE patients (contralateral > ipsilateral). Greater ipsilateral mesiotemporal activation was correlated with greater postsurgical decline of visual memory recall performance. Mesiotemporal asymmetry correlated with Wada test lateralization of memory functions.
Richardson et al.	2004	10 lTLE patients with HS	Incidental verbal encoding task	Relatively greater ipsilateral mesiotemporal activation (in proportion to contralateral activation) was linked to a more severe decline of postsurgical verbal memory. Presurgical fMRI activation asymmetries were the only significant predictor for postsurgical verbal memory changes.
Janszky et al.	2005	16 rTLE patients	Recall of an individual walk through the patient's everyday environment (Roland's Hometown Walk)	Patients with greater ipsilateral mesiotemporal activation (in proportion to the contralateral activation) showed a greater postsurgical non-verbal memory decline.
Wagner et al.	2007	11 lTLE patients, 10 rTLE patients	Verbal encoding and recall	Patients with a postsurgical decline of verbal learning performance showed greater functional connectivity between the ipsilateral hippocampus and the superior temporal gyrus and frontal cortical regions.
Powell et al.	2007	7 lTLE patients, 8 rTLE patients (all with mesial pathology, most with HS)	Incidental verbal and non-verbal encoding task (words, scenes, faces)	lTLE patients with relatively greater mesiotemporal activation had the most severe decline in verbal memory. rTLE patients with relatively greater mesiotemporal activation had the most severe decline in non-verbal memory.
Frings et al.	2008	12 lTLE patients, 10 rTLE patients (all with mesial pathology)	Encoding and recall of object locations in a virtual environment	Hippocampal activation asymmetries in lTLE and rTLE patients (contralateral > ipsilateral). The greater the presurgical ipsilateral hippocampal activation the greater the postsurgical verbal memory decline (in lTLE and rTLE patients).

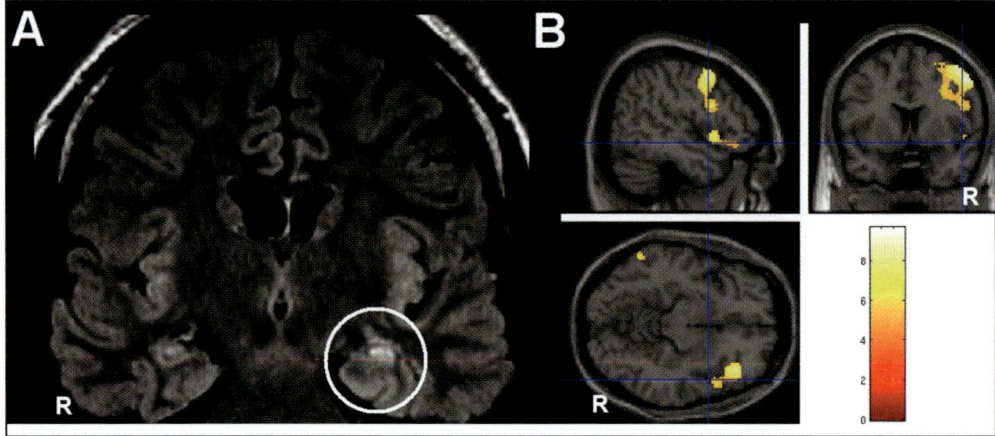

Figure 1. Patient with left-sided hippocampal sclerosis (A, circle) with partially conflicting lateralizing signs. Periictal signs lateralizing to the left hemisphere were left-sided eyelid blinking and postictal nose wiping with the left hand. Signs implicating the non-dominant hemisphere were automatisms with preserved responsiveness and dysprosodia. Language fMRI offered a solution showing right-sided dominance for language (B, note that on these fMRI maps the right side of the image is the right side of the patient). In this case the left hemisphere is the non-dominant hemisphere. This information facilitated the decision for surgery.

Although the results of these few studies are promising, studies with larger patient cohorts should be conducted to test the reliability and validity of memory fMRI. Furthermore, for clinical application, prediction of post-surgical memory should be demonstrated in individual cases.

All of the above fMRI tasks assessed episodic memory (*e.g.* learning or recall of lists of words or pictures). This is a pragmatic approach, particularly in the clinical setting, as these tasks do not require individual stimulus preparation. Addis *et al.* (2007) used individualised stimuli when assessing autobiographical memory retrieval in a small group of presurgical left-sided TLE patients. In accordance with previous studies (Lah *et al.*, 2008; Noulhiane *et al.*, 2007; Viskontas *et al.*, 2000), the patients had (mildly) reduced autobiographical memory function on the behavioural level. fMRI results showed reduced temporal activation related to retrieval within the left hippocampus, the right temporal pole and the posterior temporal lobe bilaterally. They further reported decreased strength of connectivity involving the left hippocampus. In contrast, connectivity between the left extra-hippocampal structures, such as the left retrosplenial and medial prefrontal cortex, was increased, possibly reflecting intrahemispheric reorganisation. These results: (a) confirm the possibility of activating anterior and mesial temporal lobe structures with an autobiographical fMRI memory task in TLE patients; and (b) suggest that alterations of neural correlates of autobiographical memory retrieval may reflect memory deterioration and/or compensatory mechanisms. A future direction may be to test whether autobiographical fMRI memory tasks can reliably inform about anterior temporal integrity or even predict postsurgical memory outcome.

The recent results from Binder *et al.* indicate that postsurgical memory outcome in TLE patients can be predicted using fMRI activation induced by a language fMRI task (requiring semantic decisions[1]) (Binder *et al.*, 2009; see also Binder *et al.*, 2008). Under their

---

1. Note that some authors used similar tasks declared as memory fMRI (see *Tables I and II*).

fMRI activation conditions, patients listened to animal names and had to decide whether the animals are found in the United States and whether or not the animal is "used" by humans. The authors calculated lateralization indices of supra-threshold activated voxel in frontal, temporal and parietal lateral brain regions associated with language processing. The whole brain as well as the frontal lateralization index correlated significantly with the postsurgical verbal learning changes (r = -0.39 and r = -0.41, respectively). Using a simple word generation fMRI task, we also demonstrated that a postsurgical memory loss in patients with left-sided TLE can be predicted from this non-invasive presurgical test (Labudda et al., 2010).

■ Non-memory fMRI tasks to assess functional integrity of the anterior temporal lobe

As mentioned above, the most important aim for the application of fMRI in presurgical diagnosis is to assess the functional integrity of the mesial temporal lobe structures which are to be resected. The anterior temporal lobe is not only associated with memory and language function but also with affective processes. In ATL, as well as other surgical techniques such as selective amygdalo-hippocampectomy or apical temporal lobe resection, the ipsilateral amygdala is removed. The bilateral twin structures called amygdala are involved in numerous emotional functions, such as fear conditioning, recognition of a variety of emotional stimuli (e.g. pictures of scenes or faces), and higher-order affective processes such as social cognition or theory of mind (Costafreda et al., 2008; Siegal & Varley, 2002). Some studies suggest that fMRI tasks using emotional stimuli are helpful to lateralize the side of seizure onset. Schacher et al. (2006) used an fMRI paradigm consisting of film sequences of fearful faces as the activation condition to clearly lateralise the side of seizure onset in mesial TLE patients. In contrast to symmetric bilateral activation in healthy subjects, TLE patients exhibited stronger activation within the amygdala contralateral to the side of seizure onset. In contrast, Batut et al. (2006) did not observe any amygdala activation in patients with right-sided TLE compared to healthy subjects when watching photographs of negative faces. Patients with left-sided TLE showed increased activation within the left amygdala. In contrast, Bonelli et al. (2009) was again unable to identify significant amygdala activation in presurgical patients with left-sided mesial TLE but was able to identify significant bilateral amygdala activation in right-sided TLE patients in a fearful face paradigm.

Overall, it is still unclear whether affective fMRI tasks are helpful for testing the functional integrity of anterior temporal lobe structures in TLE patients. Moreover, it is not at all clear whether activation induced by emotional fMRI tasks can be predictive (e.g. for potential postsurgical changes in emotion processing itself) or whether this temporo-anterior activation can serve as a surrogate marker, even for postsurgical memory changes.

■ Language lateralization and localization

In more than 90% of the normal population, language functions are specifically linked to the left hemisphere. Only about 5% have bilateral language organisation. The main anatomical landmark of language function within the left hemisphere is the frontal operculum, also known as Broca's area. This frontal region is particularly associated with speech production (expressive language components). Posterior temporal lobe structures, such as the angular and supramarginal gyrus, are mainly involved in receptive speech. Binder et al. (2008) and Bartha et al. (2005b) also reported hippocampal activation induced by language fMRI tasks in TLE patients. Whether the hippocampus is directly involved in speech is unclear, as the authors used a semantic decision task which was associated with long-term semantic memory retrieval.

In patients with TLE, atypical language organisation, i.e. bilateral or right-sided language dominance, is much more frequent, specifically in those patients with neuronal damage within the left hemisphere (Möddel et al., 2009). In a large sample, only 77% of right-handed epilepsy patients with left-sided mesial TLE (including hippocampal sclerosis) had left-sided language dominance, 16% had a bilateral and 7% a right-sided language pattern. In the study of Springer et al. (1999), the rate of atypical language representation in TLE patients was similar; 22% of their patients (n = 50) had atypical language representation (6% with bilateral and 6% with right-sided speech dominance). Spinger et al. identified factors which were associated with atypical language representation; early brain injury, as well as early age at onset, were linked to a higher probability of atypical language organisation. Another factor that may determine the degree of language lateralization is the severity of left mesiotemporal pathology; Janszky et al. (2006) reported that higher frequencies of interictal epileptic activity correlated with left-right shift of speech dominance measured by language fMRI in left-sided mesial TLE patients. Compared to epilepsy patients with extratemporal focal epilepsy and healthy subjects, language dominance was less lateralized in groups of patients with left-sided hippocampal sclerosis (Weber et al., 2006). These results point to the potential relevance of left hippocampal damage and/or disturbed left-sided fronto-temporal networks for language reorganisation. Aside from language shift from the left to the right hemisphere, intrahemispheric reorganisation has also been observed (Cousin et al., 2009). A resting state fMRI study demonstrated reduced connectivity between language areas in patients with left-sided TLE, possibly reflecting subtle presurgical language difficulties in these patients (Waites et al., 2006). Single case descriptions have further suggested the presence of crossed language organisation in epilepsy patients with temporal lobe lesion, e.g. typical left-sided activation within the frontal language area but right-sided temporolateral language activation (Ries et al., 2004). In single cases with mesial TLE and right-sided speech lateralization prior to surgery, it has been demonstrated that language dominance may shift back to the left hemisphere after surgery (Helmstaedter et al., 2006).

Determination of language dominance is also an important issue in the presurgical diagnostic process as some TLE patients (particularly those with seizure onset in the speech-dominant hemisphere) exhibit language deficits after ATL. However, complex language dysfunction, such as ongoing aphasia, are rare. Bartha et al. (2005a) investigated TLE patients with a detailed battery of tests in order to assess language functions such as spontaneous speech, language comprehension, naming, reading, writing and verbal fluency. They reported that four out of 23 patients with TLE had postsurgical language deficits in more than one domain. The most prominent language deficit observed in TLE patients was a deterioration in confrontation naming (Schefft et al., 2003), i.e. the ability to spontaneously generate the name of a presented object or person. These deficits may involve the inability to name animals or famous faces (Drane et al., 2008), and are most severe in patients after left-sided ATL (Glosser et al., 2003). Of the few longitudinal studies of postsurgical changes in verbal functions in individuals, Bartha et al. (2004) reported that four of 10 patients with left-sided TLE showed a significant decline of linguistic function. For seizure onset outside the left temporal lobe, patients with a higher age at seizure onset appeared to be at risk for such postsurgical decline in language function.

In these patients intra- or inter-hemispheric language reorganisation is more unlikely, compared to patients with early onset. To determine language lateralization, different fMRI tasks or combinations of tasks were proposed. To identify brain regions associated with expressive aspects of language, phonological or semantic word fluency, tasks were performed frequently. In the activation condition for these tasks, subjects had to silently generate as many words as possible beginning with specific initial letters (phonological fluency) or words belonging to predefined categories (semantic fluency), respectively. The technical effort needed to conduct these language tasks is small. The initial letters or categories could be given verbally to the patient via intercom. Despite the noise of the MR scanner, passive listening to spoken sentences or stories is sometimes used to identify language areas associated with receptive language. Neural correlates are usually located in temporoparietal regions (Wernicke's area, superior temporal gyrus, supramarginal gyrus). To localize both language components, more complex fMRI language tasks (*e.g.* rhyming tasks, semantic or syntactic decision tasks) or combinations of these tasks can be applied. Numerous studies with relatively small epilepsy patient groups (n < 25, most of which included TLE patients and some with exclusively TLE patients) have reported high concordance between language lateralization with fMRI and the Wada test (Adcock *et al.*, 2003; Benson *et al.*, 1999; Binder *et al.*, 1996; Gaillard *et al.*, 2002, 2004; Rutten *et al.*, 2002; Sabbah *et al.*, 2003; Spreer *et al.*, 2002; Yetkin *et al.*, 1998). However, some other studies did not confirm this (for word generations, refer to Woermann *et al.*, 2003; for semantic decisions, refer to Benke *et al.*, 2006; Wellmer *et al.*, 2008). In general, concordance between fMRI and Wada test language lateralization was higher for activity related to frontal speech compared to temporal language activation (Benke *et al.*, 2006; Deblaere *et al.*, 2004; Spreer *et al.*, 2002). It remains unclear whether the mean discrepancy between fMRI and the Wada test, of about 10% to 15%, results from an overestimation of bilateral language representation by fMRI or from an underestimation of bilateral language organisation by the Wada test.

Reproducibility of fMRI language lateralization by means of fMRI appears to be good (retest reliability: r > 0.80), particularly for frontal language activation (Fernandez *et al.*, 2003). Factors which are reported to reduce the reproducibility of fMRI language tasks include performing tasks following a recent cluster of epileptic seizures (Jayakar *et al.*, 2002) and the use of some anticonvulsive drugs such as topiramate (Jansen *et al.*, 2006). The reproducibility of fMRI is particularly weak regarding the exact localization of speech related areas. The concordance of language associated activation, between two separate fMRI language investigations with the same task, was only about 42% to 49% in a small group of 12 patients with focal epilepsy (Fernandez *et al.*, 2003). This reflects a general problem of fMRI; in particular, when bilateral activation or large clusters of activation are found, it remains unclear whether all of this activation is in fact essential for a function.

A recent paper by Suarez *et al.* (2009) emphasized another problem of language fMRI analyses; the calculation of laterality indices by means of counting supra-theshold voxels. It was demonstrated in neurological patients (but also in healthy subjects, see Ruff *et al.*, 2008) that lateralization indices can vary considerably depending on the threshold selected for voxel counting. A threshold-independent method was suggested for the calculation of lateralization indices. In their study, they significantly improved the concordance between Wada test language lateralization, electro-cortical stimulation lateralization (in 3 of 14 patients) and fMRI lateralization indices based on inferior frontal and supramarginal activation when using their threshold-independent approach, compared to the normal threshold-dependent method of creating a lateralization index.

There is only one reported study, that by Sabsevitz et al. (2003), which investigated whether presurgical fMRI language activations are predictive for postsurgical alterations of language functions. This study reported that the laterality index of temporal language activity correlated with postsurgical changes in naming performance. The stronger the fMRI activation within the left temporal lobe prior to surgery, the larger was the postsurgical decline in naming performance. Using DTI, Powell et al. (2008) demonstrated that in seven patients with left-sided mesial TLE, greater left-lateralization of fibre tracts (tracked from the inferior frontal gyri) was linked to a greater decline of naming after surgery.

■ Limitations of fMRI in epilepsy

For a discussion of general physiological and technical principles, as well as the limitations of BOLD-based fMRI, refer to e.g. Haller and Bartsch (2009), van Eijsden et al. (2009) or Logothetis (2003). In TLE, limitations of fMRI can be related to the patient. Beyond the well-known exclusion criteria for MRI (e.g. magnetic implants), other phenomena such as agoraphobia, learning disabilities, stimulus-related movements, epileptic seizures prior to or during the investigation, and pharmacological influences may reduce fMRI signal acquisition or even make it impossible to perform fMRI (Jayakar et al., 2002; Jokeit et al., 2001). Whether neurovascular coupling at the physiological basis of the BOLD effect is influenced by epilepsy-specific factors (e.g. propagating EEG activity, underlying brain pathology), is still unknown. Multicentre studies to standardise the application of clinical fMRI are seldom reported and have not yet been conducted in the field of epilepsy, language or memory.

Functional MRI is considered to be helpful for the identification of the so-called "eloquent cortex" (cortical regions which underlie a specific function). As outlined in this chapter, the resection of areas shown to be eloquent (e.g. for memory or language components) may be linked to a disruption of function. Removing the so-called "nociferous cortex" (epileptogenic tissue which has no function but impairs the function of other areas) might have a positive effect on cognitive abilities (Shin et al., 2009). Nociferous mesiotemporal cortex might appear less active, if not even "silent", in cognitive fMRI. The view that some of the temporal lobe regions which are to be resected are "silent" during language or memory fMRI investigations, may, however, be an error (overview in Devinsky, 2005). It cannot be excluded that these regions support other important functions. It is known that the temporal lobes support further functions which are normally not assessed prior to epilepsy surgery, neither by neuropsychological tests nor by cognitive fMRI. The temporal pole as well as the amygdala are crucially involved in different aspects of emotion processing, such as recognising anger, fearful faces and emotional music or in social functioning (Blair et al., 1999; Costafreda et al., 2008). Longitudinal studies should be conducted to first show whether these or other functions decrease in TLE patients after surgery, and secondly, if this is the case, to test whether specific fMRI tasks are helpful to predict the risk of such postsurgical deterioration.

References

- Adcock JE, Wise RG, Oxbury JM, Oxbury SM, Matthews PM. Quantitative fMRI assessment of the differences in lateralization of language-related brain activation in patients with temporal lobe epilepsy. *Neuroimage* 2003; 18: 423-38.
- Addis DR, Moscovitch M, McAndrews MP. Consequences of hippocampal damage across the autobiographical memory network in left temporal lobe epilepsy. *Brain* 2007; 130: 2327-42.
- Bartha L, Bauer G, Trinka E. Interictal language functions in temporal lobe epilepsy. *J Neurol Neurosurg Psychiatry* 2005a; 76: 808-14.
- Bartha L, Mariën P, Brenneis C, Trieb T, Kremser C, Ortler M, et al. Hippocampal formation involvement in a language-activation task in patients with mesial temporal lobe epilepsy. *Epilepsia* 2005b; 46: 1754-63.
- Bartha L, Trinka E, Ortler M, Donnemiller E, Felber S, Bauer G, et al. Linguistic deficits following left selective amygdalohippocampectomy: a prospective study. *Epilepsy Behav* 2004; 5: 348-57.
- Batut AC, Gounot D, Namer IJ, Hirsch E, Kehrli P, Metz-Lutz MN. Neural responses associated with positive and negative emotion processing in patients with left *versus* right temporal lobe epilepsy. *Epilepsy Behav* 2006; 9: 415-23.
- Batut AC, Gounot D, Namer IJ, Hirsch E, Kehrli P, Metz-Lutz MN. Language lateralization in temporal lobe epilepsy: a comparison between fMRI and the Wada Test. *Epilepsia* 2006; 47: 1308-16.
- Baxendale S, Thompson P, Harkness W, Duncan J. The role of the intracarotid amobarbital procedure in predicting verbal memory decline after temporal lobe resection. *Epilepsia* 2007; 48: 546-52.
- Benson RR, FitzGerald DB, LeSueur LL, Kennedy DN, Kwong KK, Buchbinder BR, et al. Language dominance determined by whole brain functional MRI in patients with brain lesions. *Neurology* 1999; 52: 798-809.
- Binder JR, Sabsevitz DS, Swanson SJ, Hammeke TA, Raghavan M, Mueller WM. Use of preoperative functional MRI to predict verbal memory decline after temporal lobe epilepsy surgery. *Epilepsia* 2008; 49: 1377-94.
- Binder JR, Swanson SJ, Hammeke TA, Morris GL, Mueller WM, Fischer M et al. Determination of language dominance using functional MRI: a comparison with the Wada test. *Neurology* 1996; 46: 978-84.
- Binder JR, Swanson SJ, Sabsevitz DS, Hammeke TA, Raghavan M, Mueller WM. A comparison of two fMRI methods for predicting verbal memory decline after left temporal lobectomy: Language lateralization *versus* hippocampal activation asymmetry. *Epilepsia* 2010; 51: 618-26.
- Blair RJ, Morris JS, Frith CD, Perrett DI, Dolan RJ. Dissociable neural responses to facial expressions of sadness and anger. *Brain* 1999; 122: 883-93.
- Bonelli SB, Powell HW, Yogarajah M, Thompson PJ, Symms MR, Koepp MJ, et al. Preoperative amygdala fMRI in temporal lobe epilepsy. *Epilepsia* 2009; 50: 217-27.
- Chelune GJ. Hippocampal adequacy *versus* functional reserve: predicting memory functions following temporal lobectomy. *Arch Clin Neuropsychol* 1995; 10: 413-32.
- Costafreda SG, Brammer MJ, David AS, Fu CH. Predictors of amygdala activation during the processing of emotional stimuli: A meta-analysis of 385 PET and fMRI studies. *Brain Res Rev* 2008; 58: 57-70.
- Cousin E, Baciu M, Pichat C, Kahane P, Le Bas JF. Functional MRI evidence for language plasticity in adult epileptic patients: Preliminary results. *Neuropsychiatr Dis Treat* 2009; 4: 235-56.
- Deblaere K, Boon PA, Vandemaele P, Tieleman A, Vonck K, Vingerhoets G, et al. MRI language dominance assessment in epilepsy patients at 1.0 T: region of interest analysis and comparison with intracarotid amytal testing. *Neuroradiology* 2004; 46: 413-20.

- Detre J, Maccotta L, King D, Aslop DC, Glosser G, D'Esposito M, et al. Functional MRI lateralization of memory in temporal lobe epilepsy. Neurology 1998; 50: 926-32.
- Devinsky O. The myth of silent cortex and the morbidity of epileptogenic tissue: implications for temporal lobectomy. Epilepsy Behav 2005; 7: 383-9.
- Doss RC, Chelune GJ, Naugle RI. WMS-III performance in epilepsy patients following temporal lobectomy. J Int Neuropsychol Soc 2004; 10: 173-9.
- Drane DL, Ojemann GA, Aylward E, Ojemann JG, Johnson LC, Silbergeld DL, et al. Category-specific naming and recognition deficits in temporal lobe epilepsy surgical patients. Neuropsychologia 2008; 46: 1242-55.
- Dupont S, Van de Moortele PF, Samson S, Hasboun D, Poline JB, Adam C, et al. Episodic memory in left temporal lobe epilepsy: a functional MRI study. Brain 2000; 123: 1722-32.
- Eichenbaum H, Lipton PA. Towards a functional organization of the medial temporal lobe memory system: role of the parahippocampal and medial entorhinal cortical areas. Hippocampus 2008; 18: 1314-24.
- Elsharkawy AE, Alabbasi AH, Pannek H, Oppel F, Schulz R, Hoppe M, et al. Long-term outcome after temporal lobe epilepsy surgery in 434 consecutive adult patients. J Neurosur 2009; 110: 1135-46.
- Feigenbaum JD, Morris RG. Allocentric versus egocentric spatial memory after unilateral temporal lobectomy in humans. Neuropsychology 2004; 18: 462-72.
- Fernandez G, Specht K, Weis S, Tendolkar I, Reuber M, Fell J et al. Intrasubject reproducibility of presurgical language lateralization and mapping using fMRI. Neurology 2003; 60: 969-75.
- Frings L, Wagner K, Halsband U, Schwarzwald R, Zentner J, Schulze-Bonhage A et al. Lateralization of hippocampal activation differs between left and right temporal lobe epilepsy patients and correlates with postsurgical verbal learning decrement. Epilepsy Res 2008; 78: 161-70.
- Gaillard WD, Balsamo L, Xu B, Grandin CB, Braniecki SH, Papero PH, et al. Language dominance in partial epilepsy patients identified with an fMRI reading task. Neurology 2002; 59: 256-65.
- Gaillard WD, Balsamo L, Xu B, McKinney C, Papero PH, Weinstein S, et al. fMRI language task panel improves determination of language dominance. Neurology 2004; 63: 1403-8.
- Gleissner U, Helmstaedter C, Schramm J, Elger CE. Memory outcome after selective amygdalohippocampectomy: a study in 140 patients with temporal lobe epilepsy. Epilepsia 2002; 43: 87-95.
- Glosser G, Salvucci AE, Chiaravalloti ND. Naming and recognizing famous faces in temporal lobe epilepsy. Neurology 2003; 61: 81-6.
- Golby AJ, Poldrack RA, Illes J, Chen D, Desmond JE, Gabrieli JD, et al. Memory lateralization in medial temporal lobe epilepsy assessed by functional MRI. Epilepsia 2002; 43: 855-63.
- Griffin S, Tranel D. Age of seizure onset, functional reorganization, and neuropsychological outcome in temporal lobectomy. J Clin Exp Neuropsychol 2007; 29: 13-24.
- Haller S, Bartsch AJ. Pitfalls in fMRI. Eur Radiol 2009; 19: 2689-70.
- Hamer HM, Morris HH, Mascha EJ, Karafa MT, Bingaman WE, Bej MD, et al. Complications of invasive video-EEG monitoring with subdural grid electrodes. Neurology 2002; 58: 97-103.
- Helmstaedter C, Fritz NE, González Pérez PA, Elger CE, B. W. Shift-back of right into left hemisphere language dominance after control of epileptic seizures: evidence for epilepsy driven functional cerebral organization. Epilepsy Res 2006; 70: 257-62.
- Jansen JF, Aldenkamp AP, Marian Majoie HJ, Reijs RP, de Krom MC, Hofman PA, et al. Functional MRI reveals declined prefrontal cortex activation in patients with epilepsy on topiramate therapy. Epilepsy Behav 2006; 9: 181-5.
- Janszky J, Jokeit H, Kontopoulou K, Mertens M, Ebner, Pohlmann-Eden B, et al. Functional MRI predicts memory performance after right mesiotemporal epilepsy surgery. Epilepsia 2005; 46: 244-50.

- Janszky J, Mertens M, Janszky I, Ebner A, Woermann FG. Left-sided interictal epileptic activity induces shift of language lateralization in temporal lobe epilepsy: an fMRI study. *Epilepsia* 2006; 47: 921-7.
- Janszky J, Ollech I, Jokeit H, Kontopoulou K, Mertens M, Pohlmann-Eden B, et al. Epileptic activity influences the lateralization of mesiotemporal fMRI activity. *Neurology* 2004; 63: 1813-7.
- Jayakar P, Bernal B, Santiago Medina L, Altman N. False lateralization of language cortex on functional MRI after a cluster of focal seizures. *Neurology* 2002; 58: 490-2.
- Jokeit H, Okujava M, Woermann FG. Memory fMRI lateralizes temporal lobe epilepsy. *Neurology* 2001; 57: 1786-93.
- Labudda K, Mertens M, Aengenendt J, Ebner A, Woermann FG. Presurgical language fMRI activation correlates with postsurgical verbal memory decline in left-sided temporal lobe epilepsy. *Epilepsy Res* 2010; 92: 258-61.
- Lah S, Lee T, Grayson S, Miller L. Changes in retrograde memory following temporal lobectomy. *Epilepsy Behav* 2008; 13: 391-6.
- LoGalbo A, Sawrie S, Roth DL, Kuzniecky R, Knowlton R, Faught E, et al. Verbal memory outcome in patients with normal preoperative verbal memory and left mesial temporal sclerosis. *Epilepsy Behav* 2005; 6: 337-41.
- Logothetis NK. The underpinnings of the BOLD functional magnetic resonance imaging signal. *J Neurosci* 2003; 23: 3963-71.
- Möddel G, Lineweaver T, Schuele SU, Reinholz J, Loddenkemper T. Atypical language lateralization in epilepsy patients. *Epilepsia* 2009; 50: 1506-16.
- Moscovitch M, Nadel L, Winocur G, Gilboa A, Rosenbaum RS. The cognitive neuroscience of remote episodic, semantic and spatial memory. *Curr Opin Neurobiol* 2006; 16: 179-90.
- Noulhiane M, Piolino P, Hasboun D, Clemenceau S, Baulac M, Samson S. Autobiographical memory after temporal lobe resection: neuropsychological and MRI volumetric findings. *Brain* 2007; 130: 3184-99.
- Piolino P, Desgranges B, Eustache F. Episodic autobiographical memories over the course of time: cognitive, neuropsychological and neuroimaging findings. *Neuropsychologia* 2009; 47: 2314-29.
- Powell HW, Parker GJ, Alexander DC, Symms MR, Boulby PA, Barker GJ, et al. Imaging language pathways predicts postoperative naming deficits. *J Neurol Neurosurg Psychiatry* 2008; 79: 327-30.
- Powell HW, Richardson MP, Symms MR, Boulby PA, Thompson PJ, Duncan JC, et al. Preoperative fMRI predicts memory decline following anterior temporal lobe resection. *J Neurol Neurosurg Psychiatry* 2007; 79: 686-93.
- Richardson MP, Strange BA, Thompson PJ, Baxendale S, Duncan JS, Dolan RJ. Pre-operative verbal memory fMRI predicts postoperative memory decline after left temporal lobe resection. *Brain* 2004; 127: 2419-26.
- Ries ML, Boop FA, Griebel ML, Zou P, Phillips NS, Johnson SC, et al. Functional MRI and Wada determination of language lateralization: a case of crossed dominance. *Epilepsia* 2004; 45: 85-9.
- Ruff IM, Petrovich Brennan NM, Peck KK, Hou BL, Tabar V, Brennan CW, et al. Assessment of the language laterality index in patients with brain tumor using functional MR imaging: effects of thresholding, task selection, and prior surgery. *Am J Neuroradiol* 2008; 29: 528-35.
- Rutten GJ, Ramsey NF, van Rijen PC, Alpherts WC, van Veelen CW. FMRI-determined language lateralization in patients with unilateral or mixed language dominance according to the Wada test. *Neuroimage* 2002; 17: 447-60.
- Sabbah P, Chassoux F, Leveque C, Landre E, Baudoin-Chial S, Devaux B, et al. Functional MR imaging in assessment of language dominance in epileptic patients. *Neuroimage* 2003; 18: 460-67.

- Sabsevitz DS, Swanson JM, Hammeke TA, Spanaki MV, Possing ET, Morris GL, et al. Use of preoperative functional neuroimaging to predict language deficits from epilepsy. Neurology 2003; 60: 1788-92.
- Schacher M, Haemmerle B, Woermann FG, Okujava M, Huber D, Grunwald T, et al. Amygdala fMRI lateralizes temporal lobe epilepsy. Neurology 2006; 66: 81-7.
- Schaefer M, Heinze HJ, Rotte M. Verbal memory encoding in patients with left-sided hippocampal sclerosis. Neuroreport 2006; 17: 1219-23.
- Schefft BK, Marc Testa S, Dulay MF, Privitera MD, Yeh HS. Preoperative assessment of confrontation naming ability and interictal paraphasia production in unilateral temporal lobe epilepsy. Epilepsy Behav 2003; 4: 161-8.
- Shin MS, Lee S, Seol SH, Lim YJ, Park EH, Sergeant JA, et al. Changes in neuropsychological functioning following temporal lobectomy in patients with temporal lobe epilepsy. Neurol Res 2009; 31: 692-701.
- Siegal M, Varley R. Neural systems involved in "theory of mind". Nat Rev Neurosci 2002; 3: 463-71.
- Spreer J, Arnold S, Quiske A, Wohlfarth R, Ziyeh S, Altenmüller D, et al. Determination of hemisphere dominance for language: comparison of frontal and temporal fMRI activation with intracarotid amytal testing. Neuroradiology 2002; 44: 467-74.
- Springer JA, Binder JR, Hammeke TA, Swanson SJ, Frost JA, Bellgowan PS, et al. Language dominance in neurologically normal and epilepsy subjects: a functional MRI study. Brain 1999; 122: 2033-46.
- Suarez RO, Whalen S, Nelson AP, Tie Y, Meadows ME, Radmanesh A, et al. Threshold-independent functional MRI determination of language dominance: a validation study against clinical gold standards. Epilepsy Behav 2009; 16: 288-97.
- van Eijsden P, Hyder F, Rothman DL, Shulman RG. Neurophysiology of functional imaging. Neuroimage 2009; 45: 1047-54.
- Viskontas IV, McAndrews MP, Moscovitch M. Remote episodic memory deficits in patients with unilateral temporal lobe epilepsy and excisions. J Neurosci 2000; 20: 5853-7.
- Waites AB, Briellmann RS, Saling MM, Abbott DF, Jackson GD. Functional connectivity networks are disrupted in left temporal lobe epilepsy. Ann Neurol 2006; 59: 335-43.
- Weber B, Wellmer J, Reuber M, Mormann F, Weis S, Urbach H, et al. Left hippocampal pathology is associated with atypical language lateralization in patients with focal epilepsy. Brain 2006; 129: 346-51.
- Wellmer J, Weber B, Weis S, Klaver P, Urbach H, Reul J, et al. Strongly lateralized activation in language fMRI of atypical dominant patients-implications for presurgical work-up. Epilepsy Res 2008; 80: 67-76.
- Wiebe S, Blume WT, Girvin JP, Eliasziw M, Effectiveness and Efficiency of Surgery for Temporal Lobe Epilepsy Study Group. A randomized, controlled trial of surgery for temporal-lobe epilepsy. N Engl J Med 2001; 345: 311-8.
- Woermann FG, Jokeit H, Luerding R, Freitag H, Schulz R, Guertler S, et al. Language lateralization by Wada test and fMRI in 100 patients with epilepsy. Neurology 2003; 61: 699-701.
- Yetkin FZ, Swanson S, Fischer M, Akansel G, Morris G, Mueller W, et al. Functional MR of frontal lobe activation: comparison with Wada language results. Am J Neuroradiol 1998; 19: 1095-8.

The role of the Wada test and functional transcranial Doppler sonography in the presurgical diagnosis of mesial temporal lobe epilepsy

Tobias Loddenkemper[1], Anja Haag[2]

[1] *Pediatric Epilepsy Center, Children's Hospital Boston, Harvard Medical School, Boston, USA*
[2] *Epilepsy Center Hessen, Department of Neurology, University Hospitals Giessen and Marburg GmbH & Philipps-University Marburg, Marburg, Germany*

Localization of eloquent cortical areas is crucial for the prediction of outcome and functional deficits after epilepsy surgery. As well as localization by structural lesion and cortical stimulation, intracarotid amobarbital testing is one of the most established techniques to lateralize language (Wada, 1949; Wada & Rasmussen, 1960). The procedure was expanded to test for memory lateralization and predict global aphasia prior to temporal lobectomy by Milner in 1962 (Milner *et al.*, 1962). Intracarotid amobarbital testing for the prediction of minor verbal and figural memory deficits after temporal lobectomy is now routinely used (Helmstaedter *et al.*, 2004; Loring *et al.*, 1995). Several recent publications suggest a re-evaluation of indications for intracarotid amobarbital testing, particularly in patients with temporal lobe epilepsy (Haag *et al.*, 2008; Baxendale *et al.*, 2008a; Loddenkemper, 2008b).

▪ Frequency and prevalence of Wada testing in patients undergoing presurgical evaluation for mesial temporal lobe epilepsies

The frequency of Wada tests in all presurgical evaluations is declining. In a survey in 1993, 85% of all epilepsy centres performed Wada tests on all of their patients undergoing presurgical work-up (Rausch *et al.*, 1993). In a survey of 26 European epilepsy centres, Haag *et al.* noted a decline of Wada tests from 56% in 2000 to 35% in 2005 (Haag *et al.*, 2008). Helmstaedter reported a similar decline from 70% in 1988 to less than 10% in 2004 at an epilepsy centre in Bonn, Germany (Helmstaedter, 2008), which compares with a similar decline from 99% in 1997 to 20% in 2007 at an epilepsy centre in Cleveland in the United States (Loddenkemper, 2008b).

Only one previous study has focused on the frequency of Wada tests in temporal lobe epilepsy (TLE); Baxendale *et al.* (2008a). In this survey of 92 epilepsy centres in 31 countries, 12% stated that they perform Wada tests in every case, 17.4% in more than

95% of cases, 10.9% in around 75% of cases, 9.8% in around 50% of cases, 14.1% in around 25% of cases, 22.8% in less than 5% of cases and 13% never. For the purpose of this chapter, we reviewed Wada testing in 777 temporal lobectomy patients prior to epilepsy surgery at the Cleveland Clinic, from 1997 to 2007, and noted a decline from 81% in 1997 to 14% in 2007 (*Figure 1*).

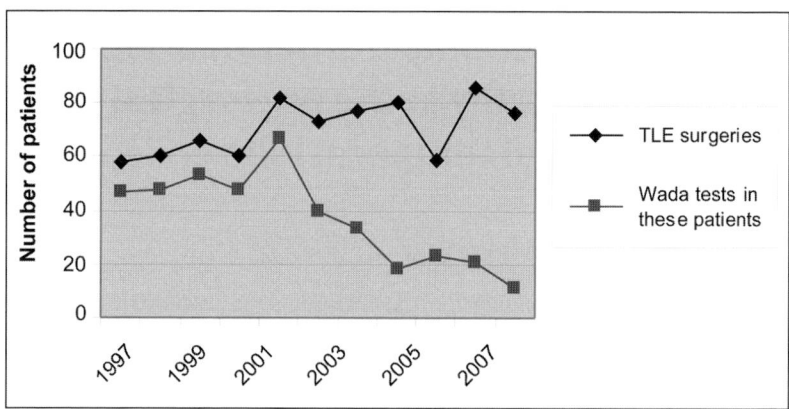

Figure 1. Decline of Wada tests in patients with temporal lobe epilepsy (TLE) at Cleveland clinic over the last decade.

Wada test indications in mesial temporal lobe epilepsy

The decline in Wada testing frequency may be related to the lack of absolute indications. Four major indications have been identified previously, including language lateralization, seizure focus lateralization, seizure outcome prediction, and prediction of memory decline and global amnesia after surgery (Baxendale *et al.*, 2008a). Seizure outcome prediction by Wada testing is rare and is usually not the only indication for Wada testing.

Seizure focus lateralization

Based on the survey by Baxendale *et al.*, the majority of epileptologists (89.1%) were either very confident or fairly confident to exclude the Wada test from presurgical work-up in order to localize the seizure focus in TLE patients, suggesting that this is a clinically less important indication.

Language lateralization

In mesial temporal lobe epilepsy (MTLE), language lateralization is rarely necessary for patients undergoing anterior temporal lobectomy to the vein of Labbé or resection of the mesial temporal structures, as primary language areas such as Broca's and Wernicke's area are not affected. Naming difficulties for patients with lesions of the secondary basal temporal speech area (Lüders' area) are usually transient. In the survey by Baxendale *et al.*, 66.3% of epileptologists indicated that they felt confident excluding the Wada test from their presurgical diagnostic test arsenal. Early left hemispheric brain lesions can result in atypical (*e.g.* bilateral or right hemispheric) language dominance (Möddel *et al.*, 2004). This is more probable if the lesion is very broad or is located in primary language areas (Helmstaedter *et al.*, 1997; Woods *et al.*, 1988), but has also been reported in smaller, more localized lesions such as MTLE in the setting of hippocampal atrophy and sclerosis

(Helmstaedter et al., 1997; Brazdil et al., 2005). Higher rates of atypical non-left hemispheric language representation have been reported in left TLE (Knake et al., 2003), which can be associated with corresponding interhemispheric memory reorganisation and thus may protect against postoperative memory decline (Kim et al., 2003).

Memory deficit prevention

According to the survey of Baxendale et al. (2008a), many epileptologists still use Wada testing for the prediction of global amnesia or minor memory deficits after surgery in temporal lobe epilepsy surgery candidates. Memory deficit prediction may be a remaining benefit of Wada testing in MTLE (Lineweaver et al., 2006).

Potential benefits of Wada testing in mesial temporal lobe epilepsy

Prediction of global amnesia after surgery for mesial temporal lobe epilepsy

The incidence of global amnesia after temporal lobectomy was estimated at 1 in 218 patients and the positive predictive value was estimated at 25% (Rausch & Langfitt, 1991).

A review of previously reported test results, involving true positives (patients who developed amnesia after a temporal lobectomy following a positive Wada memory test), false positives (patients who did not develop amnesia after temporal lobectomy, despite a positive Wada test), false negatives (patients who become amnesic, despite a negative Wada test) and true negatives (patients who did not demonstrate amnesia on Wada testing and did well after surgery), has assisted in elucidating Wada test validity (Goldstein & Gilliam, 2006; Simkins-Bullock, 2000; Baxendale et al., 2008c).

A review of the few previously reported true positive cases of patients, who underwent intracarotid amobarbital testing predicting memory loss and who subsequently underwent temporal lobectomy and suffered global amnesia, showed that all had contralateral hippocampal lesions (Baxendale et al., 2008b; Simkins-Bullock, 2000). True negatives are usually not reported because the outcome is expected.

Only a few cases of false negative test results, with no memory failure based on the intracarotid amobarbital procedure (IAP) but subsequent global amnesia after surgery, have been reported (Dodrill, 2006; Simkins-Bullock, 2000) of which only one was well described (Barr et al., 1992). Speculation of the possible reasons for failure in this case include the presentation of objects relatively late during the test and previous ipsilateral neocortical temporal lobe epilepsy surgery, potentially facilitating reorganisation (Barr et al., 1992).

Several authors have reported false positive Wada memory test results (Kubu et al., 2000a; Novelly & Williamson, 1989; Simkins-Bullock, 2000), and based on these, patients may be unnecessarily excluded from epilepsy surgery. Due to the low prevalence of postoperative amnesia, Simkins-Bullock (2000) reported: "it is difficult to demonstrate that the IAP is able to improve significantly our predictive abilities beyond what we would obtain should we simply state that no patient is at risk for amnesia following surgery".

Prediction of material-specific memory change following surgery for mesial temporal lobe epilepsy

Based on the model of functional reserve of the contralateral hippocampus and the model of functional adequacy of the ipsilateral hippocampus, prediction of minor memory deficits after temporal lobectomy was attempted based on Wada test results. Multivariate regression studies have found that Wada memory test results provide unique information which can assist in predicting memory outcome after surgery (Lineweaver et al., 2006). It is unclear, however, whether the benefits of this additional predictive value outweigh the risks of the procedure. Others have found, in a review of 15 studies, that the IAP was not an indicator for material-specific memory loss (Goldstein & Gilliam, 2006).

■ Potential risks of Wada testing

Major complications during the Wada test were seen in 1.09% of patients, including 0.36% with permanent deficit in the survey by Haag et al. (2008). Another retrospective single centre series found complications in up to 10.9% of patients and lasting deficits after intracarotid amobarbital testing in up to 0.6% (Loddenkemper et al., 2008b). In this series, complications included encephalopathy (7.2%), seizures (1.2%), strokes (0.6%), transient ischaemic attacks (0.6%), localized haemorrhage at the catheter insertion site (0.6%), carotid artery dissections (0.4%), allergic reaction to contrast (0.3%), bleeding from the catheter insertion site (0.1%), and infection (0.1%) (Loddenkemper et al., 2008b).

Variability

In addition, the variability of procedural protocols between different centres, as well as the variability within the same centre, specifically for memory test results, raises concerns about the validity, reliability and predictive value of the test results (Schulze-Bonhage et al., 2004; Loddenkemper et al., 2007a; 2007b; 2008a). Additional concerns include unblinded observers, fluctuating cooperation, the memory testing paradigm due to limited memory testing time during inactivation, potential crossover of barbiturate, and incomplete and variable inactivation of brain regions responsible for memory function. The vascular supply to the hippocampus consists mainly of PCA and lenticulostriate arteries, whereas Wada testing inactivates MCA territory and anterior circulation. A review of 1,190 patients at the Cleveland Clinic revealed that up to 4% of procedures were repeated (Loddenkemper et al., 2007a). Obtundation and the inability to test for memory were the most frequent reasons for repetition. In this series, language lateralization was always reproduced. However, repeat memory test results did not correlate well and memory lateralization was not reproducible in up to 63% of patients (Loddenkemper et al., 2007a).

■ Alternative techniques to assess language and memory lateralization

The availability of alternative non-invasive testing techniques for language and memory localization and the prediction of postoperative outcome and deficits by non-invasive tests may sway decision-making further from Wada testing. Due to the risks of morbidity and methodological concerns (Haag et al., 2008; Loddenkemper et al., 2007a; Rausch et al., 1993; Simkins-Bullock, 2000) non-invasive functional imaging methods for language and memory testing are increasingly considered as routine preoperative tests in patients with MTLE. Non-invasive functional imaging techniques have a lower morbidity, are frequently less expensive, and can easily be repeated if necessary. Due to the non-invasive nature of these tests, normative data from healthy volunteers can be collected without ethical objections.

However, most non-invasive imaging tools (apart from repetitive transcranial magnetic stimulation [rTMS]), are activation based and do not produce a temporary functional loss, which leads to reduced content validity. In particular, for localizing functional imaging methods (such as functional magnetic resonance imaging [fMRI]), consideration should be given to whether all activated brain areas are crucial for the preservation of the cognitive function in question when results are interpreted.

Alternative language (assessment) imaging techniques

fMRI is the most widely used, non-invasive, functional imaging alternative technique for language localization (Binder et al., 1996; Richardson et al., 2004) and the technique is described elsewhere in this book in detail. Unlike Wada testing, fMRI provides localizing language information in addition to lateralization. Activation paradigms with mainly frontal activation of Broca's area have been shown to have higher concordance with Wada test lateralization than paradigms targeting temporal language areas (Wernicke's area) (Benke et al., 2006; Swanson et al., 2007). In several patients with TLE and left-sided language dominance based on Wada-testing, fMRI did not show reliable language lateralization (Woermann et al., 2003; Benke et al., 2006). The combination of different language paradigms may enhance concordance with Wada testing and may be superior to single paradigm lateralization (Gaillard et al., 2004).

Functional transcranial Doppler sonography

Functional transcranial Doppler sonography (fTCD) is based on the assumption that cognitive activity results in increased regional cerebral blood flow in functional relevant brain areas, referred to as "neurovascular coupling". Comparable to event-related potentials, fTCD usually involves continuous measurement of cerebral blood flow velocity (CBFV) in homologous basal brain arteries, while a cognitive task is performed repeatedly. Alternating periods of cognitive activation and resting are recorded. Increase in CBFV during activation relative to the resting condition is compared bilaterally. A relative functional dominance is postulated for the hemisphere with greater increase in CBFV.

Hemispheric lateralization of various cognitive functions has been investigated by fTCD, including visual function (Sturzenegger et al., 1996), attention (Floel et al., 2002), visuospatial function (Floel et al., 2001), motor function (Matteis et al., 2001), music perception (Matteis et al., 1997), calculation (Vingerhoets & Stroobant, 2002), and language lateralization (Silvestrini et al., 1994; Knecht et al., 1996). fTCD for language lateralization has shown highly concordant results with Wada testing (Rihs et al., 1999; Knake et al., 2003) and fMRI (Deppe et al., 2000).

Functional transcranial Doppler sonography language lateralization: technique and paradigm

CBFV of the medial cerebral arteries (MCAs) is continuously measured at a depth of 50-54 mm with two 2 MHz-transducer probes attached to a headband and placed at the temporal skull windows, using a commercially available transcranial Doppler ultrasonic device which provides a monitoring (i.e. continuous recording) function. The patient is seated comfortably in front of a computer screen and silent word generation is used for language testing. Previous fMRI studies have supported the notion that this paradigm leads to predominantly frontal activation (Lehericy et al., 2000). Twenty epochs of continuous CBFV are recorded. Each epoch consists of a resting phase (32.5 sec.) and an activation phase (27.5 sec.). In order to control for frequently right-hemispheric attention- and preparation-related regional cerebral blood flow changes, the activation phase starts with a cueing tone and the language activation period starts five seconds after the cueing tone (Knecht et al., 1996). A letter is then presented for 2.5 seconds on a computer screen. The patient is instructed to silently generate as many words as possible starting with the letter. After 15 seconds another tone is heard and the patient is instructed to articulate some of the words they had previously generated for five seconds in order to increase motivation and compliance. A third tone signals the end of the activation phase and initiates the next resting period. The instructions for this time period are to stop generating words and relax while imagining a night sky. The simulation computer is synchronized with the Doppler machine and an analogue marker at the beginning of each activation phase permits off-line analysis of signals.

The data analysis of event-related CBFV changes is completed with the software Average® (Deppe et al., 1997). Normalisation of spectral-envelope curves of the Doppler-signal is mainly performed by heart-cycle integration. CBFV relative to the mean CBFV is then computed by averaging all measurement points per artery and then employed for further analysis (rCBFV). Mean rCBFV throughout the activation phase is compared to the mean rCBFV during the baseline period (Figure 2).

For calculation of the laterality index (LI), the time point of maximum difference between left and right rCBFV during the activation phase (t_{max}) is specified. An LI is calculated separately for each epoch from the difference of the areas under the curves for the time period, one second before to one second after t_{max}. The mean LI of all epochs and its standard error, indicating variability over the 20 task repetitions, serve as measures of hemispheric dominance. Generally, a positive LI represents left-hemispheric dominance, while right-hemispheric dominance is represented by a negative LI. Knecht et al. (1998) suggested classifying left and right hemispheric dominance, as soon as the obtained LI deviates more than two standard errors from zero.

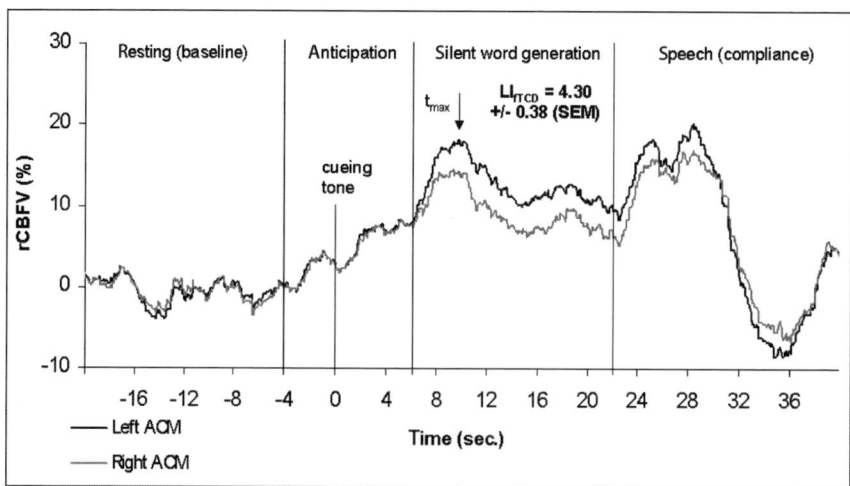

Figure 2. Averaged relative change in cerebral blood flow velocity (rCBFV) over 20 task repetitions compared to baseline CBFV during language assessment by fTCD.
MCA: Middle cerebral artery; tmax: time point of maximum difference in left-right rCBFV throughout word generation; LI: laterality index; SEM: standard error of the mean LI over task repetitions.

fTCD is non-invasive, easy to apply and well-tolerated. Despite high temporal resolution, its spatial resolution is relatively low, and it is currently only used for lateralizing cognitive function. Since movement is only minimally restricted and the word generation paradigm is easy to complete, fTCD can be conducted in most patients, even in children and many mentally challenged patients. However, a sufficient temporal bone window is required in order to allow good quality measurement of CBFV. An insufficient temporal bone window is found in 10-20% of the population (Widder & Görtler, 2004).

Magnetoencephalography

Breier et al. confirmed agreement between magnetic source imaging and Wada testing in 26 epilepsy patients during a word recognition task (Breier et al., 1999) and this paradigm was later validated in 100 adult patients (Papanicolaou et al., 2004) and in patients between the age of eight and 17 years old (Breier et al., 2001). Other paradigms for language lateralization include analysis of spatiotemporal distribution of oscillatory changes on magnetoencephalography (MEG) and comparison of these results with Wada testing during a silent reading paradigm (Hirata et al., 2004). In this study, a silent reading paradigm was compared to Wada test results in 20 patients during presurgical work-up for epilepsy surgery and the results were concordant with Wada testing in 19 of 20 cases (Hirata et al., 2004). Additional paradigms previously used comparisons of tones and vowels (Gootjes et al., 1999; Kirveskari et al., 2006).

Repetitive transcranial magnetic stimulation

The first language study using repetitive transcranial magnetic stimulation (rTMS) was performed in patients undergoing presurgical evaluation for epilepsy surgery (Pascual-Leone et al., 1991). rTMS was delivered and speech arrest was induced during a counting paradigm in six patients after stimulation of the left hemisphere (Pascual-Leone et al., 1991). This was concordant with Wada testing. In subsequent studies speech arrest was only induced in 14 of 21 (Jennum et al., 1994) and 7 of 14 patients (Michelucci et al., 1994), however, these lower rates may have been, in part, related to the stimulation paradigm and variability between studies (Epstein et al., 1996). More recent detailed studies have been able to delineate possible negative motor and motor strip stimulation effects in the precentral region from actual stimulation of Broca's area, rekindling the hope of replacing Wada testing (Stewart et al., 2001; Aziz-Zadeh et al., 2005). Further paradigms also provide insight into the localization of grammar, including syntax and verbs (Devlin and Watkins, 2007).

Other techniques

Other non-invasive techniques for language lateralization and localization include positron emission tomography (PET) (Hunter et al., 1999), single photon emission computed tomography (SPECT) (Borbely et al., 2003), near infrared spectroscopy (NIRS) (Watanabe et al., 1998), event-related potentials (ERP) (Gerschlager et al., 1998), and volumetric analysis of structural MRI (Foundas et al., 1996).

Alternative methods for the prognosis of memory decline

Neuropsychological testing

Preoperative neuropsychological testing is performed in order to provide information about epilepsy and lesion-associated functional deficits. In MTLE, memory deficits can be found to predominantly affect intended learning (Helmstaedter, 2004). However, verbal memory deficits in left TLE are more consistently described than figural memory deficits in right TLE (Kubu et al., 2000b). Similarly, verbal memory decline after left temporal lobe resection has been more frequently reported than figural memory decline after right temporal lobe resection (Loring et al., 1995; Gleissner et al., 2004).

Studies have identified several risk factors for postoperative memory decline in MTLE, which can be derived from neuropsychological test results. Higher preoperative memory performance (i.e. lack of a lesion-associated functional deficit) bears a higher risk of memory decline, while higher IQ, better attention and higher language function (as a precondition for good compensation) ameliorate postoperative memory deficits (Helmstaedter, 2004).

Demographics and structural imaging

Apart from neuropsychological test results, demographic data and clinical characteristics as well as structural imaging findings contribute to prognosis of memory change after surgery. Older age at onset as well as older age at surgical treatment increases the risk of postoperative memory deterioration (Hermann et al., 1995). Resections within the language-dominant hemisphere bear a higher risk of postoperative memory decline. A clear unilateral mesial temporal lesion without additional pathology on MRI diminishes the risk for postoperative memory loss (Stroup et al., 2003). Moreover, structural MRI data on hippocampal volumes can add substantial information and can assist in the prediction of neuropsychological outcome (Lineweaver et al., 2006).

Multivariate approach to memory prognosis after mesial temporal resection

Recent studies have used a multivariate approach for risk assessment of postoperative memory loss (Chelune & Najm, 2001; Baxendale et al., 2006; Stroup et al., 2003) including neuropsychological test results, demographic data and structural MRI. While Chelune & Najm (2001) found independent prognostic value of the Wada test in memory outcome prediction in all patients, Baxendale et al. (2007) noted that Wada test results only contributed in patients with left TLE. Binder and colleagues (Binder et al., 2008) demonstrated the added value of fMRI language lateralization in predicting verbal memory decline in left TLE patients, while neither Wada language nor memory asymmetry had further predictive power. Likewise, Lineweaver et al. (2006) did not find that the Wada test had independent predictive value for memory loss but could not rule out minimal additive predictive value. Differences in these studies may also be explained by differences in Wada test protocols and by additional demographic, neuropsychological and imaging variables which were considered in the analysis.

Functional imaging

Due to the low incidence of global amnesia after unilateral temporal lobe resection (Simkins-Bullock, 2000), functional imaging studies have focused on the prediction of more frequently observed material-specific memory decline.

Functional magnetic resonance imaging

Functional magnetic resonance imaging (fMRI) has been also used to lateralize memory function in TLE patients, mostly using encoding paradigms of different types of stimuli (Detre et al., 1998; Golby et al., 2002; Rabin et al., 2004; Branco et al., 2006). Few studies with small patient numbers have investigated memory lateralization, in comparison to the Wada test, and these have shown either good concordance (Detre et al., 1998; Golby et al., 2002; Rabin et al., 2004; Branco et al., 2006) or a substantial number of mismatches, especially in left TLE patients (Rabin et al., 2004). Some studies also demonstrated a predictive value of memory fMRI on postoperative verbal memory change after left temporal lobe resection (Rabin et al., 2004; Richardson et al., 2004; 2006). To date, no standardized memory fMRI protocol exists, despite promising initial pilot series. This therefore limits the comparability of studies. Further investigation providing clinically applicable criteria for risk estimation (e.g. normative data, cut-off-scores) is needed in order to predict memory decline on an individual basis. Memory fMRI is, however, likely be widely implemented in the presurgical work-up of MTLE patients in the coming years (Powell et al., 2004).

Positron emission tomography

Several PET studies suggest a correlation between interictal temporal glucose hypometabolism and Wada test memory lateralization (Hong et al., 2000). In addition, this may also be predictive of postoperative memory decline after left temporal lobe resection (Griffith et al., 2000). Thus, temporal glucose metabolism can probably be used as a complementary indirect measure of functional integrity.

Diffusion tensor imaging

Interestingly, some recent diffusion tensor imaging (DTI) studies have demonstrated a correlation between preoperative memory and mean fractional anisotropy of mesial temporal white matter connections in left TLE patients, which may also provide complementary information to structural MRI regarding the prognosis of memory decline (Yogarajah et al., 2008; Diehl et al., 2008).

Other imaging techniques such as SPECT, rTMS, fTCD or NIRS play currently only a minor or negligible role in memory assessment in epilepsy patients (Pelletier et al., 2007). Some of these methods comprise general limitations (e.g. low spatial resolution of fTCD), and therefore have, at this point, only limited ability to capture memory-associated neuronal activity at a resolution needed for individual risk evaluation.

Alternative seizure focus lateralization techniques

Interictal PET and ictal SPECT are discussed elsewhere in this book in detail. Although these are activation techniques, they frequently add supportive data during the presurgical decision-making process. In addition, functional transcranial Doppler ultrasound has also been described as an ictal and interictal diagnostic tool in patients with epilepsy. Diehl and colleagues were the first to describe transcranial Dopplersonographic changes with generalised epileptiform discharges and photoparoxysmal response (Diehl et al., 1998b; 1998a). Knake et al. were the first to lateralize a seizure focus by means of fTCD in concordance with SPECT and EEG in two patients with TLE (Knake et al., 2004).

■ Suggestion for a presurgical algorithm of language and memory determination in mesial temporal lobe epilepsy

Considering all risks, benefits, and available alternatives to language and memory assessment in patients with MTLE, a revision of the standard algorithm of presurgical epilepsy work-up seems warranted. Currently, non-invasive assessment of the eloquent area is frequently followed by Wada testing (Abou-Khalil, 2007) (Figure 3).

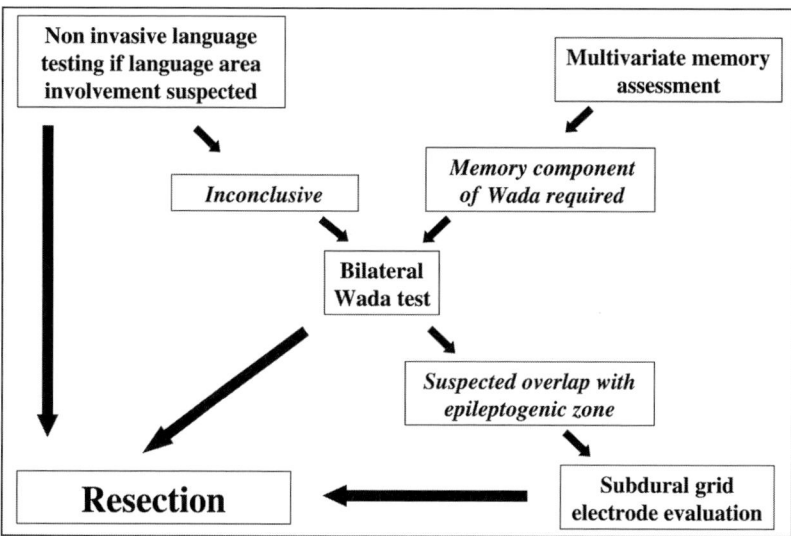

Figure 3. Previous algorithm for presurgical determination of language and memory (modified after Loddenkemper, *Epilepsy & Behavior* 2008, with permission).

We suggest a revision of this presurgical algorithm is required in order to omit and ultimately discontinue and replace Wada testing in the presurgical diagnostic work-up of patients with MTLE *(Figure 4)*. Non-invasive imaging techniques may well provide sufficient information on language and memory assessment. The risks of Wada testing, with serious and lasting complications in 0.6% of patients and minor complications in 11%, may well outweigh the risk of rare cases of global amnesia (one series estimated 0.45% [Rausch & Langfitt, 1991]) and minor material-specific memory deficits. All previously reported patients with global amnesia after ipsilateral temporal lobectomy had a structural lesion in the contralateral temporal lobe that, in hindsight, may have indicated poor memory outcome (Baxendale et al., 2008b). In addition, minor postoperative memory problems may be predicted with almost equal certainty by a multivariate non-invasive preoperative approach including neuropsychological testing and structural MRI (Baxendale et al., 2006), or possibly additional imaging techniques, such as diffusion tensor imaging and functional MRI.

Selection criteria for omission of Wada testing may include consideration of previous results, reliability and availability of non-invasive mapping techniques, localization of the epileptogenic zone and underlying aetiology or structural lesions, baseline function as well as age and cooperation.

■ Conclusions

Wada testing in MTLE adds but limited additional data for the presurgical decision-making process. Recent surveys suggest that many epileptologists no longer regard Wada testing as part of the standard work-up in most patients with isolated MTLE. Wada testing may be omitted on a case-by-case basis if comfort levels, experience and availability of alternative and less invasive techniques permit. Consideration of demographic and clinical variables, as well as structural and functional MRI data, alternative mapping techniques, and neuropsychological test results may assist in this decision-making process. Usually,

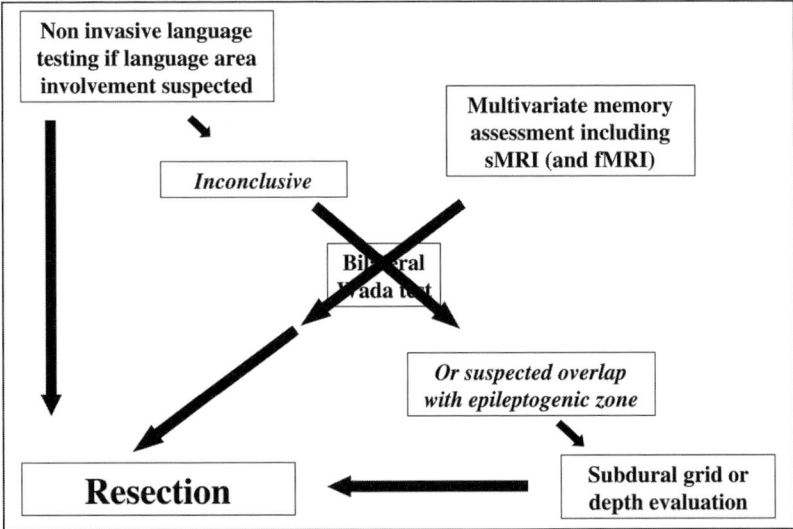

Figure 4. Potential alternative algorithm for presurgical assessment of eloquent cortex in TLE (modified after Loddenkemper, *Epilepsy & Behavior* 2008, with permission).

there is no indication for language testing in MTLE unless major language reorganisation is suspected. Non-invasive mapping techniques can only approximate cortical function. Patient counselling, including all risks, benefits, and alternatives of presurgical diagnostic options and possible consequences of MTLE surgery, is crucial. Epilepsy surgery for MTLE should not be withheld based on memory Wada test results alone, since information on validity and reliability of the memory Wada component remains limited.

References

- Abou-Khalil B. An update on determination of language dominance in screening for epilepsy surgery: the Wada test and newer noninvasive alternatives. *Epilepsia* 2007; 48: 442-55.
- Aziz-Zadeh L, Cattaneo L, Rochat M, Rizzolatti G. Covert speech arrest induced by rTMS over both motor and nonmotor left hemisphere frontal sites. *J Cogn Neurosci* 2005; 17: 928-38.
- Barr WB, Schaul N, Decker R, Lantos G. Postoperative amnesia after "passing" memory testing during the intracarotid amobarbital procedure. *Epilepsia* 1992; 33: 138.
- Baxendale S, Thompson P, Harkness W, Duncan J. Predicting memory decline following epilepsy surgery: a multivariate approach. *Epilepsia* 2006; 47: 1887-94.
- Baxendale S, Thompson P, Harkness W, Duncan J. The role of the intracarotid amobarbital procedure in predicting verbal memory decline after temporal lobe resection. *Epilepsia* 2007; 48: 546-52.
- Baxendale S, Thompson PJ, Duncan JS. The role of the Wada test in the surgical treatment of temporal lobe epilepsy: an international survey. *Epilepsia* 2008a; 49: 715-20.
- Baxendale SA, Thompson PJ, Duncan JS. Evidence-based practice: a reevaluation of the intracarotid amobarbital procedure (Wada test). *Arch Neurol* 2008b; 65: 841-5.
- Benke T, Koylu B, Visani P, Karner E, Brenneis C, Bartha L, *et al.* Language lateralization in temporal lobe epilepsy: a comparison between fMRI and the Wada Test. *Epilepsia* 2006; 47: 1308-19.

- Binder JR, Sabsevitz DS, Swanson SJ, Hammeke TA, Raghavan M, Mueller WM. Use of preoperative functional MRI to predict verbal memory decline after temporal lobe epilepsy surgery. *Epilepsia* 2008; 49: 1377-94.
- Binder JR, Swanson SJ, Hammeke TA, Morris GL, Mueller WM, Fischer M, et al. Determination of language dominance using functional MRI: a comparison with the Wada test. *Neurology* 1996; 46: 978-84.
- Borbely K, Gjedde A, Nyary I, Czirjak S, Donauer N, Buck A. Speech activation of language dominant hemisphere: a single-photon emission computed tomography study. *Neuroimage* 2003; 20: 987-94.
- Branco D M, Suarez R O, Whalen S, O'Shea J P, Nelson A P, da Costa J C, Golby A J. Functional MRI of memory in the hippocampus: Laterality indices may be more meaningful if calculated from whole voxel distributions. *Neuroimage* 2006; 32: 592-602.
- Brazdil M, Chlebus P, Mikl M, Pazourkova M, Krupa P, Rektor I. Reorganization of language-related neuronal networks in patients with left temporal lobe epilepsy - an fMRI study. *Eur J Neurol* 2005; 12: 268-75.
- Breier JI, Simos PG, Wheless JW, Constantinou JE, Baumgartner JE, Venkataraman V, Papanicolaou AC. Language dominance in children as determined by magnetic source imaging and the intracarotid amobarbital procedure: a comparison. *J Child Neurol* 2001; 16: 124-30.
- Breier JI, Simos PG, Zouridakis G, Wheless JW, Willmore LJ, Constantinou JE, et al. Language dominance determined by magnetic source imaging: a comparison with the Wada procedure. *Neurology* 1999; 53: 938-45.
- Chelune G, Najm I. Risk factors associated with postsurgical decrements in memory. In: Lüders H, Comair Y (eds.) *Epilepsy Surgery*, 2nd ed. Philadelphia: Lippincott Williams and Wilkins, 2001, pp. 497-504.
- Deppe M, Knecht S, Henningsen H, Ringelstein EB. AVERAGE: a Windows program for automated analysis of event related cerebral blood flow. *J Neurosci Methods* 1997; 75: 147-54.
- Deppe M, Knecht S, Papke K, Lohmann H, Fleischer H, Heindel W, et al. Assessment of hemispheric language lateralization: a comparison between fMRI and fTCD. *J Cereb Blood Flow Metab* 2000; 20: 263-8.
- Detre JA, Maccotta L, King D, Alsop DC, Glosser G, D'Esposito M, et al. Functional MRI lateralization of memory in temporal lobe epilepsy. *Neurology* 1998; 50: 926-32.
- Devlin J T, Watkins K E. Stimulating language: insights from TMS. *Brain* 2007; 130: 610-22.
- Diehl B, Busch R M, Duncan J S, Piao Z, Tkach J, Lüders HO. Abnormalities in diffusion tensor imaging of the uncinate fasciculus relate to reduced memory in temporal lobe epilepsy. *Epilepsia* 2008, 49: 1409-18.
- Diehl B, Knecht S, Deppe M, Young C, Stodieck SR. Cerebral hemodynamic response to generalized spike-wave discharges. *Epilepsia* 1998a; 39: 1284-9.
- Diehl B, Stodieck SR, Diehl RR, Ringelstein EB. The photic driving EEG response and photoreactive cerebral blood flow in the posterior cerebral artery in controls and in patients with epilepsy. *Electroencephalogr Clin Neurophysiol* 1998b; 107: 8-12.
- Dodrill CB. The Wada test is not a useful predictor of material-specific memory change following temporal lobe surgery for epilepsy. In: Miller JW, Silbergeld DL (eds). *Epilepsy Surgery: Principles and Controversies*. New York: Taylor & Francis, 2006, pp. 233-8.
- Epstein CM, Lah JJ, Meador K, Weissman JD, Gaitan LE, Dihenia B. Optimum stimulus parameters for lateralized suppression of speech with magnetic brain stimulation. *Neurology* 1996; 47: 1590-3.
- Floel A, Knecht S, Lohmann H, Deppe M, Sommer J, Drager B, et al. Language and spatial attention can lateralize to the same hemisphere in healthy humans. *Neurology* 2001; 57: 1018-24.

- Floel A, Lohmann H, Breitenstein C, Drager B, Buyx A, Henningsen H, Knecht S. Reproducibility of hemispheric blood flow increases during line bisectioning. *Clin Neurophysiol* 2002; 113: 917-24.
- Foundas AL, Leonard CM, Gilmore RL, Fennell EB, Heilman KM. Pars triangularis asymmetry and language dominance. *Proc Natl Acad Sci USA* 1996; 93: 719-22.
- Gaillard WD, Balsamo L, Xu B, McKinney C, Papero PH, Weinstein S, et al. fMRI language task panel improves determination of language dominance. *Neurology* 2004; 63: 1403-8.
- Gerschlager W, Lalouschek W, Lehrner J, Baumgartner C, Lindinger G, Lang W. Language-related hemispheric asymmetry in healthy subjects and patients with temporal lobe epilepsy as studied by event-related brain potentials and intracarotid amobarbital test. *Electroencephalogr Clin Neurophysiol* 1998; 108: 274-82.
- Gleissner U, Helmstaedter C, Schramm J, Elger CE. Memory outcome after selective amygdalohippocampectomy in patients with temporal lobe epilepsy: one-year follow-up. *Epilepsia* 2004; 45: 960-2.
- Golby AJ, Poldrack RA, Illes J, Chen D, Desmond JE, Gabrieli JD. Memory lateralization in medial temporal lobe epilepsy assessed by functional MRI. *Epilepsia* 2002; 43: 855-63.
- Goldstein J, Gilliam F. The Wada test may not always be needed prior to mesial temporal resection. In: Miller JW, Silbergeld DL (eds). *Epilepsy Surgery: Principles and Controversies*. New York: Taylor & Francis, 2006, pp. 243-6.
- Gootjes L, Raij T, Salmelin R, Hari R. Left-hemisphere dominance for processing of vowels: a whole-scalp neuromagnetic study. *Neuroreport* 1999; 10: 2987-91.
- Griffith HR, Perlman SB, Woodard AR, Rutecki PA, Jones JC, Ramirez LF, et al. Preoperative FDG-PET temporal lobe hypometabolism and verbal memory after temporal lobectomy. *Neurology* 2000; 54: 1161-5.
- Haag A, Knake S, Hamer HM, Boesebeck F, Freitag H, Schulz R, et al. The Wada test in Austrian, Dutch, German, and Swiss epilepsy centers from 2000 to 2005: a review of 1,421 procedures. *Epilepsy Behav* 2008; 13: 83-9.
- Helmstaedter C. Neuropsychological aspects of epilepsy surgery. *Epilepsy Behav* 2004; 5 (Suppl 1): S45-S55.
- Helmstaedter C. The role of the Wada test ub tge surgical treatment of temporal lobe epilepsy: An international perspective – commentary on Baxendale et al. *Epilepsia* 2008; 49: 720-2.
- Helmstaedter C, Kurthen M, Linke DB, Elger CE. Patterns of language dominance in focal left and right hemisphere epilepsies: relation to MRI findings, EEG, sex, and age at onset of epilepsy. *Brain Cogn* 1997; 33: 135-50.
- Hermann BP, Seidenberg M, Haltiner A, Wyler AR. Relationship of age at onset, chronologic age, and adequacy of preoperative performance to verbal memory change after anterior temporal lobectomy. *Epilepsia* 1995; 36: 137-45.
- Hirata M, Kato A, Taniguchi M, Saitoh Y, Ninomiya H, Ihara A, et al. Determination of language dominance with synthetic aperture magnetometry: comparison with the Wada test. *Neuroimage* 2004; 23: 46-53.
- Hong SB, Roh SY, Kim SE, Seo DW. Correlation of temporal lobe glucose metabolism with the Wada memory test. *Epilepsia* 2000; 41: 1554-9.
- Hunter KE, Blaxton TA, Bookheimer SY, Figlozzi C, Gaillard WD, Grandin C, Anyanwu A, Theodore WH. 15)O water positron emission tomography in language localization: a study comparing positron emission tomography visual and computerized region of interest analysis with the Wada test. *Ann Neurol* 1999; 45: 662-5.
- Jennum P, Friberg L, Fuglsang-Frederiksen A, Dam M. Speech localization using repetitive transcranial magnetic stimulation. *Neurology* 1994; 44: 269-73.
- Kim H, Yi S, Son EI, Kim J. Material-specific memory in temporal lobe epilepsy: effects of seizure laterality and language dominance. *Neuropsychology* 2003; 17: 59-68.

- Kirveskari E, Salmelin R, Hari R. Neuromagnetic responses to vowels vs. tones reveal hemispheric lateralization. *Clin Neurophysiol* 2006; 117: 643-8.
- Knake S, Haag A, Hamer HM, Dittmer C, Bien S, Oertel WH, Rosenow F. Language lateralization in patients with temporal lobe epilepsy: a comparison of functional transcranial Doppler sonography and the Wada test. *Neuroimage* 2003; 19: 1228-32.
- Knake S, Haag A, Pilgramm G, Reis J, Klein KM, Hoeffken H, et al. Ictal functional TCD for the lateralization of the seizure onset zone–a report of two cases. *Epilepsy Res* 2004; 62: 89-93.
- Knecht S, Deppe M, Ebner A, Henningsen H, Huber T, Jokeit H, Ringelstein EB. Noninvasive determination of language lateralization by functional transcranial Doppler sonography: a comparison with the Wada test. *Stroke* 1998; 29: 82-6.
- Knecht S, Henningsen H, Deppe M, Huber T, Ebner A, Ringelstein EB. Successive activation of both cerebral hemispheres during cued word generation. *Neuroreport* 1996; 7: 820-4.
- Kubu CS, Girvin JP, McLachlan RS, Pavol M, Harnadek MC. Does the intracarotid amobarbital procedure predict global amnesia after temporal lobectomy? *Epilepsia* 2000a; 41: 1321-9.
- Kubu CS, Lineweaver T, Chelune G. The role of neuropsychological assessment in the presurgical evaluation of epilepsy surgery candidates. In: Rosenow F, Lüders H (eds). *Presurgical Assessment of the Epilepsies with Clinical Neurophysiology and Functional Imaging.* Amsterdam: Elsevier, 2000b, pp. 245-56.
- Lehericy S, Cohen L, Bazin B, Samson S, Giacomini E, Rougetet R, et al. Functional MR evaluation of temporal and frontal language dominance compared with the Wada test. *Neurology* 2000; 54: 1625-33.
- Lineweaver TT, Morris HH, Naugle RI, Najm IM, Diehl B, Bingaman W. Evaluating the contributions of state-of-the-art assessment techniques to predicting memory outcome after unilateral anterior temporal lobectomy. *Epilepsia* 2006; 47: 1895-903.
- Loddenkemper T, Morris HH, Lineweaver T, Kellinghaus C. Repeated intracarotid amobarbital tests. *Epilepsia* 2007a; 48: 553-8.
- Loddenkemper T, Morris HH, Lineweaver T, Kellinghaus C. Wada test reliability (Response to Haber et al.). *Epilepsia* 2007b; 48: 1816-7.
- Loddenkemper T. Quo vadis Wada? *Epilepsy Behav* 2008a; 13: 1-2.
- Loddenkemper T, Morris H H, Moddel G. Complications during the Wada test. *Epilepsy Behav* 2008b; 13: 551-3.
- Loring DW, Meador KJ, Lee GP, King DW, Nichols ME, Park YD, et al. Wada memory asymmetries predict verbal memory decline after anterior temporal lobectomy. *Neurology* 1995; 45: 1329-33.
- Matteis M, Caltagirone C, Troisi E, Vernieri F, Monaldo BC, Silvestrini M. Changes in cerebral blood flow induced by passive and active elbow and hand movements. *J Neurol* 2001; 248: 104-8.
- Matteis M, Silvestrini M, Troisi E, Cupini LM, Caltagirone C. Transcranial doppler assessment of cerebral flow velocity during perception and recognition of melodies. *J Neurol Sci* 1997; 149: 57-61.
- Michelucci R, Valzania F, Passarelli D, Santangelo M, Rizzi R, Buzzi AM, et al. Rapid-rate transcranial magnetic stimulation and hemispheric language dominance: usefulness and safety in epilepsy. *Neurology* 1994; 44: 1697-700.
- Milner B, Branch C, Rasmussen T. Study of short-term memory after intracarotid injection of sodium Amytal. *Trans Am Neurol Assoc* 1962; 87: 224-6.
- Möddel G, Loddenkemper T, Lineweaver T, Dinner D. Atypical language representation in epilepsy patients: neuropsychological and imaging features. *Epilepsia* 2004; 45: 184.
- Novelly RA, Williamson PD. Incidence of false-positive memory impairment in the intracarotid Amytal procedure. *Epilepsia* 1989; 30: 711.
- Papanicolaou AC, Simos PG, Castillo EM, Breier JI, Sarkari S, Pataraia E, et al. Magnetocephalography: a noninvasive alternative to the Wada procedure. *J Neurosurg* 2004; 100: 867-76.

- Pascual-Leone A, Gates JR, Dhuna A. Induction of speech arrest and counting errors with rapid-rate transcranial magnetic stimulation. *Neurology* 1991; 41: 697-702.
- Pelletier I, Sauerwein HC, Lepore F, Saint-Amour D, Lassonde M. Non-invasive alternatives to the Wada test in the presurgical evaluation of language and memory functions in epilepsy patients. *Epileptic Disord* 2007; 9: 111-26.
- Powell HW, Koepp MJ, Richardson MP, Symms MR, Thompson PJ, Duncan JS. The application of functional MRI of memory in temporal lobe epilepsy: a clinical review. *Epilepsia* 2004; 45: 855-63.
- Rabin ML, Narayan VM, Kimberg DY, Casasanto DJ, Glosser G, Tracy JI, French JA, et al. Functional MRI predicts post-surgical memory following temporal lobectomy. *Brain* 2004; 127: 2286-98.
- Rausch R, Langfitt JT. Memory evaluation during the intracarotid amobarbital procedure. In: Lüders H (ed). *Epilepsy Surgery*. New York: Raven Press, 1991, pp. 507-14.
- Rausch R, Silfvenius H, Wieser HG, Dodrill CB, Meador KJ, Jones-Gotman M. Intraarterial amobarbital procedures. In: Engel J Jr (ed). *Surgical Treatment of the Epilepsies*. 2nd ed. New York: Raven Press, 1993, pp. 341-57.
- Richardson MP, Strange BA, Duncan JS, Dolan RJ. Memory fMRI in left hippocampal sclerosis: optimizing the approach to predicting postsurgical memory. *Neurology* 2006; 66: 699-705.
- Richardson MP, Strange BA, Thompson PJ, Baxendale SA, Duncan JS, Dolan RJ. Pre-operative verbal memory fMRI predicts postoperative memory decline after left temporal lobe resection. *Brain* 2004; 127: 2419-26.
- Rihs F, Sturzenegger M, Gutbrod K, Schroth G, Mattle HP. Determination of language dominance: Wada test confirms functional transcranial Doppler sonography. *Neurology* 1999; 52: 1591-6.
- Schulze-Bonhage A, Quiske A, Loddenkemper T, Dinner DS, Wyllie E. Validity of language lateralization by unilateral intracarotid Wada test. *J Neurol Neurosurg Psychiatry* 2004; 75: 1367-8.
- Silvestrini M, Cupini LM, Matteis M, Troisi E, Caltagirone C. Bilateral simultaneous assessment of cerebral flow velocity during mental activity. *J Cereb Blood Flow Metab* 1994; 14: 643-8.
- Simkins-Bullock J. Beyond speech lateralization: a review of the variability, reliability, and validity of the intracarotid amobarbital procedure and its nonlanguage uses in epilepsy surgery candidates. *Neuropsychol Rev* 2000; 10: 41-74.
- Stewart L, Walsh V, Frith U, Rothwell JC. TMS produces two dissociable types of speech disruption. *Neuroimage* 2001; 13: 472-8.
- Stroup E, Langfitt J, Berg M, McDermott M, Pilcher W, Como P. Predicting verbal memory decline following anterior temporal lobectomy (ATL). *Neurology* 2003; 60: 1266-73.
- Sturzenegger M, Newell DW, Aaslid R. Visually evoked blood flow response assessed by simultaneous two-channel transcranial Doppler using flow velocity averaging. *Stroke* 1996; 27: 2256-61.
- Swanson S J, Sabsevitz D S, Hammeke T A, Binder J R. Functional magnetic resonance imaging of language in epilepsy. *Neuropsychol Rev* 2007; 17: 491-504.
- Vingerhoets G, Stroobant N. Reliability and validity of day-to-day blood flow velocity reactivity in a single subject: an fTCD study. *Ultrasound Med Biol* 2002; 28: 197-202.
- Wada J. A new method for the determination of the side of cerebral speech dominance: a preliminary report on the intracarotid injection of Amytal in man. *Igaku Seibutsugaku* 1949; 14: 221-2.
- Wada J, Rasmussen T. Intracarotid injection of sodium Amytal for the lateralization of cerebral speech dominance: experimental and clinical observations. *J Neurosurg* 1960; 17, 266-82.
- Watanabe E, Maki A, Kawaguchi F, Takashiro K, Yamashita Y, Koizumi H, Mayanagi Y. Non-invasive assessment of language dominance with near-infrared spectroscopic mapping. *Neurosci Lett* 1998; 256: 49-52.

- Widder B, Görtler M. *Doppler- und Duplexsonographie der hirnversorgenden Arterien*. Hamburg: Springer Verlag, 2004.
- Woermann FG, Jokeit H, Luerding R, Freitag H, Schulz R, Guertler S, *et al*. Language lateralization by Wada test and fMRI in 100 patients with epilepsy. *Neurology* 2003; 61: 699-701.
- Woods RP, Dodrill CB, Ojemann GA. Brain injury, handedness, and speech lateralization in a series of amobarbital studies. *Ann Neurol* 1988; 23: 510-8.
- Yogarajah M, Powell HW, Parker GJ, Alexander DC, Thompson PJ, Symms MR, *et al*. Tractography of the parahippocampal gyrus and material specific memory impairment in unilateral temporal lobe epilepsy. *Neuroimage* 2008; 40: 1755-64.

PET and ictal SPECT in mesial temporal lobe epilepsy

Wim Van Paesschen[1], Karolien Goffin[2], Koen Van Laere[2]

[1] Department of Neurology, University Hospital Leuven, Leuven, Belgium
[2] Division of Nuclear Medicine, University Hospital Leuven, Leuven, Belgium

Mesial temporal lobe epilepsy (MTLE) is a common focal epilepsy syndrome which has been extensively studied within the setting of presurgical evaluation for intractable epilepsy. The most common cause of intractable MTLE is hippocampal sclerosis (HS) (Van Paesschen et al., 1997). The amygdala is another important structure which can be involved in MTLE. The neuropathology of epileptic lesions confined to the amygdala is more varied, and includes small tumours which have a predilection for the amygdala, vascular lesions, amygdala sclerosis, and cortical dysplasia (Van Paesschen et al., 1996). The nature of these lesions and the extent of resection determines seizure outcome after epilepsy surgery.

Positron emission tomography (PET) and single photon emission computed tomography (SPECT) are functional imaging modalities that provide information on the ictal onset and functional deficit zones, and seizure propagation. These imaging modalities are commonly used in the presurgical evaluation of patients with refractory MTLE. Combined with electrophysiological and structural data, these techniques allow a non-invasive presurgical evaluation in a majority of patients with refractory MTLE, and are particularly useful in patients with MTLE and discordant seizure semiology, EEG or morphological data (Uijl et al., 2007; Zaknun et al., 2008).

A presurgical evaluation starts with a complete seizure history, physical and neurological examination, routine scalp electroencephalography (EEG), and high-resolution magnetic resonance imaging (MRI) of the brain to assess structural abnormalities. These investigations are complemented by video-EEG monitoring, which allows evaluation of the clinical features of seizures, interictal and ictal EEG, ictal SPECT, interictal 2-[^{18}F]fluoro-2-deoxy-d-glucose (FDG) PET and neuropsychological examination. The aim of the presurgical evaluation of patients with refractory MTLE is to localize and determine whether a patient has a single epileptogenic zone. The epileptogenic zone is the cortical region which is indispensable for the generation of seizures and has to be removed in order to render a patient seizure-free. It is a theoretical construct and is defined in terms of different cortical zones (Rosenow & Lüders, 2001). The irritative zone is the region of cerebral cortex producing interictal spikes. The seizure onset zone is the region from which the seizures actually originate. Ictal SPECT is the only imaging modality that can define, in a reliable and consistent manner, the ictal onset zone. The symptomatogenic zone is the (sub)cortical region, producing ictal symptoms. The epileptic lesion can be visualized on morphological imaging, such as MRI. The functional deficit zone is the part of the cortex with an abnormal function between seizures, due to morphological or The functional deficit zone, or both. Interictal FDG-PET provides information on regions of cortex displaying decreased glucose metabolism, which usually contain at least the ictal onset zone. Epilepsy surgery provides best results when the different cortical zones are concordant, *i.e.* point towards the same cortical region, provided that there is no overlap with eloquent cortex.

Single photo emission computed tomography

SPECT studies in focal epilepsy have been carried out with blood flow tracers. Two commonly used tracers are ^{99m}Tc-hexamethylene propylene amine (^{99m}Tc-HMPAO) (Ceretec®) and ^{99m}Tc-ethyl cysteinate dimer (^{99m}Tc-ECD, Neurolite®) (Oku et al., 1997). These lipophilic amines rapidly cross the blood-brain barrier (around 85% of brain uptake on the first pass). Once inside the brain, they form a hydrophilic compound which is trapped within cells and prevents washout. Cerebral uptake is complete within two minutes and redistribution during the first hours postinjection is small, thus the activity in the brain remains essentially constant. Radioligand uptake is considered proportional to regional perfusion at the time of administration and its distribution is not affected by subsequent changes in cerebral blood flow or pharmacological intervention. Given the long physical half-life of ^{99m}Tc and these kinetics, static SPECT scans can be acquired up to 180 minutes after their intravenous administration. Ictal SPECT is a safe, non-invasive procedure that can be completed on a routine basis in the epilepsy monitoring unit, provided appropriately trained medical staff are employed as part of a structured multidisciplinary program. Several methods for rapid and safe ictal injection have been described (Herrendorf et al., 1999; Smith et al., 1999; Vanbilloen et al., 1999).

SPECT is now often used for the presurgical evaluation of patients with intractable focal epilepsy. The localizing value of SPECT performed with cerebral perfusion imaging agents in patients with focal epilepsy is based on cerebral metabolic and perfusion coupling. An interictal SPECT is obtained when the ligand is injected between seizures. Interictal SPECTs in focal epilepsy have shown areas of low perfusion in a proportion of patients, mainly with TLE. The usefulness of interictal SPECT for preoperative seizure focus localization, however, is limited due to a low sensitivity (McNally et al., 2005; Rowe et al., 1991b). It is now recommended that an interictal SPECT is obtained in order to compare the ictal SPECT, and obtain subtraction ictal SPECT co-registered to MRI (SISCOM), *i.e.* an analysis technique comparing ictal and interictal studies and co-registering to MRI (Zubal et al., 1995). The difference images are thresholded, usually at two standard deviations, to highlight regions of hyperperfusion. SISCOM has improved localization and visualization of the region of hyperperfusion (O'Brien et al., 1998).

Ictal perfusion patterns in mesial temporal lobe epilepsy

The sequence of perfusion changes in temporal lobe complex focal seizures has been well documented (Newton et al., 1995). During the ictus, there is hyperperfusion of the anterior temporal lobe *(Figures 1 and 2)*. Also, the ipsilateral insula and basal ganglia are often

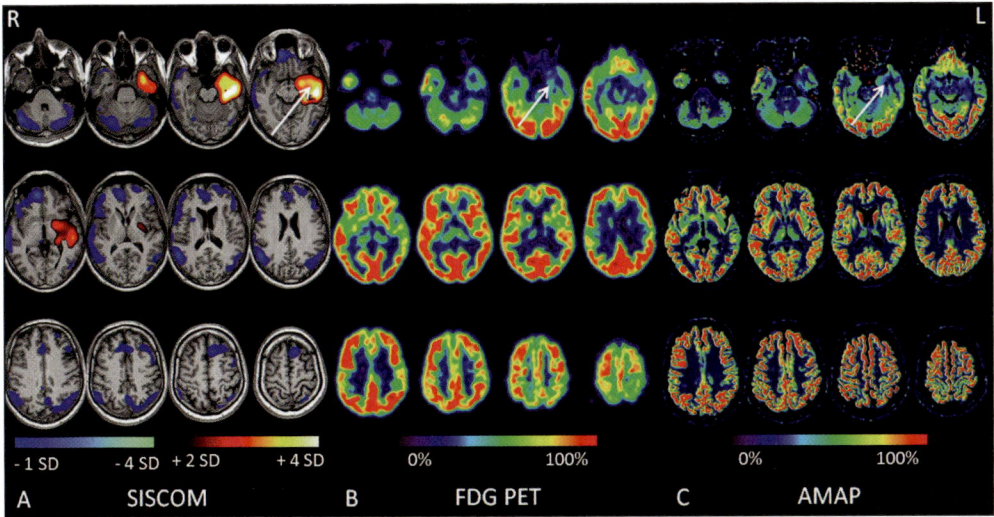

Figure 1. Ictal SPECT and interictal FDG PET in left MTLE-HS: axial sections.
Patient was a 32 year old man with left MTLE-HS. The epilepsy started at age 4 years. He had on average 5 complex focal seizures per month. Interictal and ictal EEG showed epileptic activity in the left temporal lobe. He has remained seizure free for more than 5 years after a standard temporal lobectomy including hippocampus and amygdala. **A.** SISCOM showed a cluster of hyperperfusion (orange-red) in the left temporal lobe (white arrow). The ictal SPECT injection was given during a complex focal seizure that lasted 67 seconds, with initiation of the injection 27 seconds after seizure onset. Hypoperfusion (blue) was present in frontoparietal lobes, cerebellum and contralateral temporal lobe. **B.** FDG PET showed asymmetric temporal lobe hypometabolism, which was more pronounced on the left (white arrow). **C.** AMAP reconstruction of FDG PET images showed asymmetric temporal lobe hypometabolism, which was more pronounced on the left (white arrow). All images **(A-C)** were coregistered. R: right; L: left; SD: standard deviation.

involved (Kaiboriboon *et al.*, 2005). Up to two minutes postictally, there is hyperperfusion of the mesial temporal structures with hypoperfusion of lateral temporal structures, and from two to 15 minutes postictally, hypoperfusion of the whole temporal lobe, *i.e.* postictal switch (Newton *et al.*, 1992b; Rowe *et al.*, 1991a). A return to normal is seen after 10-30 minutes. Sensitivity of ictal SPECT localization in patients with temporal lobe complex focal seizures, relative to diagnostic evaluation, has been reported to be around 97%, and for postictal SPECT studies, around 75% (Leveille *et al.*, 1992). The sensitivity of ictal SPECT localization during simple focal seizures is lower compared with studies during complex focal seizures (Shin *et al.*, 2002; Van Paesschen *et al.*, 2000). Ictal hyperperfusion patterns also depend on interictal spikes, and semiological and EEG progression after ictal SPECT injection (Kim *et al.*, 2007; Shin *et al.*, 2002; Wichert-Ana *et al.*, 2004). In patients with dystonic posturing during seizures, basal ganglia hyperperfusion in the hemisphere opposite the side of the dystonic posturing has been observed (Joo *et al.*, 2004; Mizobuchi *et al.*, 2001; 2004; Newton *et al.*, 1992a; Shin *et al.*, 2002). Secondary generalised tonic-clonic seizures show multilobar hyperfusion (Shin *et al.*, 2002).

Few studies have addressed perfusion patterns according to underlying aetiology of TLE. Ho *et al.* (1995; 1996) described hyperperfusion in the ipsilateral mesial and lateral temporal regions in patients with HS and patients with foreign-tissue lesions in the mesial temporal lobe. In patients with foreign-tissue lesions in the lateral temporal lobe, hyperperfusion was seen bilaterally in the temporal lobes with predominant changes in the region of the lesion. Different pathways of seizure propagation could explain these perfusion patterns.

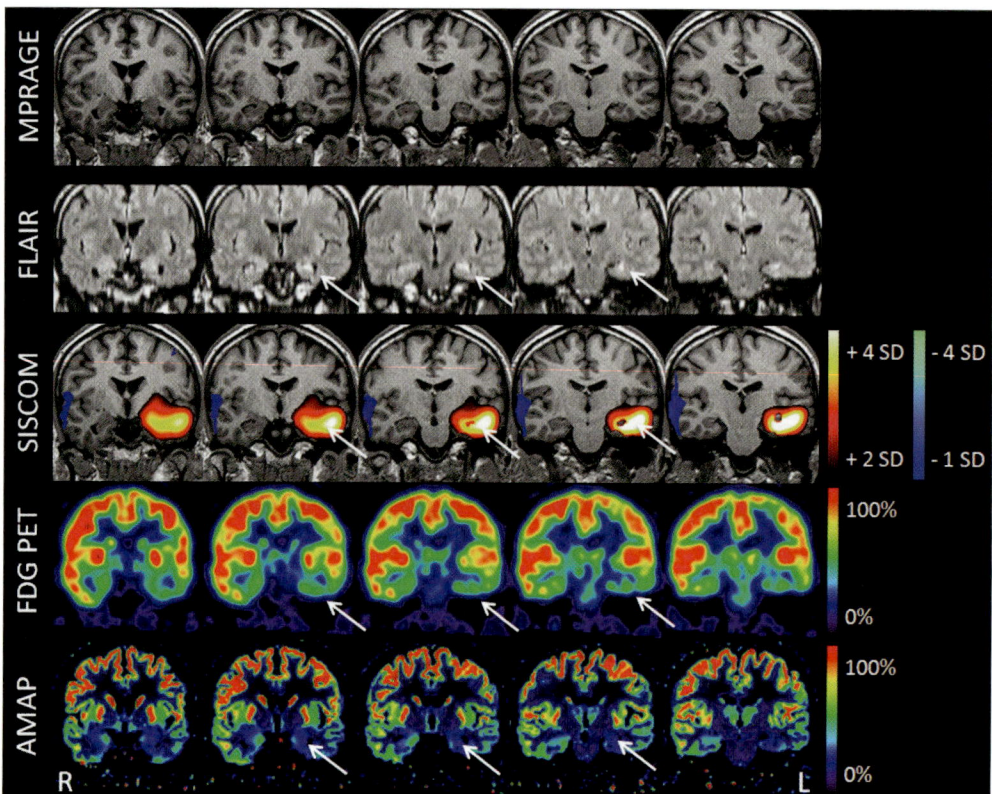

Figure 2. MRI, ictal SPECT and interictal FDG PET in left MTLE-HS: coronal sections.
The clinical details were the same as in *Figure 1*. MPRAGE showed an atrophic left hippocampus, and FLAIR an increased signal in the left hippocampus (white arrows), consistent with left HS. SISCOM showed a cluster of hyperperfusion in the left temporal lobe (white arrows) and hypoperfusion (blue) in the contracterai temporal lobe. FDG PET showed asymmetric temporal lobe hypometabolism, which was more pronounced on the left (white arrows). AMAP reconstruction of FDG PET images showed similar asymmetric temporal lobe hypometabolism, which was more pronounced on the left with pronounced hypometabolism in the left hippocampus (white arrows). All images were coregistered. R: right; L: left; SD: standard deviation.

False lateralizations due to rapid seizure spread in MTLE are uncommon. Rapid propagation to the contralateral temporal lobe has been reported in around 1% of cases (Ho et al., 1995). In these cases, early ictal SPECT can demonstrate seizure onset in the ipsilateral temporal lobe before seizure propagation has occurred (Van Paesschen et al., 2000). Patients with refractory MTLE-HS can present clinically with extratemporal seizures due to rapid seizure spread. Early ictal SPECT can demonstrate this propagation, obviating the need for invasive EEG studies.

Systematic perfusion changes during complex focal seizures in patients with MTLE-HS have been studied using statistical parametric mapping (SPM) of ictal-interictal SPECT difference images (Blumenfeld et al., 2004; Nelissen et al., 2006; Tae et al., 2005; Van Paesschen et al., 2003) or composite SPECT (Kaiboriboon et al., 2005; Nelissen et al., 2006). SPM identifies regions with statistically significant increased or decreased perfusion during the ictal phase compared with the interictal phase. In patients with MTLE-HS, ipsilateral temporal lobe hyperperfusion is present throughout a complex focal seizure, and disappears in the postictal period. Several regions outside the epileptic temporal lobe show ictal hypoperfusion *(Figures 1 and 2)*. Ipsilateral, as well as contralateral frontal lobe hypoperfusion, is present during both the ictal and postictal period. Contralateral cerebellar hypoperfusion occurs in the early ictal period and hyperperfusion in midline cerebellar structures during the postictal period. Ipsilateral parietal lobe hypoperfusion is a late ictal phenomenon, and has been observed in ictal SPECTs with injection times ranging from 60 to 90 seconds. Bilateral medial thalamic hyperperfusion is present postictally (Van Paesschen, 2004). Ictal frontal lobe hypoperfusion may represent an inhibitory process in view of the presence of a crossed cerebellar diaschisis. Crossed cerebellar diaschisis is due to deactivation of Purkinje cells caused by a decrease in excitatory input due to suppression of electrical activity in the contralateral frontal cortex (Gold & Lauritzen, 2002). Furthermore, these SPECT findings corroborate optical imaging experiments, which showed a decrease in optical signal together with a decrease in neuronal activity in cortex surrounding an epileptic focus, consistent with ictal surround inhibition (Schwartz & Bonhoeffer, 2001). Impaired consciousness in temporal lobe complex focal seizures may result from focal abnormal activity in temporal and subcortical networks linked to widespread hypoperfusion/impaired function of the association cortices (Blumenfeld *et al.*, 2004).

Ictal SPECT in the presurgical evaluation of mesial temporal lobe epilepsy

In patients with refractory unilateral MTLE and a lesion on MRI, with concordant or non-lateralizing ictal EEG or concordant interictal EEG, it has been suggested that other investigations, such as ictal SPECT and PET provide little additional information in the presurgical evaluation (Cendes *et al.*, 2000; Kilpatrick *et al.*, 2003). Ictal perfusion SPECT, however, is an effective diagnostic modality for correctly identifying seizure origin in TLE, and may provide complementary information to ictal EEG and MRI in an individual patient (Simons *et al.*, 2004). Lee *et al.* (2000) reported ictal SPECT findings in 68 patients with TLE who underwent successful temporal lobectomy. Correct lateralization of ictal SPECT occurred in 10 of 14 patients with non-lateralized ictal EEG. They concluded that ictal SPECT is an independent and confirmatory presurgical evaluation technique. In a study of 74 patients with TLE who underwent epilepsy surgery, Zaknun *et al.* (2008) demonstrated the add-on value of ictal SPECT by its ability to correctly localize 17 of 22 (77%) seizure foci, undetected by ictal EEG, and 8 of 10 (80%) seizure foci undetected by MRI.

■ Positron emission tomography

PET is used to realise the *in vivo* study of cerebral metabolic and neurochemical processes. In epilepsy, cerebral glucose metabolism has been studied extensively using ^{18}Fluoro-2-deoxyglucose (FDG). Among PET receptor ligands, ^{11}C-Flumazenil (FMZ), which binds to the central benzodiazepine receptor, has been studied most extensively in MTLE-HS (Duncan, 1997).

FDG-PET

Methodology

FDG PET is usually evaluated visually *(Figures 1 and 2)*. In addition, an objective, pixel-wise comparison of the patient's image to an age-matched reference database can be performed in an automated way, resulting in z-score images which can be displayed as three-dimensional stereotactic surface projections *(Figure 3)*. Such an automated analysis

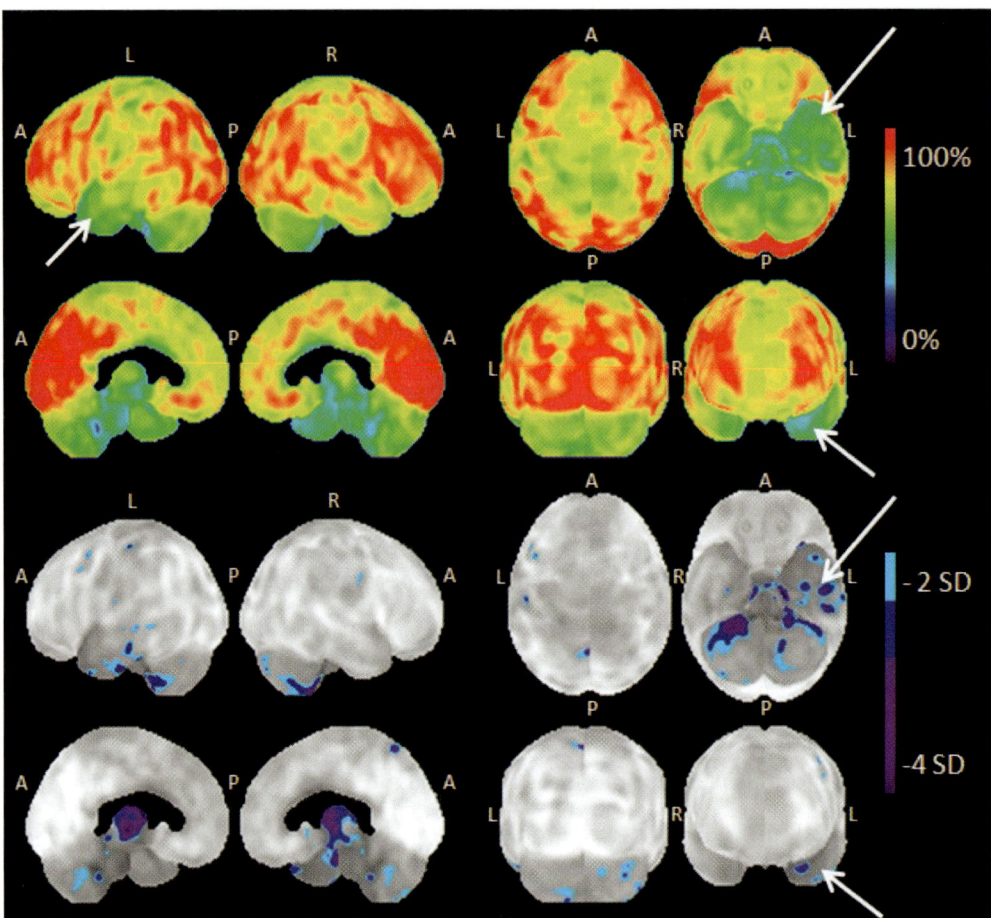

Figure 3. Three-dimensional stereotactic surface projection analysis of FDG PET images in left MTLE-HS. The clinical details were the same as in *Figure 1*. FDG-PET images showed an asymmetric temporal lobe hypometabolism, which was more pronounced on the left (top, white arrows). Comparison of the patient's data to a database of healthy volunteers showed hypometabolism in the left temporal lobe (bottom, white arrows). A: anterior; P: posterior; L: left; R: right; SD: standard deviation.

is especially useful in patients with extratemporal epilepsy (Drzezga et al., 1999). In patients with TLE, automated quantification of the maximal metabolic asymmetry in the temporal lobes has been reported (Lin et al., 2007). An anatomy-corrected asymmetry index (ACAI) that highlights inter-hemispheric metabolic asymmetry in FDG images may be particularly useful in the evaluation of FDG-PET images of patients with MTLE (Zhou et al., 2008) (*Figure 4*).

Measuring small brain structures, such as the cortical ribbon, will lead to an underestimation of the tracer activity due to the limited resolution (approximately 4-5 mm) of current PET scanners. This partial volume effect (PVE) can lead to spurious hypometabolic regions, resulting in an increased amount of false-positively predicted hypometabolic regions. Moreover, if the finite spatial resolution of the imaging system is not accounted for, a possible spill-over of activity to neighbouring regions can occur, leading to a misinterpretation of the extent of hypometabolic regions. Several algorithms are available for

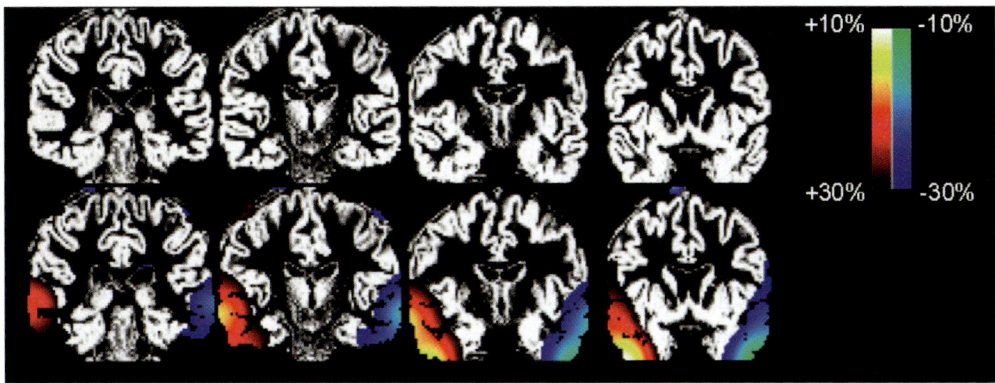

Figure 4. Anatomy-corrected asymmetry Index (ACAI) map of FDG-PET image. The clinical details were the same as in *Figure 1*. The anatomical information was obtained from an MPRAGE MRI image which was segmented into gray matter (GM), white matter (WM) and CSF. The segmentation of GM was used as the prior information in the ACAI algorithm (top row). FDG and MRI images were coregistered and wrapped to the MNI space. Image pre-processing was done in SPM2 with the standard parameter settings. The ACAI map was calculated using a Gaussian kernel with a FWHM of 11 voxels, and showed an asymmetry index of around 30% in the temporal lobes. The left temporal lobe was more hypometabolic compared with the right.

partial volume correction, both post-hoc (*e.g.* PVEOut [Quarantelli *et al.*, 2004]) or during reconstruction, *e.g.* an anatomy-based maximum a posteriori iterative reconstruction algorithm (A-MAP) (Baete *et al.*, 2004b). We have shown that partial volume correction improves the detection accuracy of small hypometabolic lesions in FDG PET images of the brain in a human observer study, compared to post-smoothed maximum-likelihood reconstruction (ML-EM) (Baete *et al.*, 2004a).

FDG-PET and ictal onset zone in mesial temporal lobe epilepsy

The majority of FDG-PET studies have been carried out during the interictal state. Interictal FDG-PET scans are characterised by a localised depression in cerebral glucose consumption which correlates anatomically with EEG spike foci (Hong *et al.*, 2002; Kuhl *et al.*, 1980) and EEG delta slowing (Erbayat *et al.*, 2005) in patients with TLE. FDG-PET studies have demonstrated hypometabolic regions in MTLE, including the ipsilateral mesial-lateral temporal lobe in 90-95% of patients, the contralateral mesial-lateral temporal lobe in 10-40%, the ipsilateral thalamus in 60-70% (Khan *et al.*, 1997), the ipsilateral basal ganglia in 40-50% (Dupont *et al.*, 1998), the ipsilateral insula in 40-60% (Bouilleret *et al.*, 2002; Dupont *et al.*, 2003), ipsilateral basal frontal lobe in 20-30% (Van Bogaert *et al.*, 2000), ipsilateral parietal lobe in 20-30% and ipsilateral occipital lobe in 0-4% (Henry *et al.*, 1990; 1993; Ho *et al.*, 1995; Spencer, 1994). Identical FDG-PET abnormalities, however, are present in MTLE-HS, MTLE with alien tissue lesions, MTLE with developmental lesions, MTLE with dual pathology, MTLE with "no pathology" and in neocortical TLE (Spanaki *et al.*, 2000). Kim *et al.* (2003) reported that the hypometabolism was more prominent in the lateral temporal than medial temporal structures in TLE, and that a relatively preserved medial temporal lobe glucose metabolism was suggestive of lateral TLE, rather than medial TLE. Diehl *et al.* (2003) reported that HS with concurrent temporal neocortical microscopic cortical dysplasia was associated with more prominent lateral metabolic dysfunction compared with isolated HS. Interictal temporal lobe hypometabolism has been shown to be uncoupled from perfusion, *i.e.* hypometabolism can be associated with a normal perfusion pattern (Fink *et al.*, 1996; Gaillard *et al.*, 1995;

Lee *et al.*, 2001; Zubal *et al.*, 2000). Interictal FDG-PET hypometabolism, therefore, is more sensitive for the lateralization of TLE than interictal PET or SPECT-based perfusion studies (Spencer, 1994; Theodore *et al.*, 1994).

Several FDG-PET studies were previously performed before HS could be reliably detected by MRI, and included patients with TLE of different aetiologies. Prediction of seizure outcome on the basis of PET data is an important issue in patients with uncontrolled focal seizures as PET results may influence patient selection for surgery. In patients with TLE, temporal hypometabolism on FDG-PET predicts successful temporal lobectomy even when surface EEG and MRI are non-localising (Dupont *et al.*, 2000; Manno *et al.*, 1994; Radtke *et al.*, 1993; Theodore *et al.*, 1992; Uijl *et al.*, 2007; Wong *et al.*, 1996). Multilobar hypometabolism (Theodore *et al.*, 1997), or extratemporal hypometabolism (Manno *et al.*, 1994), in particular hypometabolism in the contralateral cerebral cortex or bilateral temporal lobe (Benbadis *et al.*, 1995; Blum *et al.*, 1998; Choi *et al.*, 2003; Koutroumanidis *et al.*, 2000; Swartz *et al.*, 1992), has been reported to be associated with a greater likelihood of postsurgical seizure activity. In the study of Newberg and colleagues (2000), patients with relative contralateral thalamic hypometabolism were not seizure-free postoperatively. In MTLE-HS, however, extent and severity of hypometabolism appeared not to be related to surgical outcome (Lee *et al.*, 2002). In 38 patients with unilateral MTLE-HS, who were rendered seizure-free after surgery, the anterior half of the temporal lobes and thalami were the most asymmetric regions using z-score parametric FDG-PET (Wong *et al.*, 2007).

FDG-PET can provide additional information in the presurgical evaluation of patients with refractory TLE which is independent of results from other investigations, such as high resolution MRI. Carne *et al.* (2004) reported good surgical results in patients with MR-negative refractory TLE and unilateral temporal hypometabolism, and suggested that MR-negative, PET-positive TLE represents a surgically remediable syndrome distinct from MTLE-HS. In the largest series to date, Lee and colleagues (2005) reported their experience using FDG-PET of surgical outcome in 89 patients with refractory focal epilepsy and normal MRI. Thirty-five had frontal lobe epilepsy, 31 neocortical TLE, 11 occipital lobe epilepsy, 11 parietal lobe epilepsy and one multifocal epilepsy. Forty-seven percent of patients remained seizure-free for more than two years after surgery and 80% had a seizure reduction of at least 90%. Diagnostic sensitivity of FDG-PET as analyzed by SPM was 44%. FDG-PET localisation was greatest in neocortical TLE and significantly related to seizure-free outcome. This study confirmed the usefulness of lateralized hypometabolism in MR-negative TLE. Uijl and colleagues (2008) reported that FDG-PET was most useful in patients with TLE when MRI was normal or did not show unilateral temporal lobe abnormalities, and when ictal EEG results were not concordant with MRI findings or seizure semiology. O'Brien and colleagues (2008) reported that FDG-PET is cost-effective in the presurgical evaluation, particularly when used in patients with non-localising or non-concordant video-EEG monitoring or MRI results.

FDG-PET hypometabolism in areas remote from the ictal onset zone in mesial temporal lobe epilepsy

The underlying neurobiology of FDG-PET hypometabolism is not well understood, and has been ascribed to factors such as neuronal loss, diaschisis, inhibitory processes or reduction in synaptic density. Interictal FDG-PET provides information on regions of cortex displaying decreased glucose metabolism, which usually contain at least the ictal onset zone (Akimura *et al.*, 1999; Nelissen *et al.*, 2006; Rosenow & Lüders, 2001). In

MTLE-HS, hypometabolism may extend to the ipsilateral frontal and parietal cortex, as well as to subcortical structures such as the ipsilateral basal ganglia and thalamus, and the contralateral cerebellar lobe (Henry et al., 1990). MTLE-HS is characterized by neuronal loss and gliosis in the hippocampus. There is, however, no relationship between the degree of interictal PET hypometabolism and the amount of hippocampal gliosis or cell loss (Foldvary et al., 1999). Furthermore, temporal lobe hypometabolism has been observed in the absence of HS or any other identifiable pathology (Carne et al., 2004; Lee et al., 2005), suggesting that hippocampal atrophy is not a major determinant of hypometabolism. Using relative FDG-PET data normalised to white matter activity, we correlated interictal FDG-PET metabolism and ictal SPECT perfusion changes in MTLE-HS (Nelissen et al., 2006). Surprisingly, we found that *interictal PET hypometabolism* was greatest in the ipsilateral frontal lobe, and that this region coincided with the area of greatest *ictal SPECT hypoperfusion*, consistent with a seizure-related dynamic process. Crossed cerebellar diaschisis suggested that ipsilateral frontal lobe hypoperfusion/metabolism represented strong inhibition during complex focal seizures (Van Paesschen et al., 2003). We formulated the hypothesis of "surround inhibition", which is a dynamic (*i.e.* seizure-related) process, present in seizure propagation pathways, and a defence mechanism against seizure propagation. It is characterized by interictal hypometabolism and ictal hypoperfusion, and may be responsible for interictal and ictal functional deficits, which may be reversible upon cessation of seizure activity (Van Paesschen et al., 2007). In this hypothesis, some interneurons in the hyperperfused temporal lobe undergo active synaptic inhibition with downstream decreased synaptic activity in the ipsilateral frontal lobe, which is the most common route of spread of mesial temporal lobe seizures (Lieb et al., 1991). This hypothesis may explain why ipsilateral frontal lobe excitability, as measured by transcranial magnetic stimulation in patients with refractory TLE, strongly correlates with time to next seizure (Wright et al., 2006). Witte and colleagues (Witte et al., 1994) reported PET findings of a patient who had a seizure during PET scanning and documented that the transition from interictal to ictal activity was accompanied by the development of a hypermetabolic epileptic focus and the dynamic enlargement of surrounding hypometabolism.

FDG-PET hypometabolism in areas remote from the ictal onset has been related to neuropsychological and psychiatric dysfunction in MTLE. Jokeit and colleagues (Jokeit et al., 1997) reported a correlation between prefrontal metabolic asymmetry with frontal lobe cognitive deficits in patients with TLE. Takaya and colleagues (Takaya et al., 2006) compared cognitive functions and interictal cerebral glucose metabolism between 11 patients with MTLE and frequent seizures and 10 patients with MTLE and rare seizures. The frequent-seizure group had more executive set-shifting impairment which correlated with glucose hypometabolism in the prefrontal cortices. These results suggested that frequent seizures in MTLE are associated with hypofunction of the prefrontal cortex. Salzberg and colleagues (Salzberg et al., 2006) reported that only patients with TLE and a history of depression, at any time preoperatively, showed focal hypometabolism in the ipsilateral orbitofrontal cortex. Chassoux et al. (2004) performed FDG-PET studies in 50 patients with refractory MTLE-HS and found correlations between electroclinical characteristics and patterns of FDG-hypometabolism, suggesting that hypometabolism may be related to ictal discharge generation and spread pathways. Unilateral dystonic posturing during complex focal seizures has been associated with hypometabolism in the striatal region, suggesting that the basal ganglia are involved in the generation of ictal dystonic posturing in MTLE (Dupont et al., 1998).

Several reports provide evidence that hypometabolism at a distance from the seizure focus may disappear on seizure remission. Akimura et al. (1999) described improvement in hypometabolism of ipsilateral areas remote from the ictal onset zone, mainly the frontal lobe, in patients who underwent temporal lobectomy. Spanaki and colleagues (2000) documented increases in metabolism in the ipsilateral inferior frontal lobe and thalamus after temporal lobectomy for intractable TLE. Joo et al. (2005) compared pre- and postoperative FDG-PET scans in patients with MTLE-HS who were rendered seizure-free after surgery. Increases in FDG metabolism after surgery were seen in the propagation pathways of ictal and interictal epileptic discharges, e.g. temporal stem white matter, inferior precentral gyrus and anterior cingulate gyrus in the ipsilateral hemisphere, suggesting that hypometabolism in these regions was functional, seizure-related and reversible. On the other hand, decreases were seen in brain structures with afferents from resected anterior mesial temporal structures.

A key question is whether disappearance of FDG-PET hypometabolism at a distance from the ictal onset zone after (postsurgical) seizure remission correlates with neuropsychological and neuropsychiatric improvement, which is common after successful epilepsy surgery (Helmstaedter et al., 2003; Wiebe et al., 2001). In the presurgical assessment, attention is focused on eloquent cortex and loss of function after epilepsy surgery. It is equally important to counsel the patients in order for them to understand what they could gain in terms of cerebral functioning after successful epilepsy surgery. Studies correlating neuropsychological and neuropsychiatric improvements with disappearance of FDG-PET hypometabolism in the frontal lobes in MTLE have not been performed, and are warranted.

γ-amino-butyric acid (GABA) receptor and flumazenil PET in mesial temporal lobe epilepsy

GABA is the main inhibitory neurotransmitter in the brain and maintains the inhibitory tone that counterbalances neuronal excitation. Evidence from experimental and clinical studies indicates that GABA plays an important role in the mechanism and treatment of epilepsy (Treiman, 2001). GABA acts on two types of receptors: $GABA_A$ and $GABA_B$. Imaging of the $GABA_A$ receptor can be performed using either [^{11}C] or [^{18}F] labelled flumazenil (FMZ). FMZ binds to the central benzodiazepine receptor and has been shown to be reduced in the affected hippocampus in patients with MTLE-HS in more than 90% of cases, and to a lesser extent in the ipsilateral thalamus and insula (Hand et al., 1997; Juhasz et al., 1999; Koepp et al., 1996; 1997a; 1997b; Ryvlin et al., 1998). In vivo FMZ-PET has been shown to correlate with ex vivo FMZ autoradiography in HS (Koepp et al., 1997b). The area of decreased FMZ binding was often smaller than that of glucose hypometabolism (Ryvlin et al., 1998). Debets et al. (1997) reported that FMZ-PET was not superior to FDG-PET in the presurgical evaluation of TLE. In the study of Ryvlin et al. (1998), FMZ-PET did not prove superior to FDG-PET in assessing the extent of the ictal onset zone, as defined by intracranial EEG recordings. However, in MTLE-HS, FMZ-PET abnormalities delineated the site of seizure onset precisely, whenever coextensive with FDG-PET abnormalities. Extrahippocampal neocortical changes of central benzodiazepine receptor binding in MTLE due to HS have been reported (Hammers et al., 2001). The changes which can be seen in FMZ binding, as is the case for the changes in glucose metabolism, are dynamic. A test-retest FMZ PET study in patients with TLE revealed a significant effect of the duration of the interictal period on FMZ binding with lower maximal FMZ binding related to shorter interictal periods, implying that a FMZ PET scan should be obtained as soon as possible following a seizure for best results (Bouvard et al., 2005).

Opioid receptor in mesial temporal lobe epilepsy

There is evidence for the existence of an endogenous anticonvulsant mechanism in humans modulated by an anticonvulsant substance with opioid characteristics. Endogenous opioids are thought to play a dynamic role in the termination of seizures (Tortella & Long, 1985), since high frequency firing is required for their endogenous release (Wagner et al., 1990). Interictal PET studies in patients with TLE using [^{11}C] carfentanyl (Frost et al., 1988; Mayberg et al., 1991), selective for the δ opioid peptide receptor, or [^{11}C]methylnaltrindole (Madar et al., 1997), selective for the δ opioid peptide receptor, have shown increased binding in the lateral temporal neocortex on the side of the epileptogenic focus in patients with TLE.

Hammers and colleagues (2007) showed that changes in the opioid system are seizure-related. In a longitudinal study, each patient with TLE was scanned twice using the non-subtype selective opioid receptor PET radioligand [^{11}C] diprenorphine; one scan was performed within hours of a seizure. There was an increase of opioid receptor availability in the temporal pole and fusiform gyrus ipsilateral to the seizure focus, and this increase correlated negatively with the time since the last seizure, compatible with an early increase and gradual return to baseline. This study emphasized the possible important role of the opioid system in seizure control.

5-hydroxytryptamine-1A (5-HT1A) receptor in mesial temporal lobe epilepsy

Serotonin has been reported to play a role in the pathophysiology of epilepsy. The 5-hydroxytryptamine-1A (5-HT$_{1A}$) receptor is one of several subtypes of serotonin receptors. Central 5-HT$_{1A}$ receptors are found in high density in the brainstem raphe nuclei, hippocampus and temporal neocortex. The predominant effect of serotonin may be 5-HT$_{1A}$ receptor-mediated inhibition of epileptic activity. Toczek and colleagues (2003) used [^{18}F]FCWAY, a selective 5-HT$_{1A}$ receptor antagonist, to study this receptor in patients with TLE and demonstrated reduced serotonin receptor binding in temporal lobe epileptic foci, which remained significant after partial volume correction (Giovacchini et al., 2005). Merlet et al. (2004a; 2004b) confirmed decreased 5-HT$_{1A}$ receptor binding in the epileptic temporal lobe of patients with TLE using the 5-HT$_{1A}$ receptor antagonist [^{18}F]MPPF, and reported a significantly greater decrease in the ictal onset zone. Savic and colleagues (2004) reported a reduction of 5-HT$_{1A}$ receptor binding in TLE, not only in the hippocampus but also its limbic connections using [^{11}C]WAY-100 635 PET. Ito and co-authors (2007) also used [^{11}C]WAY-100 635 PET and found decreased 5-HT$_{1A}$ receptor binding predominantly in ipsilateral mesial temporal lobe structures but also in the contralateral side in patients with non-lesional TLE. A relationship between hippocampal 5-HT$_{1A}$ binding and depressive symptoms in patients with TLE was reported (Theodore et al., 2007). TLE and comorbid major depressive disorder was associated with a significantly more pronounced reduction in 5-HT$_{1A}$ receptor binding, extending into non-lesional limbic brain areas outside the epileptic focus (Hasler et al., 2007).

In conclusion, over the past 20 years it has been shown that metabolic and receptor PET, as well as ictal SPECT, play an important role in the functional characterisation, prognosis and treatment follow-up of patients with MTLE, which remains relevant today.

References

- Akimura T, Yeh HS, Mantil JC, Privitera MD, Gartner M, Tomsick TA. Cerebral metabolism of the remote area after epilepsy surgery. *Neurol Med Chir* 1999; 39: 16-25.
- Baete K, Nuyts J, Van Laere K, Van Paesschen W, Ceyssens S, De Ceuninck L, et al. Evaluation of anatomy based reconstruction for partial volume correction in brain FDG-PET. *Neuroimage* 2004a; 23: 305-17.
- Baete K, Nuyts J, Van Paesschen W, Suetens P, Dupont P. Anatomical-based FDG-PET reconstruction for the detection of hypo-metabolic regions in epilepsy. *IEEE Trans Med Imaging* 2004b; 23: 510-9.
- Benbadis SR, SO NK, Antar MA, Barnett GH, Morris HH. The value of PET scan (and MRI and Wada test) in patients with bitemporal epileptiform abnormalities. *Arch Neurol* 1995: 52: 1062-8.
- Blum DE, Ehsan T, Dungan D, Karis JP, Fisher RS. Bilateral temporal hypometabolism in epilepsy. *Epilepsia* 1998; 39: 651-9.
- Blumenfeld H, McNally KA, Vanderhill SD, Paige AL, Chung R, Davis K, et al.. Positive and negative network correlations in temporal lobe epilepsy. *Cereb Cortex* 2004; 14: 892-902.
- Bouilleret V, Dupont S, Spelle L, Baulac M, Samson Y, Semah F. Insular cortex involvement in mesiotemporal lobe epilepsy: a positron emission tomography study. *Ann Neurol* 2002; 51: 202-8.
- Bouvard S, Costes N, Bonnefoi F, Lavenne F, Mauguiere F, Delforge J, Ryvlin P. Seizure-related short-term plasticity of benzodiazepine receptors in partial epilepsy: a [11C]flumazenil-PET study. *Brain* 2005; 128: 1330-43.
- Carne RP, O'Brien TJ, Kilpatrick CJ, MacGregor LR, Hicks RJ, Murphy MA. MRI-negative PET-positive temporal lobe epilepsy: a distinct surgically remediable syndrome. *Brain* 2004; 127: 2276-85.
- Cendes F, Li LM, Watson C, Andermann F, Dubeau F, Arnold DL. Is ictal recording mandatory in temporal lobe epilepsy? Not when the interictal electroencephalogram and hippocampal atrophy coincide. *Arch Neurol* 2000; 57: 497-500.
- Chassoux F, Semah F, Bouilleret V, Landre E, Devaux B, Turak B, et al. Metabolic changes and electroclinical patterns in mesiotemporal lobe epilepsy: a correlative study. *Brain* 2004; 127: 164-74.
- Choi JY, Kim SJ, Hong SB, Seo DW, Hong SC, Kim BT, Kim SE. Extratemporal hypometabolism on FDG PET in temporal lobe epilepsy as a predictor of seizure outcome after temporal lobectomy. *Eur J Nucl Med Mol Imaging* 2003; 30: 581-7.
- Debets RM, Sadzot B, van Isselt JW, Brekelmans GJ, Meiners LC, van Huffelen AO, et al. Is 11C-flumazenil PET superior to 18FDG PET and 123I-iomazenil SPECT in presurgical evaluation of temporal lobe epilepsy? *J Neurol Neurosurg Psychiatry* 1997; 62: 141-50.
- Diehl B, LaPresto E, Najm I, Raja S, Rona S, Babb T, et al. Neocortical temporal FDG-PET hypometabolism correlates with temporal lobe atrophy in hippocampal sclerosis associated with microscopic cortical dysplasia. *Epilepsia* 2003; 44: 559-64.
- Drzezga A, Arnold S, Minoshima S, Noachtar S, Szecsi J, Winkler P, et al. 18F-FDG PET studies in patients with extratemporal and temporal epilepsy: evaluation of an observer-independent analysis. *J Nucl Med* 1999; 40: 737-46.
- Duncan JS. Imaging and epilepsy. *Brain* 1997; 120 (Pt 2): 339-77.
- Dupont S, Bouilleret V, Hasboun D, Semah F, Baulac M. Functional anatomy of the insula: new insights from imaging. *Surg Radiol Anat* 2003; 25: 113-9.
- Dupont S, Semah F, Baulac M, Samson Y. The underlying pathophysiology of ictal dystonia in temporal lobe epilepsy: an FDG-PET study. *Neurology* 1998; 51: 1289-92.

- Dupont S, Semah F, Clemenceau S, Adam C, Baulac M, Samson Y. Accurate prediction of postoperative outcome in mesial temporal lobe epilepsy: a study using positron emission tomography with 18fluorodeoxyglucose. *Arch Neurol* 2000; 57: 1331-6.
- Erbayat AE, Fessler AJ, Gallagher M, Attarian HP, Dehdashti F, Vahle VJ, et al. Correlation of severity of FDG-PET hypometabolism and interictal regional delta slowing in temporal lobe epilepsy. *Epilepsia* 2005; 46: 573-6.
- Fink GR, Pawlik G, Stefan H, Pietrzyk U, Wienhard K, Heiss WD. Temporal lobe epilepsy: evidence for interictal uncoupling of blood flow and glucose metabolism in temporomesial structures. *J Neurol Sci* 1996; 137: 28-34.
- Foldvary N, Lee N, Hanson MW, Coleman RE, Hulette CM, Friedman AH, et al.. Correlation of hippocampal neuronal density and FDG-PET in mesial temporal lobe epilepsy. *Epilepsia* 1999; 40: 26-9.
- Frost JJ, Mayberg HS, Fisher RS, Douglass KH, Dannals RF, Links JM, et al.. Mu-opiate receptors measured by positron emission tomography are increased in temporal-lobe epilepsy. *Ann Neurol* 1988; 23: 231-7.
- Gaillard WD, Fazilat S, White S, Malow B, Sato S, Reeves P, et al. Interictal metabolism and blood flow are uncoupled in temporal lobe cortex of patients with complex partial epilepsy. *Neurology* 1995; 45: 1841-7.
- Giovacchini G, Toczek MT, Bonwetsch R, Bagic A, Lang L, Fraser C, et al. 5-HT 1A receptors are reduced in temporal lobe epilepsy after partial-volume correction. *J Nucl Med* 2005; 46: 1128-35.
- Gold L, Lauritzen M. Neuronal deactivation explains decreased cerebellar blood flow in response to focal cerebral ischemia or suppressed neocortical function. *Proc Natl Acad Sci USA* 2002; 99: 7699-704.
- Hammers A, Asselin MC, Hinz R, Kitchen I, Brooks DJ, Duncan JS, Koepp MJ. Upregulation of opioid receptor binding following spontaneous epileptic seizures. *Brain* 2007; 130: 1009-16.
- Hammer A, Koepp MJ, Labbe C, Brooks DJ, Thom M, Cunningham VJ, Duncan JS. Neocortical abnormalities of [11C]-flumazenil PET in mesial temporal lobe epilepsy. *Neurology* 2001; 56: 897-906.
- Hand KS, Baird VH, Van Paesschen W, Koepp MJ, Revesz T, Thom M., et al. Central benzodiazepine receptor autoradiography in hippocampal sclerosis. *Br J Pharmacol* 1997; 122: 358-64.
- Hasler G, Bonwetsch R, Giovacchini G, Toczek MT, Bagic A, Luckenbaugh DA, et al. 5-HT1A receptor binding in temporal lobe epilepsy patients with and without major depression. *Biological Psychiatry* 2007; 62: 1258-64.
- Helmstaedter, C., Kurthen, M., Lux, S., Reuber, M., Elger, C.E.,. Chronic epilepsy and cognition: a longitudinal study in temporal lobe epilepsy. *Ann Neurol* 2003; 54: 425-32.
- Henry TR, Mazziotta JC, Engel J, Jr. Interictal metabolic anatomy of mesial temporal lobe epilepsy. *Arch Neurol* 1993; 50: 582-9.
- Henry TR, Mazziotta JC, Engel J, Jr, Christenson PD, Zhang JX, Phelps ME, Kuhl DE. Quantifying interictal metabolic activity in human temporal lobe epilepsy. *J Cereb Blood Flow Metab* 1990; 10: 748-57.
- Herrendorf G, Steinhoff BJ, Bittermann HJ, Mursch K, Meller J, Becker W. An easy method to accelerate ictal SPECT. *J Neuroimaging* 1999; 9: 129-30.
- Ho SS, Berkovic SF, Berlangieri SU, Newton MR, Egan GF, Tochon-Danguy HJ, McKay WJ. Comparison of ictal SPECT and interictal PET in the presurgical evaluation of temporal lobe epilepsy. *Ann Neurol* 1995; 37: 738-45.
- Ho SS, Berkovic SF, McKay WJ, Kalnins RM, Bladin PF. Temporal lobe epilepsy subtypes: differential patterns of cerebral perfusion on ictal SPECT. *Epilepsia* 1996; 37: 788-95.

- Hong SB, Han HJ, Roh SY, Seo DW, Kim SE, Kim MH. Hypometabolism and interictal spikes during positron emission tomography scanning in temporal lobe epilepsy. *Eur Neurol* 2002; 48: 65-70.
- Ito S, Suhara T, Ito H, Yasuno F, Ichimiya T, Takano A, et al. Changes in central 5-HT(1A) receptor binding in mesial temporal epilepsy measured by positron emission tomography with [(11)C]WAY100635. *Epilepsy Res* 2007; 73: 111-8.
- Jokeit H, Seitz RJ, Markowitsch HJ, Neumann N, Witte OW, Ebner A. Prefrontal asymmetric interictal glucose hypometabolism and cognitive impairment in patients with temporal lobe epilepsy. *Brain* 1997; 120 (Pt 12): 2283-94.
- Joo EY, Hong SB, Han HJ, Tae WS, Kim JH, Han SJ, et al. Postoperative alteration of cerebral glucose metabolism in mesial temporal lobe epilepsy. *Brain* 2005; 128: 1802-10.
- Joo EY, Hong SB, Lee EK, Tae WS, Kim JH, Seo DW, et al. Regional cerebral hyperperfusion with ictal dystonic posturing: ictal-interictal SPECT subtraction. *Epilepsia* 2004; 45: 686-9.
- Juhasz C, Nagy F, Watson C, da Silva EA, Muzik O, Chugani DC, et al. Glucose and [11C]flumazenil positron emission tomography abnormalities of thalamic nuclei in temporal lobe epilepsy. *Neurology* 1999; 53: 2037-45.
- Kaiboriboon K, Bertrand ME, Osman MM, Hogan RE. Quantitative analysis of cerebral blood flow patterns in mesial temporal lobe epilepsy using composite SISCOM. *J Nucl Med* 2005; 46: 38-43.
- Khan N, Leenders KL, Hajek M, Maguire P, Missimer J, Wieser HG. Thalamic glucose metabolism in temporal lobe epilepsy measured with 18F-FDG positron emission tomography (PET). *Epilepsy Res* 1997; 28: 233-43.
- Kilpatrick C, O'Brien T, Matkovic Z, Cook M, Kaye A. Preoperative evaluation for temporal lobe surgery. *J Clin Neurosci* 2003; 10: 535-9.
- Kim JH, Im KC, Kim JS, Lee SA, Lee JK, Khang SK, Kang JK. Ictal hyperperfusion patterns in relation to ictal scalp EEG patterns in patients with unilateral hippocampal sclerosis: a SPECT study. *Epilepsia* 2007; 48: 270-7.
- Kim YK, Lee DS, Lee SK, Kim SK, Chung CK, Chang KH, et al. Differential features of metabolic abnormalities between medial and lateral temporal lobe epilepsy: quantitative analysis of (18)F-FDG PET using SPM. *J Nucl Med* 2003; 44: 1006-12.
- Koepp MJ, Labbe C, Richardson MP, Brooks DJ, Van Paesschen W, Cunningham VJ, Duncan JS. Regional hippocampal [11C]flumazenil PET in temporal lobe epilepsy with unilateral and bilateral hippocampal sclerosis. *Brain* 1997a; 120 (Pt 10): 1865-76.
- Koepp MJ, Richardson MP, Brooks DJ, Poline JB, Van Paesschen W, Friston KJ, Duncan JS. Cerebral benzodiazepine receptors in hippocampal sclerosis. An objective *in vivo* analysis. *Brain* 1996; 119 (Pt 5): 1677-87.
- Koepp MJ, Richardson MP, Labbe C, Brooks DJ, Cunningham VJ, Ashburner J, et al. 11C-flumazenil PET, volumetric MRI, and quantitative pathology in mesial temporal lobe epilepsy. *Neurology* 1997b; 49: 764-73.
- Koutroumanidis M, Hennessy MJ, Seed PT, Elwes RD, Jarosz J, Morris RG, et al. Significance of interictal bilateral temporal hypometabolism in temporal lobe epilepsy. *Neurology* 2000; 54: 1811-21.
- Kuhl DE, Engel J, Jr, Phelps ME, Selin C. Epileptic patterns of local cerebral metabolism and perfusion in humans determined by emission computed tomography of 18FDG and 13NH3. *Ann Neurol* 1980; 8: 348-60.
- Lee DS, Lee JS, Kang KW, Jang MJ, Lee SK, Chung JK, Lee MC. Disparity of perfusion and glucose metabolism of epileptogenic zones in temporal lobe epilepsy demonstrated by SPM/SPAM analysis on 15O water PET, [18F]FDG-PET, and [99mTc]-HMPAO SPECT. *Epilepsia* 2001; 42: 1515-22.
- Lee SK, Lee DS, Yeo JS, Lee JS, Kim YK, Jang MJ, et al. FDG-PET images quantified by probabilistic atlas of brain and surgical prognosis of temporal lobe epilepsy. *Epilepsia* 2002; 43: 1032-8.

- Lee SK, Lee SH, Kim SK, Lee DS, Kim H. The clinical usefulness of ictal SPECT in temporal lobe epilepsy: the lateralization of seizure focus and correlation with EEG. *Epilepsia* 2000; 41: 955-62.
- Lee SK, Lee SY, Kim KK, Hong KS, Lee DS, Chung CK. Surgical outcome and prognostic factors of cryptogenic neocortical epilepsy. *Ann Neurol* 2005; 58: 525-32.
- Leveille J, Demonceau G, Walovitch RC. Intrasubject comparison between technetium-99m-ECD and technetium-99m-HMPAO in healthy human subjects. *J Nucl Med* 1992; 33: 480-4.
- Lieb JP, Dasheiff RM, Engel J, Jr. Role of the frontal lobes in the propagation of mesial temporal lobe seizures. *Epilepsia* 1991; 32: 822-37.
- Lin TW, de Aburto MA, Dahlbom M, Huang LL, Marvi MM, Tang M, et al. Predicting seizure-free status for temporal lobe epilepsy patients undergoing surgery: prognostic value of quantifying maximal metabolic asymmetry extending over a specified proportion of the temporal lobe. *J Nucl Med* 2007; 48: 776-82.
- Madar I, Lesser RP, Krauss G, Zubieta JK, Lever JR, Kinter CM, et al. Imaging of delta- and mu-opioid receptors in temporal lobe epilepsy by positron emission tomography. *Ann Neurol* 1997; 41: 358-67.
- Manno EM, Sperling MR, Ding X, Jaggi J, Alavi A, O'Connor MJ, Reivich M. Predictors of outcome after anterior temporal lobectomy: positron emission tomography. *Neurology* 1994; 44: 2331-6.
- Mayberg HS, Sadzot B, Meltzer CC, Fisher RS, Lesser RP, Dannals RF, et al. Quantification of mu and non-mu opiate receptors in temporal lobe epilepsy using positron emission tomography. *Ann Neurol* 1991; 30: 3-11.
- McNally KA, Paige AL, Varghese G, Zhang H, Novotny EJ, Jr, Spencer SS, et al.. Localizing value of ictal-interictal SPECT analyzed by SPM (ISAS). *Epilepsia* 2005; 46: 1450-64.
- Merlet I, Ostrowsky K, Costes N, Ryvlin P, Isnard J, Faillenot I, et al.. 5-HT1A receptor binding and intracerebral activity in temporal lobe epilepsy: an [18F]MPPF-PET study. *Brain* 2004a; 127: 900-13.
- Merlet I, Ryvlin P, Costes N, Dufournel D, Isnard J, Faillenot I, et al. Statistical parametric mapping of 5-HT1A receptor binding in temporal lobe epilepsy with hippocampal ictal onset on intracranial EEG. *Neuroimage* 2004b; 22: 886-96.
- Mizobuchi M, Matsuda K, Inoue Y, Sako K, Sumi Y, Chitoku S, et al. Dystonic posturing associated with putaminal hyperperfusion depicted on subtraction SPECT. *Epilepsia* 2004; 45: 948-53.
- Mizobuchi M, Sumi Y, Sako K, Nihira A, Nakagawara J. Putaminal hyperperfusion in dystonic posturing on subtracted SPECT: a case report. *Ann Nucl Med* 2001; 15: 255-7.
- Nelissen N, Van Paesschen W, Baete K, Van Laere K, Palmini A, Vanbilloen H, Dupont P. Correlations of interictal FDG-PET metabolism and ictal SPECT perfusion changes in human temporal lobe epilepsy with hippocampal sclerosis. *Neuroimage* 2006; 32: 684-95.
- Newberg AB, Alavi A, Berlin J, Mozley PD, O'Connor M, Sperling M. Ipsilateral and contralateral thalamic hypometabolism as a predictor of outcome after temporal lobectomy for seizures. *J Nucl Med* 2000; 4: 1964-8.
- Newton MR, Berkovic SF, Austin MC, Reutens DC, McKay WJ, Bladin PF. Dystonia, clinical lateralization, and regional blood flow changes in temporal lobe seizures. *Neurology* 1992a; 42: 371-7.
- Newton MR, Berkovic SF, Austin MC, Rowe CC, McKay WJ, Bladin PF. Postictal switch in blood flow distribution and temporal lobe seizures. *J Neurol Neurosurg Psychiatry* 1992b; 55: 891-4.
- Newton MR, Berkovic SF, Austin MC, Rowe CC, McKay WJ, Bladin PF. SPECT in the localisation of extratemporal and temporal seizure foci. *J Neurol Neurosurg Psychiatry* 1995; 59: 26-30.

- O'Brien TJ, Miles K, Ware R, Cook MJ, Binns DS, Hicks RJ. The cost-effective use of 18F-FDG PET in the presurgical evaluation of medically refractory focal epilepsy. *J Nucl Med* 2008; 49: 931-7.
- O'Brien TJ, So EL, Mullan BP, Hauser MF, Brinkmann BH, Bohnen NI, et al. Subtraction ictal SPECT co-registered to MRI improves clinical usefulness of SPECT in localizing the surgical seizure focus. *Neurology* 1998; 50: 445-54.
- Oku N, Matsumoto M, Hashikawa K, Moriwaki H, Ishida M, Seike Y, et al. Intra-individual differences between technetium-99m-HMPAO and technetium-99m-ECD in the normal medial temporal lobe. *J Nucl Med* 1997; 38: 1109-11.
- Quarantelli M, Berkouk K, Prinster A, Landeau B, Svarer C, Balkay L, et al. Integrated software for the analysis of brain PET/SPECT studies with partial-volume-effect correction. *J Nucl Med* 2004; 45: 192-201.
- Radtke RA, Hanson MW, Hoffman JM, Crain BJ, Walczak TS, Lewis DV, et al. Temporal lobe hypometabolism on PET: predictor of seizure control after temporal lobectomy. *Neurology* 1993; 43: 1088-92.
- Rosenow F, Lüders H. Presurgical evaluation of epilepsy. *Brain* 2001; 124: 1683-700.
- Rowe CC, Berkovic SF, Austin MC, McKay WJ, Bladin PF. Patterns of postictal cerebral blood flow in temporal lobe epilepsy: qualitative and quantitative analysis. *Neurology* 1991a; 41: 1096-103.
- Rowe CC, Berkovic SF, Austin MC, Saling M, Kalnins RM, McKay WJ, Bladin PF. Visual and quantitative analysis of interictal SPECT with technetium-99m-HMPAO in temporal lobe epilepsy. *J Nucl Med* 1991b; 32: 1688-94.
- Ryvlin P, Bouvard S, Le BD, De Lamerie G, Gregoire MC, Kahane P, et al. Clinical utility of flumazenil-PET *versus* [18F]fluorodeoxyglucose-PET and MRI in refractory partial epilepsy. A prospective study in 100 patients. *Brain* 1998; 121 (Pt 11): 2067-81.
- Salzberg M, Taher T, Davie M, Carne R, Hicks RJ, Cook M, et al. Depression in temporal lobe epilepsy surgery patients: an FDG-PET study. *Epilepsia* 2006; 47: 2125-30.
- Savic I, Lindstrom P, Gulyas B, Halldin C, Andree B, Farde L. Limbic reductions of 5-HT1A receptor binding in human temporal lobe epilepsy. *Neurology* 2004; 62: 1343-51.
- Schwartz TH, Bonhoeffer T. In vivo optical mapping of epileptic foci and surround inhibition in ferret cerebral cortex. *Nat Med* 2001; 7: 1063-7.
- Shin WC, Hong SB, Tae WS, Kim SE. Ictal hyperperfusion patterns according to the progression of temporal lobe seizures. *Neurology* 2002; 58: 373-80.
- Simons PJ, Van Paesschen W, Palmini A, Dupont P, Van Driel G, Van Laere K. The development of hippocampal sclerosis in a patient with occipital lobe epilepsy and migraine. *Neurology* 2004; 62: 1024-5.
- Smith BJ, Karvelis KC, Cronan S, Porter W, Smith L, Pantelic MV, Elisevich K. Developing an effective program to complete ictal SPECT in the epilepsy monitoring unit. *Epilepsy Res* 1999; 33: 189-97.
- Spanaki MV, Kopylev L, DeCarli C, Gaillard WD, Liow K, Fazilat S, et al. Postoperative changes in cerebral metabolism in temporal lobe epilepsy. *Arch Neurol* 2000; 57: 1447-52.
- Spencer SS. The relative contributions of MRI, SPECT, and PET imaging in epilepsy. *Epilepsia* 1994; 35 (Suppl 6): S72-S89.
- Swartz BE, Tomiyasu U, Delgado-Escueta AV, Mandelkern M, Khonsari A. Neuroimaging in temporal lobe epilepsy: test sensitivity and relationships to pathology and postoperative outcome. *Epilepsia* 1992; 33: 624-34.
- Tae WS, Joo EY, Kim JH, Han SJ, Suh YL, Kim BT, et al. Cerebral perfusion changes in mesial temporal lobe epilepsy: SPM analysis of ictal and interictal SPECT. *Neuroimage* 2005; 24: 101-10.

- Takaya S, Hanakawa T, Hashikawa K, Ikeda A, Sawamoto N, Nagamine T, et al. Prefrontal hypofunction in patients with intractable mesial temporal lobe epilepsy. Neurology 2006; 67: 1674-6.
- Theodore WH, Gaillard WD, Sato S, Kufta C, Leiderman D. Positron emission tomographic measurement of cerebral blood flow and temporal lobectomy. Ann Neurol 1994; 36: 241-4.
- Theodore WH, Hasler G, Giovacchini G, Kelley K, Reeves-Tyer P, Herscovitch P, Drevets W. Reduced hippocampal 5HT1A PET receptor binding and depression in temporal lobe epilepsy. Epilepsia 2007; 48: 1526-30.
- Theodore WH, Sato S, Kufta C, Balish MB, Bromfield EB, Leiderman DB. Temporal lobectomy for uncontrolled seizures: the role of positron emission tomography. Ann Neurol 1992; 32: 789-94.
- Theodore WH, Sato S, Kufta CV, Gaillard WD, Kelley K. FDG-positron emission tomography and invasive EEG: seizure focus detection and surgical outcome. Epilepsia 1997; 38: 81-6.
- Toczek MT, Carson RE, Lang L, Ma Y, Spanaki MV, Der MG. et al.. PET imaging of 5-HT1A receptor binding in patients with temporal lobe epilepsy. Neurology 2003; 60: 749-56.
- Tortella FC, Long JB. Endogenous anticonvulsant substance in rat cerebrospinal fluid after a generalized seizure. Science 1985; 228: 1106-08.
- Treiman DM. GABAergic mechanisms in epilepsy. Epilepsia 2001; 42 (Suppl 3): 8-12.
- Uijl SG, Leijten FS, Arends JB, Parra J, van Huffelen AC, Moons KG. The added value of [18F]-fluoro-D-deoxyglucose positron emission tomography in screening for temporal lobe epilepsy surgery. Epilepsia 2007; 48: 2121-9.
- Uijl SG, Leijten FS, Arends JB, Parra J, van Huffelen AC, Moons KG. Prognosis after temporal lobe epilepsy surgery: The value of combining predictors. Epilepsia 2008; 49: 1317-23.
- Van Bogaert P, Massager N, Tugendhaft P, Wikler D, Damhaut P, Levivier M, et al. Statistical parametric mapping of regional glucose metabolism in mesial temporal lobe epilepsy. Neuroimage 2000; 12: 129-38.
- Van Paesschen W. Qualitative and quantitative imaging of the hippocampus in mesial temporal lobe epilepsy with hippocampal sclerosis. Neuroimaging Clin N Am 2004; 14: 373-400, vii.
- Van Paesschen W, Connelly A, Johnson CL, Duncan JS. The amygdala and intractable temporal lobe epilepsy: a quantitative magnetic resonance imaging study. Neurology 1996; 47: 1021-31.
- Van Paesschen W, Connelly A, King MD, Jackson GD, Duncan JS. The spectrum of hippocampal sclerosis: a quantitative magnetic resonance imaging study. Ann Neurol 1997; 41: 41-51.
- Van Paesschen W, Dupont P, Sunaert S, Goffin K, Van Laere K. The use of SPECT and PET in routine clinical practice in epilepsy. Curr Opin Neurol 2007; 20: 194-202.
- Van Paesschen W, Dupont P, Van Driel G, Vanbilloen H, Maes A. SPECT perfusion changes during complex partial seizures in patients with hippocampal sclerosis. Brain 2003; 126: 1103-11.
- Van Paesschen W, Dupont P, Van Heerden B, Vanbilloen H, Mesotten L, Maes A, et al. Self-injection ictal SPECT during partial seizures. Neurology 2000; 54: 1994-7.
- Vanbilloen H, Dupont P, Mesotten L, Mortelmans L, Verbeke K, Verbruggen A, et al. Simple design for rapid self-injection ictal SPET during aura. Eur J Nucl Med 1999; 26: 1380-1.
- Wagner JJ, Caudle RM, Neumaier JF, Chavkin C. Stimulation of endogenous opioid release displaces mu receptor binding in rat hippocampus. Neuroscience 1990; 37: 45-53.
- Wichert-Ana L, Velasco TR, Terra-Bustamante VC, Alexandre V Jr, Guarnieri R, Walz R, et al. Ictal chronology and interictal spikes predict perfusion patterns in temporal lobe epilepsy: a multivariate study. Seizure 2004; 13: 346-57.
- Wiebe S, Blume WT, Girvin JP, Eliasziw M. A randomized, controlled trial of surgery for temporal-lobe epilepsy. N Engl J Med 2001; 345: 311-8.
- Witte OW, Bruehl C, Schlaug G, Tuxhorn I, Lahl R, Villagran R, Seitz RJ. Dynamic changes of focal hypometabolism in relation to epileptic activity. J Neurol Sci 1994; 124: 188-197.

- Wong CY, Gannon J, Bong J, Wong CO, Saha GB. Computer-assisted lateralization of unilateral temporal lobe epilepsy using Z-score parametric F-18 FDG PET images. *BMC Nucl Med* 2007; 7: 5.
- Wong CY, Geller EB, Chen EQ, MacIntyre WJ, Morris HH III, Raja S, et al.. Outcome of temporal lobe epilepsy surgery predicted by statistical parametric PET imaging. *J Nucl Med* 1996; 37: 1094-100.
- Wright MA, Orth M, Patsalos PN, Smith SJ, Richardson MP. Cortical excitability predicts seizures in acutely drug-reduced temporal lobe epilepsy patients. *Neurology* 2006; 67: 1646-51.
- Zaknun JJ, Bal C, Maes A, Tepmongkol S, Vazquez S, Dupont P, Dondi M. Comparative analysis of MR imaging, Ictal SPECT and EEG in temporal lobe epilepsy: a prospective IAEA multi-center study. *Eur J Nucl Med Mol Imaging* 2008; 35: 107-15.
- Zhou L, Dupont P, Baete K, Van Paesschen W, Van Laere K, Nuyts J. Detection of inter-hemispheric metabolic asymmetries in FDG-PET images using prior anatomical information. *NeuroImage* 2009; 44: 35-42.
- Zubal IG, Avery RA, Stokking R, Studholme C, Corsi M, Dey H, et al. Ratio-images calculated from interictal positron emission tomography and single-photon emission computed tomography for quantification of the uncoupling of brain metabolism and perfusion in epilepsy. *Epilepsia* 2000; 41: 1560-6.
- Zubal IG, Spencer SS, Imam K, Seibyl J, Smith EO, Wisniewski G, Hoffer PB. Difference images calculated from ictal and interictal technetium-99m-HMPAO SPECT scans of epilepsy. *J Nucl Med* 1995; 36: 684-9.

Section V:
Treatment of mesial temporal lobe epilepsies

Antiepileptic treatment of patients with mesial temporal lobe epilepsies

Eugen Trinka

Christian Doppler Klinik, Salzburg, Austria

■ General considerations: the hidden population

Mesial temporal lobe epilepsies (MTLEs) are well recognized as one of the major drug-resistant epilepsy syndromes amenable to epilepsy surgery. Current literature therefore focuses on the surgical outcome of temporal lobe epilepsies. However, due to the natural course of the diseases and the long duration with active seizures, medical treatment remains one of the cornerstones of management for this patient group. Data from randomized controlled trials in MTLE are not available to inform the clinicians appropriately. The population of patients with MTLE is hidden in the usual randomized control trials using the classic add-on design. Due to the lack of clinical information and the non-specific inclusion criteria in these trials, it is impossible to draw any firm conclusions on the responsiveness of MTLE to a certain antiepileptic drug. Monotherapy trials should allow assessment of clinical responsiveness of MTLE from the very beginning of the disease, however, clinical stratification and syndromic classification are not precise enough, in any currently available monotherapy study, to draw any conclusion on clinical responsiveness in patients with MTLE. This striking lack of randomized control trials for this syndrome is unlikely to be overcome in the near future, due to the comparatively small number of patients with MTLE and the difficulty of precise diagnosis, at least in some cases, at disease onset. Most information is derived from selected series of patients who underwent epilepsy surgery or were stratified according to their diagnoses based on MRI (*e.g.* hippocampal sclerosis) or seizure type (complex focal seizures).

Patients with MTLE are therefore usually included in two types of trials. Firstly, add-on trials (phase III) for patients with refractory focal epilepsy; these are so-called "pivotal trials", which are necessary for the licensing of the drug. Secondly, some patients with MTLE may also be included in monotherapy trials for newly diagnosed epilepsy; these trials are either class I (or class II if less stringent criteria and study designs are used) or class III trials (such as the SANAD trial) according to the ILAE criteria. These different trials represent the two loose ends of the clinical spectrum of MTLE; on the one hand, drug-resistant MTLE is more likely to be better treated with appropriate resective surgery, and on the other, newly diagnosed patients with MTLE may respond initially well to medical treatment. Although no epidemiological studies have specifically addressed this issue, the medical outcome for the majority of patients with MTLE may well be midway between these two scenarios. At present, it is impossible to give a clear prognosis on the medical responsiveness at disease onset (even in the presence of clear-cut MTLE or dual pathology). Our understanding of medical outcome of patients with newly diagnosed MTLE is therefore incomplete. Information is only available in selected series based on MRI presence of hippocampal sclerosis or the presence of complex partial seizures. Even more biased are the results from surgical series. The only available randomised controlled trials comparing medical *vs.* surgical outcome have included only refractory patients with TLE.

■ What have we learnt from monotherapy trials in newly diagnosed focal epilepsies?

Monotherapy trials in patients with newly diagnosed epilepsy are mainly performed for regulatory purposes (Marson & Williamson, 2009). The minimum requirement for inclusion is at least two focal onset seizures. These studies do not allow for syndromic diagnosis of the patients, not even retrospectively. Therefore, we are only able to estimate the efficacy of any given AED in a population of patients with focal epilepsies. These trials have consistently shown that the seizure-free rate is between 50 and 60%.

To date, the largest reported class I trial is the seminal VA trial comparing carbamazepine, phenytoin, primidone and phenobarbital (Mattson *et al.*, 1985). In this trial, carbamazepine and phenytoin were superior to phenobarbital or primidone in terms of retention rate. In fact, the difference between the drugs in this trial was mainly due to tolerability rather than efficacy. A recent trial compared modified-release carbamazepine and levetiracetam in newly diagnosed epilepsy (Brodie *et al.*, 2007). Astonishingly, 20 years after the landmark study by Mattson and co-workers, the seizure-free rate has not improved much. The seizure-free rate after one year was 49.8%; 53% with levetiracetam and 53.3% with controlled-release carbamazepine (Brodie *et al.*, 2007). The discontinuation rate over the first year of treatment was virtually the same between levetiracetam and controlled-release carbamazepine. The conclusion of the study was that levetiracetam is not inferior to controlled-release carbamazepine in newly diagnosed epilepsy. In summary, controlled-release carbamazepine and levetiracetam are the first line treatment for newly diagnosed focal epilepsies (Brodie *et al.*, 2007; Glauser *et al.*, 2006).

Randomised controlled trials are generally regarded as the gold standard of evidence-based medicine. However, one may criticize that the study design does not reflect clinical practice (Marson & Williamson, 2009); the duration is usually less than one year, and the patient population is highly selected, excluding patients with psychiatric or other comorbidities. Thus, the results cannot be extended to the whole population of patients with epilepsy. Pragmatic trials may provide important information on the long-term effects of treatments for epilepsy and are more reflective of the patients seen in general and specialist practices (Marson *et al.*, 2007a; 2007b; Trinka *et al.*, 2008). They also have the advantage of flexible and clinically relevant dosing schedules. The largest naturalistic study to date is the SANAD trial, which included focal (study arm A [Marson *et al.*, 2007a]) and generalised epilepsies (study arm B [Marson *et al.*, 2007b]). In arm A of the SANAD study, 1,721 patients were randomized to carbamazepine, gabapentin, lamotrigine, oxcarbazepine and topiramate. The main outcome was based on the time to treatment failure and the time to one-year remission. Again, the most effective drugs were lamotrigine and carbamazepine. Regarding retention, lamotrigine was significantly superior to carbamazepine (HR 0.78 [95% CI 0.63-0.97]), gabapentin (HR 0.65 [95% CI 0.52-0.80]) and topiramate (HR 0.64 [95% CI 0.52-0.79]). The time to one-year remission was significantly longer with carbamazepine compared to gabapentin (HR 0.75 [95% CI 0.63-0.90]). However, there was no difference compared to lamotrigine in this respect at two years (-8% to +7%). In summary, lamotrigine seems to be the best drug for focal epilepsies in the SANAD trial in terms of tolerability, but not inferior to carbamazepine (Marson et al., 2007a).

What can we learn from add-on trials of patients with refractory focal epilepsies?

We have to accept that the classic add-on trials in patients with refractory focal epilepsies are designed for regulatory purposes and do not inform the clinicians about best practice. They are usually conducted over a short time period (three months) with placebo as a comparator. The European licensing authorities (EMA) use the 50% responder rate as the primary outcome, whereas the Food and Drug Administration (FDA) of the US uses the percentage change in mean seizure frequency as the main outcome criterion. One of the many drawbacks of these types of trials is the narrow inclusion criteria (Marson & Williamson, 2009; Tlusta et al., 2008). Because of the high rate of comorbidity, most of the patients with refractory MTLE will probably not qualify for these trials (Tlusta et al., 2008). Overall, the 50% responder rates are between 6.7% and 66.7% (LaRoche & Helmers, 2004a; 2004b), the mean decrease of seizure frequency is between 17% and 59%, and only a small fraction, usually less than 10%, of patients become seizure-free.

Medical outcome of patients with mesial temporal lobe epilepsy in selected series

Cross-sectional studies from different epilepsy centres have demonstrated that the responsiveness to antiepileptic drugs is strongly associated with the aetiology of epilepsy. Semah and co-workers (1998) found only 11% of patients with hippocampal sclerosis out of 2,200 patients at the epilepsy centre in Paris in remission (defined as seizure-free for more than one year). When dual pathology was identified, only 2% patients were shown to be in remission. Compared to this low percentage, about 54% of all patients with post-stroke epilepsy were seizure-free for more than one year (Semah et al., 1998). Another group found a similar association between aetiology and responsiveness demonstrating 42% of patients with hippocampal sclerosis in remission, which was significantly less than that for any other aetiology (Stephen et al., 2001).

Hippocampal sclerosis is the only essential feature for the diagnosis of MTLE (Wieser, 2004). Selected series of patients with hippocampal sclerosis have demonstrated that there is a somewhat privileged subgroup of patients with MTLE with a more benign course than the classic group. Kim and co-workers (1999) identified 104 patients with MTLE. Hippocampal sclerosis was identified in 35%. The aetiology was meningoencephalitis in 19% and head trauma in 10%. All patients were followed at a single centre and for 38% patients, seizures became intractable. However, 37% improved with a seizure reduction of more than 50% and 25% were seizure-free for at least

24 months. In another cross-sectional study by Labate and co-workers (2006), of 101 consecutive patients with benign temporal lobe epilepsy with rare seizures during a follow-up of at least two years, 39% were shown to have hippocampal sclerosis based on MRI. Another characteristic feature of MTLE is the characteristic seizure semiology. Most of the patients suffer from complex focal seizures with or without secondary generalisation. In a combined analysis of both VA studies (No.s 118 and 264), the overall prognosis was worse if complex partial seizures were the predominating seizure type ($p < 0.0001$) (Mattson et al., 1996). In fact the prognosis was based on the predominating seizure type in patients with multiple seizure types, and again the presence of complex partial seizures complicated the prognosis which tended to be worse when complex partial seizures were present. Only 23% in one VA study (No. 118), and 26% in another VA study (No. 264) achieved a twelve-month seizure-free period, compared to 54% and 48% of patients who only had secondary generalised tonic-clonic seizures, respectively. Of note, the VA studies included newly diagnosed patients, which did not preclude these patients becoming seizure-free later in the course of their disease.

However, long-term information regarding medical prognosis of patients with MTLE is not yet available. In a cross-sectional study of 210 patients treated at our own centre, 40% of our patients were shown to be in remission and 46% were shown to have a seizure reduction of more than 50% (Trinka et al., 2001). The mean duration of seizure remission was 7.6 years (+/- 5.4 years). The patients entered remission after a mean of 15.17 years (+/- 12.3 years) of active epilepsy and 25% of the patients remained seizure-free for 6.1 years (+/- 5.4 years) after the discontinuation of antiepileptic drugs. The main predictor of a poor outcome in our study was a high seizure frequency of more than three per month at the beginning of the disease (OR 4.84 [95% CI 1.78-13.6]), mental retardation (OR 3.78 [95% CI 1.53-9.35]), and an abnormal neurological examination (OR 2.3 [95% CI 1.95-3.54]) (Trinka et al., 2001).

Data from cross-sectional studies, as well as case series and information from trials with newly diagnosed epilepsy, suggest that the natural course of epilepsy, especially MTLE, is not linear but shows periods of active devastating epilepsy which may remit for some time. Berg and co-workers (2003) investigated intermittent remissions in patients with refractory epilepsy. In a series of 234 patients who underwent presurgical evaluation between 1996 and 2001, 26% had a remission of more than one year and 8.5% had a remission of more than five years in their previous history. This led to a mean latency of 9.1 years to the presurgical evaluation (Berg et al., 2003). The same group investigated 614 children prospectively over a follow-up period of 9.7 years. The age at onset of epilepsy was 5.8 years. Twenty percent became refractory, however, 74.4% of patients entered temporary remission, which lasted 1.1 to 8.5 years. A remission period was observed more than once in 20.5% of the patients (Berg et al., 2001; Berg & Engel, Jr., 2006). This suggests that patients with refractory epilepsy show a relapsing-remitting course at a considerable rate, which could explain, at least in part, the long latency from the beginning of the disease to eventual epilepsy surgery. However neither study by Berg investigated specifically temporal lobe epilepsy patients. In a small series of 174 patients, we investigated the temporal pattern of our patients who underwent resective surgery in the Innsbruck Epilepsy Surgery Programme. We found that 14% of the temporal lobe epilepsy patients and 15% of the extratemporal lobe patients had a relapsing-remitting course, which was defined as at least two remissions lasting for more than a year. In addition, 43.8% of temporal lobe epilepsy and 42.3% of extratemporal lobe epilepsy patients followed had a secondary pharmacoresistant course, which was defined as remission for more than year once before resective surgery. The remaining 52% with temporal lobe epilepsy and 42.3% with extratemporal lobe epilepsy had a primary pharmacoresistant course (Rohracher, 2010).

Two studies have analysed the results of effects of antiepileptic drugs in apparent drug-resistant epilepsy patients. Callaghan and co-workers (2007) investigated 246 patients with refractory epilepsy who were taking more than two antiepileptic drugs and followed them for a mean duration of three years. They identified a cumulative probability for patients to enter remission for at least six months after addition of an antiepileptic drug in 40.1%. Luciano and Shorvon (2007) investigated 265 antiepileptic drug treatments in 155 patients. In their study 16% resulted in a 12-month remission and in another 21%, a 50%-decrease in seizure frequency occurred. Overall, 28% of patients were rendered seizure-free. A short duration and previous failure of a small number of antiepileptic drugs were identified as positive predictors (Luciano & Shorvon, 2007). However, over time, the chance of achieving remission may decrease. Schiller and Najjar (2008) investigated a cohort of 478 consecutive patients with newly administered antiepileptic drugs with a follow-up period of between 1.5 to 7.5 years, and analyzed the response to newly administered drug treatments in relation to treatment history. For the first antiepileptic drug, they found seizure-free rates, which decreased from 61.8% to 41.7%, to be 16.6% and 0% after 0-5 and 6-7 previous antiepileptic drug failures, respectively. In addition to the number of antiepileptic drug failures, the type of epilepsy, duration of epilepsy, and number of seizures in the six-month period prior to antiepileptic drug initiation were found to be predictive factors.

■ Conclusions

There is a lack of long-term prognostic investigations of patients with MTLE who receive only drug treatment as the form of therapy. The early drug responsiveness in these patient groups is not well defined and the apparently benign cases which can be identified in cross-sectional studies represent most likely the patients who have a relapsing-remitting course (Shorvon & Luciano, 2007; Shorvon, 1984). This intermittent course may substantially delay referral for epilepsy surgery.

Abnormal neurological examination, high seizure frequency from the outset and a poor response to antiepileptic drug treatment remain the best indicators for a poor prognosis and a primary pharmacoresistant course.

References

- Berg AT, Engel J, Jr. Hippocampal atrophy and the prognosis of epilepsy: some answers, more questions. *Neurology* 2006; 67: 12-3.
- Berg AT, Langfitt J, Shinnar S, Vickrey BG, Sperling MR, Walczak T, et al.. How long does it take for partial epilepsy to become intractable? *Neurology* 2003; 60: 186-90.
- Berg AT, Shinnar S, Levy SR, Testa FM, Smith-Rapaport S, Beckerman B. Early development of intractable epilepsy in children: a prospective study. *Neurology* 2001; 56: 1445-52.
- Brodie MJ, Perucca E, Ryvlin P, Ben Menachem E, Meencke HJ. Comparison of levetiracetam and controlled-release carbamazepine in newly diagnosed epilepsy. *Neurology* 2007; 68: 402-8.

- Callaghan BC, Anand K, Hesdorffer D, Hauser WA, French JA. Likelihood of seizure remission in an adult population with refractory epilepsy. *Ann Neurol* 2007; 62: 382-9.
- Glauser T, Ben Menachem E, Bourgeois B, Cnaan A, Chadwick D, Guerreiro C, et al. ILAE treatment guidelines: evidence-based analysis of antiepileptic drug efficacy and effectiveness as initial monotherapy for epileptic seizures and syndromes. *Epilepsia* 2006; 47: 1094-120.
- Kim WJ, Park SC, Lee SJ, Lee JH, Kim JY, Lee BI, Kim DI. The prognosis for control of seizures with medications in patients with MRI evidence for mesial temporal sclerosis. *Epilepsia* 1999; 40: 290-3.
- Labate A, Ventura P, Gambardella A, Le PE, Colosimo E, Leggio U, et al. MRI evidence of mesial temporal sclerosis in sporadic "benign" temporal lobe epilepsy. *Neurology* 2006; 66: 562-5.
- LaRoche SM, Helmers SL. The new antiepileptic drugs: clinical applications. *JAMA* 2004a; 291: 615-20.
- LaRoche SM, Helmers SL. The new antiepileptic drugs: scientific review. *JAMA* 2004b; 291: 605-14.
- Luciano AL, Shorvon SD Results of treatment changes in patients with apparently drug-resistant chronic epilepsy. *Ann Neurol* 2007; 62: 375-81.
- Marson AG, Al Kharusi AM, Alwaidh M, Appleton R, Baker GA, Chadwick DW, et al. The SANAD study of effectiveness of carbamazepine, gabapentin, lamotrigine, oxcarbazepine, or topiramate for treatment of partial epilepsy: an unblinded randomised controlled trial. *Lancet* 2007a; 369: 1000-15.
- Marson AG, Al Kharusi AM, Alwaidh M, Appleton R, Baker GA, Chadwick DW, et al. The SANAD study of effectiveness of valproate, lamotrigine, or topiramate for generalised and unclassifiable epilepsy: an unblinded randomised controlled trial. *Lancet* 2007b; 369: 1016-26.
- Marson AG, Williamson PR. Interpreting regulatory trials in epilepsy. *Curr Opin Neurol* 2009; 22: 167-73.
- Mattson RH, Cramer JA, Collins JF. Prognosis for total control of complex partial and secondarily generalized tonic clonic seizures. Department of Veterans Affairs Epilepsy Cooperative Studies No. 118 and No. 264. Group. *Neurology* 1996; 47, 68-76.
- Mattson RH, Cramer JA, Collins JF, Smith DB, Delgado-Escueta AV, Browne TR, et al. Comparison of carbamazepine, phenobarbital, phenytoin, and primidone in partial and secondarily generalized tonic-clonic seizures. *N Engl J Med* 1985; 313: 145-51.
- Rohracher A. *The natural history of pharmacoresistant epilepsies – a retrospective investigation of surgically treated patients.* [Thesis] Medical University Innsbruck, 2010.
- Schiller Y, Najjar Y. Quantifying the response to antiepileptic drugs: effect of past treatment history. *Neurology* 2008; 70: 54-65.
- Semah F, Picot MC, Adam C, Broglin D, Arzimanoglou A, Bazin B, et al. Is the underlying cause of epilepsy a major prognostic factor for recurrence? *Neurology* 1998; 51: 1256-62.
- Shorvon S, Luciano AL. Prognosis of chronic and newly diagnosed epilepsy: revisiting temporal aspects. *Curr Opin Neurol* 2007; 20: 208-12.
- Shorvon SD. The temporal aspects of prognosis in epilepsy. *J Neurol Neurosurg Psychiatry* 1984; 47: 1157-65.
- Stephen LJ, Kwan P, Brodie MJ. Does the cause of localisation-related epilepsy influence the response to antiepileptic drug treatment? *Epilepsia* 2001; 42: 357-62.
- Tlusta E, Handoko KB, Majoie M, Egberts TC, Vlcek J, Heerdink ER. Clinical relevance of patients with epilepsy included in clinical trials. *Epilepsia* 2008; 49: 1479-80.
- Trinka E, Van Paesschen W, Hallstrom Y, Yon P, Marson A.G, Muscas G, et al. The KOMET study: An open-label, randomized, parallel group trial comparing the efficacy and safety of levetiracetame with sodium valproate and carbamazepine as monotherapy in subjects with newly diagnosed epilepsy. *Epilepsia* 2008; 49 (Suppl. 8th ECE Berlin), 50.

- Trinka E, Martin F, Luef G, Unterberger I, Bauer G. Chronic epilepsy with complex partial seizures is not always medically intractable–a long-term observational study. *Acta Neurol Scand* 2001; 103: 219-25.
- Wieser HG. ILAE Commission Report. Mesial temporal lobe epilepsy with hippocampal sclerosis. *Epilepsia* 2004; 45: 695-714.

Depth electrodes (SEEG) in temporal lobe epilepsy

Massimo Cossu, Francesco Cardinale, Laura Tassi, Francesca Gozzo, Marco Schiariti, Ivana Sartori, Laura Castana, Giorgio Lo Russo

C. Munari Epilepsy Surgery Centre, Niguarda Hospital, Milan, Italy

---

Drug-resistant temporal lobe epilepsy (TLE) receives surgical attention more frequently than other forms of symptomatic localization-related epilepsy. It is not surprising, therefore, that until a few years ago, invasive EEG investigations were performed in a comparable proportion of TLE cases susceptible to surgical treatment. The extensive employment of intracranial, especially intracerebral, electrodes has undoubtedly provided essential information on the organization of the epileptogenic networks underlying TLE, and has contributed to the recognition of distinct epileptic syndromes involving the different temporal lobe structures. The ability to record ictal EEG activity from external and internal areas of the temporal lobe has, for example, enabled the differentiation between mesial and neocortical temporal lobe epilepsies. Furthermore, the main bulk of knowledge concerning the relative contribution of the different mesial and neocortical temporal lobe structures to the organization of the ictal discharge in mesial and antero-mesial TLE derives from intracerebral electrode evaluation employed according to the methodology of stereo-electro-encephalography (SEEG) (Bartolomei 1999; 2008). It is probably for these reasons, along with the availability of more advanced imaging techniques which provide additional localizing information, that the recourse to invasive recordings in patients presenting "classic" electroclinical patterns of TLE is steadily decreasing. Indeed, our experience shows that, from the beginning of the Epilepsy Surgery Program at Niguarda Hospital in 1996, of the subpopulation of cases receiving temporal lobe resection, the proportion of patients submitted for SEEG dropped from 27% to 3% (*Figure 1*). This means that most of the patients with presumed TLE may currently be offered surgery after non-invasive electroclinical evaluation, including long-term video-EEG monitoring when required, and accurate imaging by high-resolution magnetic resonance imaging (MRI). On the other hand, a small but challenging subset of patients still requires invasive SEEG monitoring before temporal lobe resection. The present chapter focuses mainly on clinical-EEG and neuroradiological features of these cases, essential points of SEEG methodology employed in presurgical evaluation and surgical results of SEEG-based temporal lobe resections.

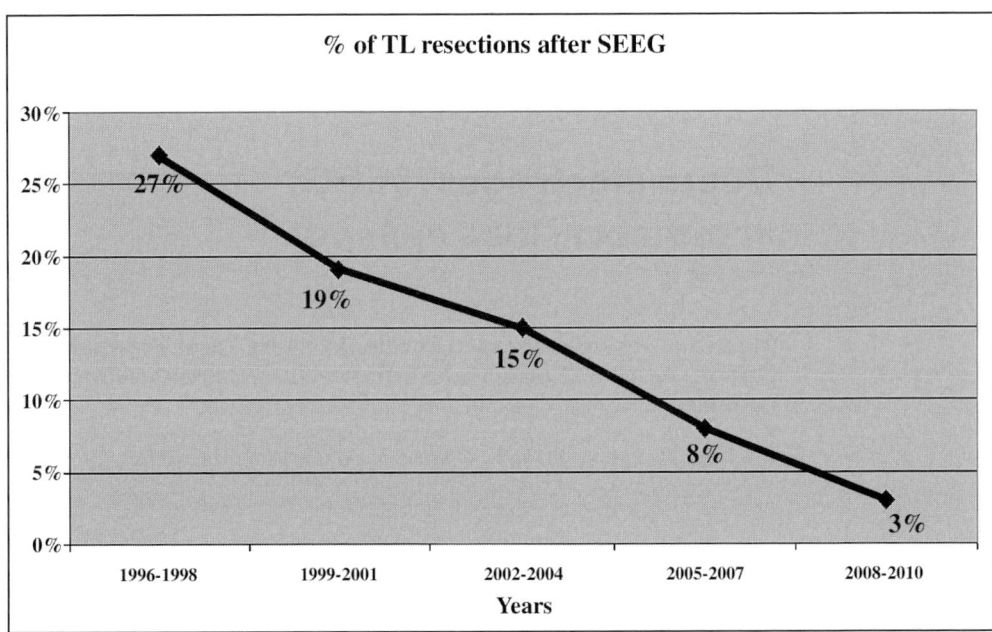

Figure 1. Percentage of SEEG evaluations in patients who received a temporal lobe resection as a function of time. In the last decade, this proportion has dropped from approximately 20% to 3%.

SEEG methodology and technique

General principles

SEEG methodology has developed alongside stereotactic techniques and the concept of the epileptogenic zone (EZ). Human stereotactic devices for recording electrical activity from deep brain structures were introduced in the early 50s (Spiegel et al., 1950). Stereotactic placement of intracerebral electrodes gained popularity and was reported for the evaluation of TLE in the early 60s (Crandall et al., 1963). Meanwhile, in the Neurosurgical Unit of the Sainte-Anne Hospital in Paris, stereotactic investigations of epileptic patients with intracerebral electrodes were inspired by a newly elaborated concept: epileptic seizures were regarded as a dynamic process with a spatial-temporal, often multidirectional, organization which is best defined by three-dimensional arrangement (Bancaud et al., 1965). The site of origin and primary organization of this dynamic process in focal epilepsies was defined as the EZ. Indeed, SEEG couples the potential of accurate stereotactic targeting of practically every intracranial structure with spatial-temporal definition of ictal discharges by tailored investigations (*i.e.* specific arrangements of intracerebral electrodes).

SEEG: indications and strategies of electrode placement

A SEEG evaluation may be required when non-invasive investigations fail to correctly localize the EZ. This is the result of a varying degree of incoherence between anatomical, electrical and clinical findings, individual to every given patient. Although this means that indications for a SEEG investigation are usually customized to the requirements of

vpsingle cases, a retrospective analysis has allowed us to recognize specific patterns of anatomo-electro-clinical incoherence (Cossu et al., 2005), which can be schematically summarized as follows:
- no definite anatomical abnormality seen on MRI, scalp ictal/interictal EEG findings are partially or fully discordant with ictal clinical semiology;
- a well documented focal abnormality seen on MRI, scalp ictal/interictal EEG findings and/or ictal clinical semiology suggest a wide involvement of extralesional areas;
- ictal clinical semiology is discordant with an apparently localizing ictal scalp EEG pattern, irrespective of MRI evidence;
- either MRI, ictal scalp EEG, or ictal clinical semiology suggest an early involvement of highly eloquent areas. Establishing the relationship between these factors and the epileptogenic zone is required and functional mapping should be performed in order to define both the prognosis of seizures following resection and the associated surgical risks;
- large focal, hemispheric, multifocal, or bilateral abnormalities seen on MRI, with ictal scalp EEG and clinical evidence of more localized/lateralized ictal onset.

Partially inconclusive, pre-SEEG data should be employed to formulate a hypothesis regarding the localization of the EZ, which needs to be verified by SEEG investigation. Thus, the arrangement of intracerebral electrodes must address the individual requirements of each case, and the SEEG strategy should be tailored according to the specific hypothesis formulated for each patient. From this point of view, SEEG differs substantially from the so called "depth electrodes", since the latter are placed in a standard fashion, usually into both hippocampi, to reveal the side of seizure origin in cases of uncertain lateralization (Diehl et al., 2000). In contrast, for SEEG investigations, coverage with intracerebral electrodes should include the region of presumed ictal onset, the areas of apparent spread of the ictal discharge, the lesion(s) demonstrated by MRI (if present) and the functionally critical structures presumably close to or embedded in either the EZ or the anatomical lesion. When seizures are believed to originate from, or propagate early to, the temporal lobe, an adequate coverage of neocortical and mesial structures should be considered. A classic arrangement of intracerebral electrodes includes placement perpendicular to the sagittal plane for sampling of external and internal cortex of the temporal pole, the middle temporal gyrus and amygdala, the middle temporal gyrus and both anterior and posterior hippocampi and parahippocampal gyrus, the anterior and posterior superior temporal gyrus, and the basal cortex including both inferior temporal and fusiform gyri at different levels. Additional electrodes may be added when, for instance, coverage of the temporal language areas in the dominant hemisphere is required. Nevertheless, SEEG investigations in presumed TLE, although focused on a "temporal lobe hypothesis", aim to verify the likelihood of early involvement of extratemporal structures configuring a so called "temporal plus" epilepsy (Ryvlin et al., 2005), as well as to disclose the spread to the temporal lobe of a discharge with an extratemporal onset. According to a hypothesis-based strategy, extratemporal coverage is therefore almost invariably required, taking into account the general concept that the propagation of an ictal discharge may follow multidirectional trajectories. As already outlined, even if standard arrangements of electrodes are not used, a retrospective review of SEEG in suspected TLE cases has allowed us to recognize some typical patterns of investigation. These patterns include coverage of the parietal-occipital lobes when posterior hemispheric involvement is suspected, targeting of the opercular and insular cortex in cases of presumed temporo-perisylvian seizures (Isnard et al., 2004), and more or less extensive investigation of the frontal lobe in selected cases of temporo-frontal or fronto-temporal epilepsies. Usually, the issue of seizure lateralization is addressed before

SEEG is considered. Nevertheless, bilateral temporal lobe coverage is needed when the side of seizure origin is unclear. Finally, investigations limited exclusively to the temporal lobe of the hemisphere dominant for language may be useful to investigate the role of the Wernicke's area in the organization of the ictal discharge. *Figures 2 to 5* provide some examples of these patterns of coverage.

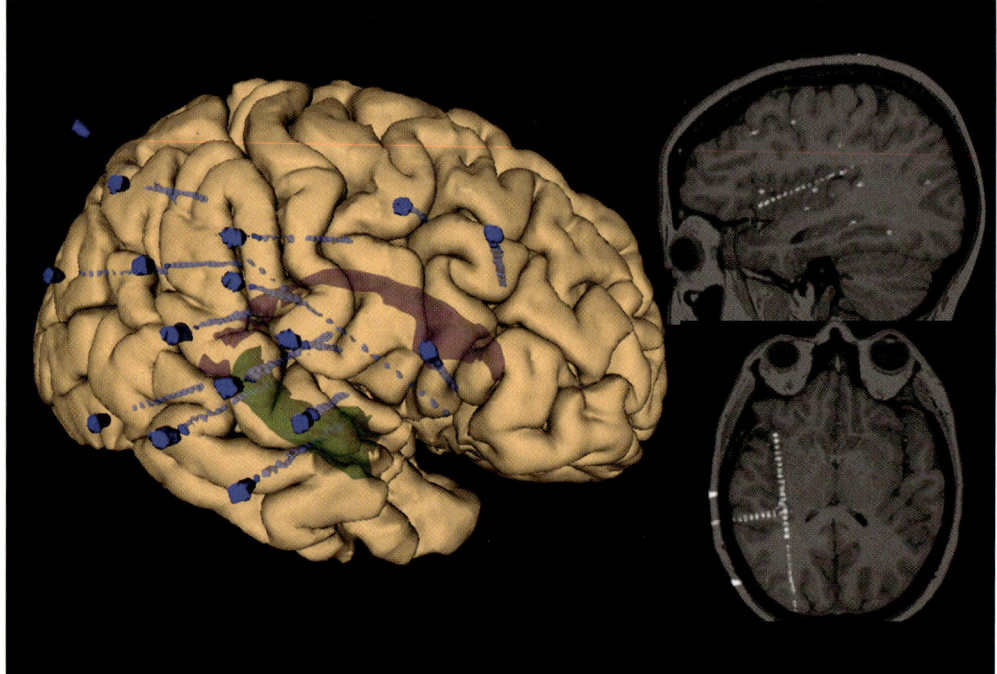

Figure 2. Example of a predominantly right temporo-perisylvian SEEG investigation.
Left: the brain model is the result of the co-registration of different volumetric data sets obtained before and after electrode placement. Violet: ventricle; green: hippocampus; blue: intracerebral electrodes. Right: two reformatted slices of co-registered volumetric T1-weighted pre-implantation MRI and post-implantation CT scan, showing the position of an intracerebral electrode sampling the insular cortex with several contacts.

SEEG: surgical technique

The key principles of the original methodology of SEEG (Talairach *et al.*, 1980) are still fully respected, although the neuroimaging employed for presurgical planning and the surgical techniques of electrode implant have been progressively updated. Some of these technical modifications, such as the use of passive robotic tools in electrode placement, have been already described (Cossu *et al.*, 2005). Multimodal preoperative neuroimaging is extensively employed, with projective angiography and ventriculography replaced by rotational angiography and MRI. Three-dimensional visualization of brain anatomy is therefore obtained by multiplanar and surface reformatting. Current informatic algorithms, such as Mutual Information, enable automatic co-registration of different datasets, as well as extensive multimodal integration of anatomical and functional information (for example, functional MRI and DTI-Fibre Tracking).

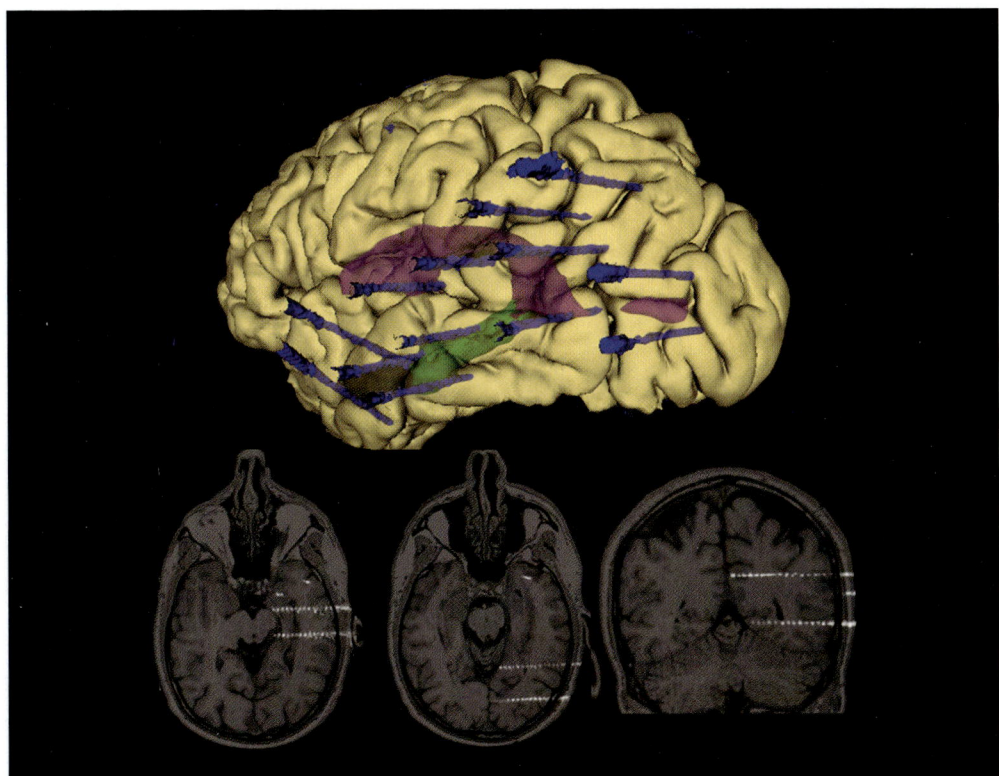

Figure 3. Example of a left temporal SEEG investigation with additional coverage of the occipital lobe.
Upper box: brain model resulting from co-registration of different data sets obtained before and after electrode placement. Colours are the same as in *Figure 2*. Lower boxes: three reformatted slices of co-registered volumetric T1-weighted pre-implantation MRI and post-implantation CT scans, showing intracerebral electrodes placed in the anterior and posterior hippocampus and in the occipital lobe.

The correct positioning of intracerebral electrodes must address two essential requirements: 1) accurate targeting of desired intracerebral structures and 2) minimizing the risk of vessel injury with consequent intracranial haemorrhage. The first requirement is addressed by employing adequate data sets of structural and, if needed, functional neuroimaging which are acquired in frameless conditions. These therefore include:
- all the appropriate sequences demonstrating the presumed epileptogenic lesion(s), if present. For example, T2-weighted Fluid Attenuation Inversion Recovery (FLAIR) sequences are particularly helpful to detect subtle cortical malformations as well as mesial temporal sclerosis (MTS), and T1-weighted Inversion Recovery (IR) sequences provide an excellent definition of the grey-white matter interface and of the gyro-sulcal cortical arrangement;
- areas of activation determined by functional MRI (fMRI), as well as Diffusion Tensor Imaging for Fibre-Tracking (DTI-FT), when functionally critical structures require special attention within the investigative strategy;
- a volumetric data set (usually FFE T1-weighted sequence in the axial plane, voxel $0.46 \times 0.46 \times 1$ mm, no gap, reconstruction matrix 560×560), which usually represents the reference data set for subsequent co-registration of other images.

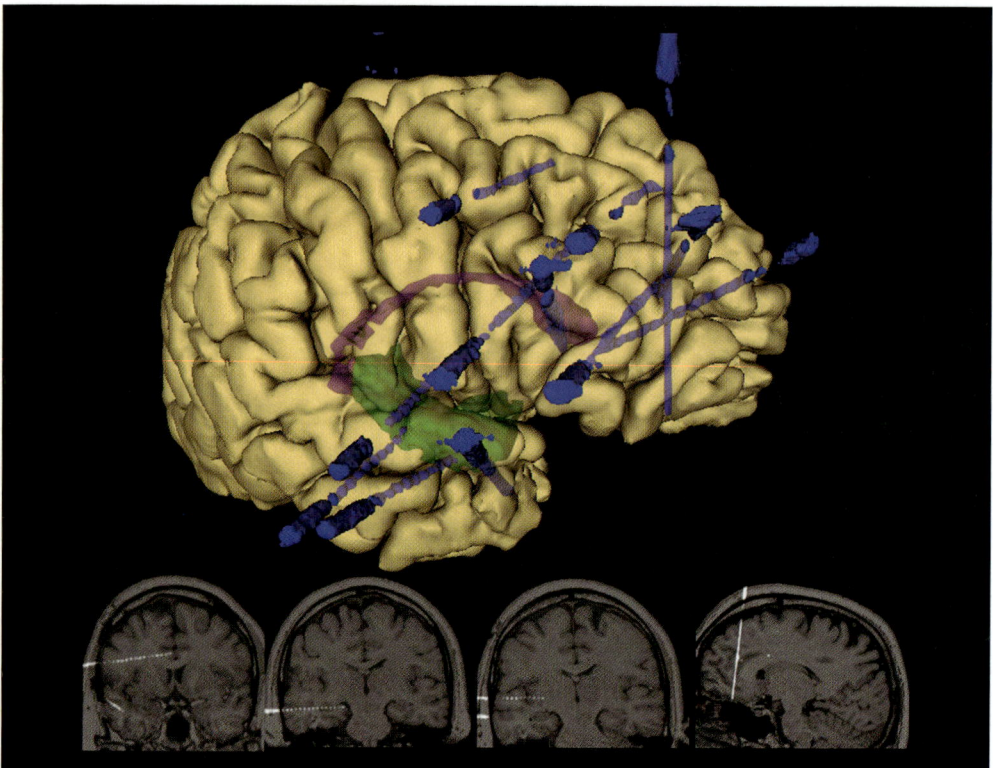

Figure 4. Example of a SEEG investigation with coverage of both the right temporal and frontal lobes.
Upper box: brain model resulting from co-registration of different data sets obtained before and after electrode placement. Colours are the same as in *Figure 2*. Lower boxes: four reformatted slices of co-registered volumetric T1-weighted pre-implantation MRI and post-implantation CT scans, showing intracerebral electrodes sampling several temporal and frontal areas, including extratemporal limbic structures as the cingulated gyrus, the insula, and the fronto-orbital cortex.

Furthermore, to minimize the risk of vascular damage, 3D brain angiography through a frameless rotational acquisition (via selective intra-arterial injection of radio-opaque contrast medium) of the pertinent intracranial vessels is obtained. The classic stereotactic 2D angiography has been progressively abandoned.

Once the image data sets are acquired, they are co-registered to the reference data set (the T1-3D sequence) and imported into the planning software (Voxim, IVS, Chemnitz, Germany). Investigation may then be prepared according to the defined strategy and planning of avascular trajectories which reach the desired targets with the accuracy of the stereotactic technique.

The trajectories of the electrodes are arranged in order to impact as many desired structures as possible. Targeting of deep-seated or mesial temporal and extratemporal structures, such as the amygdala, hippocampus, uncus, cingulated gyrus, gyrus rectus, and mesial convolutions of the frontal, parietal and occipital lobes, is feasible, as well as excellent sampling of the insular cortex by electrodes inserted through the supra or infra-sylvian opercula or by a retro-insular trajectory with a dorso-lateral entry point. Intracerebral electrodes also allow excellent coverage of deep-seated cortical malformations, such as periventricular or subcortical heterotopic clusters of grey matter.

Implantation of intracerebral electrodes is performed under general anaesthesia and following placement of the stereotactic frame. Commercially available, platinum-iridium, semi-flexible, multilead intracerebral electrodes (diameter 0.8 mm; 5 to 18 contacts of 1.5 mm length, 2 mm apart) are employed, the number of electrodes per patient averaging approximately 12 electrodes. Details of the implantation technique have been reported elsewhere (Cossu *et al.*, 2005). After placement of the electrodes, the patient is awakened from anaesthesia and moved to the recovery room.

Intensive video-EEG monitoring usually starts the day following implantation, with the purpose of recording the patient's habitual ictal manifestations. After an adequate number of seizures is obtained, the patient undergoes sessions of intracerebral electrical stimulation (see below). Mean duration of video-SEEG monitoring approximates 10 days. Once monitoring is complete, electrodes are withdrawn usually under local anaesthesia (or under sedation in less cooperative patients and children) and the patient is usually discharged the day after electrode removal.

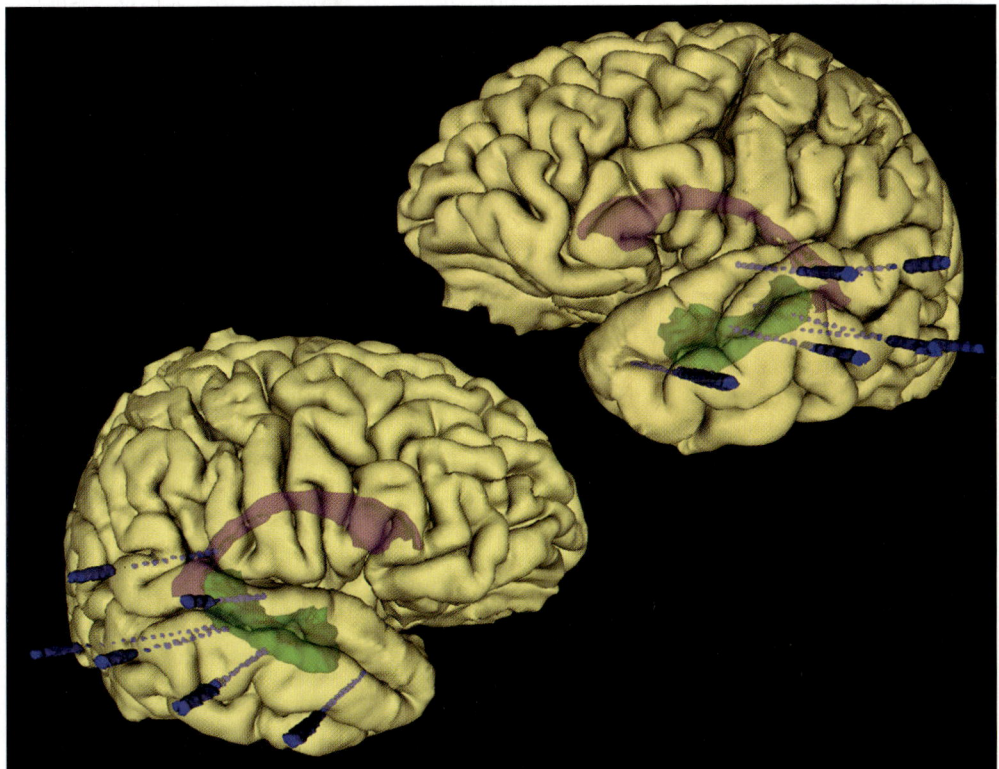

Figure 5. Example of a SEEG investigation in a case of temporal lobe epilepsy with uncertain lateralization. The two brain models show the bilateral coverage of neocortical and mesial temporal lobe structures.

The collected electroclinical data are reviewed by the epileptologist, and the EZ is defined as the region characterized by the presence of an electrical discharge of low-voltage fast activity occurring before or concomitantly with ictal clinical symptoms. The purely epileptological information is integrated with functional data to draw a complete picture of the relationships between the EZ and functionally critical areas (see below).

SEEG-guided functional mapping

The aim of high and low-frequency intracerebral electrical stimulations, delivered to pairs of contiguous contacts, is twofold; to induce habitual ictal manifestations and provide a functional map of the implanted regions (Kahane *et al.*, 1993; Munari *et al.*, 1993).

Intracerebral electrical stimulations performed for functional purposes enable the identification of regions related to different critical functions: primary somatomotor and somatosensory, visual, acoustic and speech. Positive responses consist of either objective clinical events (*e.g.* clonic jerks of circumscribed body areas, errors in naming or reading and tachyphemia) or subjective manifestations (dysesthesic sensations, positive or negative visual and acoustic phenomena) concurrent with electrical stimulations. For primary sensory-motor functions, low-frequency stimulations (frequency 1 Hz, duration of single stimulus 2-3 msec, current intensity 0.4-3 mA) are preferred. In most cases, positive responses may be obtained from stimulations both in grey and white matter, thus allowing extensive mapping of critical pathways. For this latter purpose, planning of electrode trajectories may be supported by DTI-FT imaging. Speech and visual areas are mapped using a combination of low and high-frequency (frequency 50 Hz, duration of single stimulus 1 msec, current intensity 1-3 mA) stimulations. Low-frequency stimulations are usually adequate to induce subjective acoustic changes; the effect of high frequencies is often unpleasant for the patient.

Chronic intracerebral seizure monitoring coupled with functional mapping is crucial to distinguish between patients with early ictal involvement of highly eloquent regions, for whom the impact of postoperative permanent deficits must be balanced against the severity of epilepsy, and those with later spread of the discharge to these structures, who may undergo surgery with limited surgical risks and good predictable seizure outcome. Functional mapping allows the prediction of potentially acceptable postoperative deficits, such as visual field defects in posterior temporal, occipital and parietal resections, as well as the evaluation of the risk-to-benefit ratio of excision close to more critical regions, such as sensory-motor and language areas. Although similar functional information can also be obtained from acute intraoperative electrical cortical stimulation, the following points must be stressed. First, chronic SEEG intracerebral electrical stimulation enables the mapping of both cortex and fibres to be feasible, as well as the planning of safer resections in potentially critical subcortical areas. Second, the availability of functional information before and not during surgery allows the patient to participate in the discussion of the risk-to-benefit balance in a relaxed and comfortable setting. Third, intraoperative electrocorticography only exceptionally results in spontaneous seizure recording, which is essential in evaluating the actual ictal involvement of eloquent areas.

■ SEEG-based temporal lobe resections: the Niguarda Hospital series

The analysis of the Niguarda Hospital series, in agreement with other reports (Diehl et al., 2000), reveals how the indications for invasive EEG monitoring, in cases of presumed TLE, have evolved during a 14-year-period in a single centre, fully dedicated to the surgical treatment of epilepsy. In fact, during the very early phase of the Epilepsy Surgery Program in our centre, several patients with the typical form of mesial TLE underwent a tailored temporal lobe resection after a SEEG evaluation, owing to the limited amount of specific epileptological knowledge available at the time. With the continuous advance in methods of patient selection and recognition of specific focal epileptic syndromes (Kahane et al., 2010), invasive evaluations are reserved only for more complicated cases. This explains why the number of patients who undergo SEEG-based temporal lobe resection today has considerably decreased, with the profile of these patients progressively changing over time (Diehl et al., 2000). The following review covers the period of 1996 to the present day and therefore includes also less recent cases that today would be operated on without SEEG.

Of a consecutive series of 944 cases of surgery for focal drug-resistant epilepsy, 487 patients (51.5%) received resective surgery within the anatomical limits of the temporal lobe. Sixty-five of these (13.3% of the TLE cases) had been presurgically evaluated by SEEG. Of these, 32 were male and 33 female (mean age at seizure onset was 9.5 ± 6.7 years, mean age at surgery was 30.2 ± 9.1 years, mean epilepsy duration was 20.7 ± 9.9 years). Seizure frequency was daily (more than 30/month) in 13 cases, weekly (5-30/month) in 39 cases and monthly (1-4/month) in 13 cases.

The essential anatomo-electro-clinical characteristics of the patients are detailed in *Table I*. The ability of ictal scalp EEG to identify the side and site (temporal or extratemporal) of ictal onset was considered, as well as the consistency of the ictal clinical semiology with temporal lobe onset, according to previously assessed criteria (Maillard et al., 2004). The possible occurrence of initial involvement of the temporal speech area was also recorded. For SEEG investigations, a total of 794 intracerebral electrodes were employed. The temporal lobe was covered by 463 electrodes (mean 7.1 ± 1.9/patient), whereas 331 electrodes (mean 5.1 ± 1.9/patient) were placed in extratemporal areas. The patterns of SEEG electrode arrangement are outlined in *Table II*: a temporo-perisylvian or temporo-posterior arrangement was employed in approximately three quarters of cases. Intracerebral electrodes were placed in the right hemisphere in 34 patients, in the left hemisphere in 29 and bilaterally in two cases. In the latter two cases, one side was favoured by more electrode coverage.

SEEG-based microsurgery consisted of a tailored neocortical plus mesial resection in 62 cases. In two of these cases, resection was limited to the intermediate segment of the temporal lobe. The remaining three cases received only a neocortical resection. *Table III* shows the results of histological evaluation based on the tissue specimens removed; for more than half of the cases a malformation of cortical development was found. Furthermore, MTS was more frequently associated with malformative or tumoural pathologies, rather than detected as an isolated finding.

Postoperative seizure outcome for the 64 patients with a follow-up of at least two years was assessed using the Engel scoring scale (Engel et al., 1987): 39 patients (61%) were in class I (free of disabling seizures) and 25 patients were in classes II-IV (not seizure-free). Among Class I patients, 19 (30%) were completely seizure-free since surgery (Engel Class Ia).

Table I. Anatomo-electro-clinical features of 65 patients presurgically evaluated by SEEG

	No of cases	%
MRI findings		
Lesion in TL	23	35
Lesion in TL and MTS	3	5
MTS	25	38
Normal	14	22
EEG*		
Side + TL	15	23
Side + TL + extraTL	45	69
Side + extraTL	3	5
Bilateral TL	2	3
Ictal clinical semiology		
Consistent with TL	20	31
Consistent with TL + Lang	7	11
Inconsistent with TL	38	58

* Data derived from video-EEG evaluation except for one case with only interictal EEG recording; MRI: Magnetic Resonance Imaging; MTS: mesial temporal sclerosis; TL: temporal lobe; Lang: suggestive of early involvement of the temporal speech areas.

Table II. SEEG evaluation: patterns of electrode arrangement

	No. of cases	%
TL + perisylvian/insular	26	40
TL + posterior	23	35
TL + frontal	11	17
TL + extensive extraTL	2	3
TL bilateral	2	3
TL only	1	2

TL: temporal lobe.

This concise report allows us to draw a reliable profile of the patients requiring invasive investigations for temporal lobe resection, at least in the authors' centre. In this subset of cases, we recognize a considerable proportion with uninformative MRIs, as well as poor localizing ictal scalp EEG. Furthermore, these patients present with an ictal clinical semiology, which may often resemble that of extratemporal seizures (Nobili et al., 2004; Mai et al., 2005). However, in contrast to other reports, few investigations were performed in our centre with the aim of revealing the side of seizure onset in cases with uncertain lateralization. The chance of a favourable postoperative seizure outcome was lower in patients who were scheduled to have SEEG than those who underwent surgery after non-invasive evaluations (61% and 85% of cases in Engel Class I, respectively). These figures reflect the high degree of epileptological complexity of cases which require invasive monitoring, but also demonstrate that surgery may be offered in a considerable number of these complex cases with excellent seizure outcome.

Final remarks

Invasive EEG investigation, including SEEG, is infrequently required in the presurgical work-up of patients who are subsequently scheduled for temporal lobe resection. Nevertheless, the historical role of SEEG to accumulate the available bulk of knowledge of TLE

Table III. Histology of resected specimens

	No. of cases	%
MCDs*	36	55
FCD	32	
Nodular heterotopias	4	
Tumours[†]	11	17
Hamartomas	4	
Glial-neuronal	4	
Others	3	
MTS alone	6	10
Gliotic scars	2	3
No abnormalities	10	15

MCD: malformations of cortical development; FCD: focal cortical dysplasia; MTS: mesial temporal sclerosis.
* with MTS in 19 cases; [†] with MTS in two cases.

should not be underestimated. Studies with intracerebral electrodes have provided an essential contribution to the discovery of the different subtypes of TLE (Kahane et al., 2010), demonstrating that distinct clinical patterns may be reasonably associated with specific modalities of discharge organization (Maillard et al., 2004), offering a surgical solution to a substantial proportion of patients with drug-resistant TLE without the additional risk of invasive evaluations. Nevertheless, when non-invasive investigations show incongruent results with regards to the localization of the EZ, SEEG monitoring may be mandatory to identify the region which requires surgical removal. These selected cases, however, show less favourable seizure outcome compared to those receiving surgery without the need for invasive recordings.

References

- Bartolomei F, Wendling F, Vignal JP, Kochen S, Bellanger JJ, Badier JM, et al. Seizures of temporal lobe epilepsy: identification of subtypes by coherence analysis using stereo-electro-encephalography. *Clin Neurophysiol* 1999; 110: 1741-54.
- Bartolomei F, Chauvel P, Wendling F. Epileptogenicity of brain structures in human temporal lobe epilepsy: a quantified study from intracerebral EEG. *Brain* 2008; 131: 1818-30.
- Spiegel EA, Wycis HT. Thalamic recordings in man with special reference to seizure discharges. *Electroencephalogr Clin Neurophysiol* 1950; 2: 23-39.
- Crandall PH, Walter RD, Rand RW. Clinical applications of studies on stereotactically implanted electrodes in temporal-lobe epilepsy. *J Neurosurg* 1963; 20: 827-40.
- Bancaud J, Talairach J, Bonis A, Schaub C, Szikla G, Morel P, Bordas-Ferrer M. La *stereo-electro-encephalographie dans l'epilepsie*. Paris: Masson, 1965, 321 p.
- Cossu M, Cardinale F, Castana L, Citterio A, Francione S, Tassi L, et al. Stereo-EEG in the presurgical evaluation of focal epilepsy: a retrospective analysis of 215 procedures. *Neurosurgery* 2005; 57: 706-18.
- Diehl B, Lüders HO. Temporal lobe epilepsy: when are invasive recordings needed? *Epilepsia* 2000; 41 (Suppl 3): S61-S74.

- Ryvlin P, Kahane P. The hidden causes of surgery-resistant temporal lobe epilepsy: extratemporal or temporal plus? *Curr Opin Neurol* 2005; 18: 125-7.
- Isnard J, Guénot M, Sindou M, Mauguière F. Clinical manifestations of insular lobe seizures: a stereo-electroencephalographic study. *Epilepsia* 2004; 45: 1079-90.
- Talairach J, Szikla G. Application of stereotactic concepts to the surgery of epilepsy. *Acta Neurochir* 1980; 30 (Suppl): 35-54.
- Kahane P, Tassi L, Francione S, Hoffmann D, Lo Russo G, Munari C. Manifestations électro-cliniques induites par la stimulation électrique intracérébrale par "chocs" dans les épilepsies temporales. *Neurophysiol Clin* 1993; 22: 305-26.
- Munari C, Kahane P, Tassi L, Francione, S, Hoffmann D, Lo Russo G, Benabid AL. Intracerebral low frequency electrical stimulation: a new tool for the definition of the "epileptogenic area"? *Acta Neurochir* 1993 (Suppl 58): 181-5.
- Kahane P, Bartolomei F. Temporal lobe epilepsy and hyppocampal sclerosis: Lessons from depth EEG recordings. *Epilepsia* 2010; 51 (Suppl 1): 59-62.
- Maillard L, Vignal JP, Gavaret M, Guye M, Biraben A, McGonigal A, *et al*. Semeiologic and electrophysiologic correlations in temporal lobe seizure subtypes. *Epilepsia* 2004; 45: 1590-9.
- Engel J Jr. Outcome with respect to epileptic seizures. In: Engel J Jr, ed. *Surgical Treatment of the Epilepsies*. New York: Raven Press, 1987: 553-71.
- Nobili L, Cossu M, Mai R, Tassi L, Cardinale F, Castana L, *et al*. Sleep-related hyperkinetic seizures of temporal lobe origin. *Neurology* 2004; 62: 482-5.
- Mai R, Sartori I, Francione S, Tassi L, Castana L, Cardinale F, *et al*. Sleep related hyperkinetic seizures: always a frontal onset? *Neurol Sci* 2005; 26 (Suppl 3): S220-S224.

Surgery for temporal lobe epilepsy: pros, cons and comparison between different procedures

Stephan Chabardès[1,2], Shivadatta Prabhu[1], Taner Tanriverdi[3]

[1] Grenoble institute of neurosciences, Inserm U836, Joseph-Fourier University, Grenoble, France
[2] Neurosurgery department, University Hospital, Grenoble, France
[3] Department of Neurosurgery, Montreal Neurological Institute and Hospital, McGill University, Montreal, Quebec, Canada

---

Temporal lobe epilepsy surgery is an established method to address a disease which is difficult to treat, often pharmacoresistant and debilitating, and influences the quality of life in a patient. As well as being associated with a good clinical outcome, surgery for temporal lobe epilepsy has also been proven to be cost effective compared to other therapies (King et al., 1997). In recent times, with the advancement of understanding of the pathology of temporal lobe epilepsy, improved imaging techniques (including functional MRI, SPECT and co-registration with other modalities) and a better understanding of neurophysiology based on subdural and depth electrodes, surgery has evolved into a safer option with better outcome. Tailored or selective resections have been developed in an attempt to adapt the classic anterior temporal lobectomy (ATL) to individual patients.

However, the true benefits of surgery remain to be clarified, as outlined by Penfield and Paine in 1955: *"It is not enough to know whether the surgery procedure has stopped attacks or not. We must know its effect upon the patient's ability to work, to hold a job, to study; the effect on physical and mental function, the effect on behaviour and on the happiness of the patient and friends"* (Penfield & Paine, 1955). With this in mind, we present a comprehensive review of the pros and cons of different surgical approaches for temporal lobe surgery for the treatment of epilepsy with a brief history of the development of temporal lobe surgery.

■ History of the development of temporal lobe surgery for the treatment of epilepsy

In 1928, Penfield and his surgical partner Cone at Montreal Neurological Institute first performed temporal lobe surgery on a young patient with post-traumatic epilepsy (Penfield & Cone, 1943). The patient underwent three operations with remarkable results; the patient exhibited reduced seizure activity with an eventual frequency of just four seizures in 13 years when he started taking the anticonvulsant, dilantin (Feindel et al., 2009). From 1945 to 1955, surgery was mainly directed at the convexity of the lobe and included the removal of lesions such as scars or tumours. Gibbs and Lennox in 1936 classified temporal lobe epilepsy (psychomotor epilepsy) as a disorder of the rate regulating mechanism of the brain and maintained that structural lesion was an exception (Gibbs et al., 1938). Jasper suspected the deep temporal lobe to be the origin of seizures.

Jasper and Penfield became close associates as a neurosurgeon and neurophysiologist, respectively. Penfield would often decline to operate if a structural lesion was not present after craniotomy, however, at that time no sophisticated imaging techniques were available. The success rate of just over 50% for anterolateral cortical resection led Penfield to extend surgical resection to mesial structures during secondary surgery in order to reduce spike activity on ECoG. Penfield noted that *"these structures including uncus and hippocampus were rough, tough, rubbery, yellow and hard to suck"*. Meanwhile, Gibbs and Baily at the University of Illinois performed gyrotomies at a lateral and anterior aspect to the temporal lobe (Baily & Gibbs, 1951).

In the early 1950s, Kaada demonstrated attacks of arrest of movements and automatism in animals by stimulation (Kaada, 1951). These experiments pointed to mesial and temporal lobes as the origins of epileptic activity. In 1952, Feindel and collaborators reproduced temporal lobe seizures, consisting of habitual auras and other typical symptoms, using depth electrode stimulation of the amygdala and ventral claustrum during surgery in 16 patients (Feindel et al., 1952). As a result, the functions of the amygdala and hippocampus became more evident and the way was paved for anteromesial resection. The now classic report on this technique was published by Penfield and Baldwin (1952) and other neurosurgical centres followed this more "mesial" approach. This allowed pathologists to have more specimens from mesial structures which led to a better understanding of the pathology of hippocampal sclerosis (HS) with regards to mesial temporal epilepsy. In 1954, Gastaut arranged a meeting at Marseille on the treatment of temporal lobe epilepsy where an exchange of ideas between different groups took place. Another meeting in 1958 in the USA confirmed the validity of the anteromesial surgical procedure. In 1958, Rasmussen and Jasper confirmed that electrical and clinical features of temporal lobe epilepsy could be consistently evoked by stimulation of the amygdaloid area (Rasmussen & Jasper, 1958). During the same conference in 1958, Paul Niemeyer described "selective amygdalo-hippocampectomy" (sAHE) with preservation of the temporal cortex in order to minimize cognitive dysfunction after surgery (Niemeyer, 1958). The 1960s brought a better understanding of the pathology and structures involved in temporal lobe seizures based on stereotactic apparatus and depth electrodes applied by Talairach and Bancaud at the Sainte-Anne Hospital in Paris, France (Bancaud et al., 1969; 1970).

Later, the discovery, or rather the confirmation, of hippocampal atrophy led to the description of the so called "mesial temporal lobe epilepsy syndrome" (MTLE). The focal abnormalities often observed in the atrophic hippocampus were seen as the main reason to explain epileptogenesis in these cases and a selective approach was proposed by Yasargil and Wieser who introduced "key hole" sAHE (Wieser & Yasargil, 1982). This selective approach contrasted with the more classic approach consisting of anteromesial resection, as described by Falconer (Falconer, 1958) and popularised by Spencer (Hori et al., 2007). The different surgical approaches and their relative advantages are discussed below.

Surgery for temporal lobe epilepsy

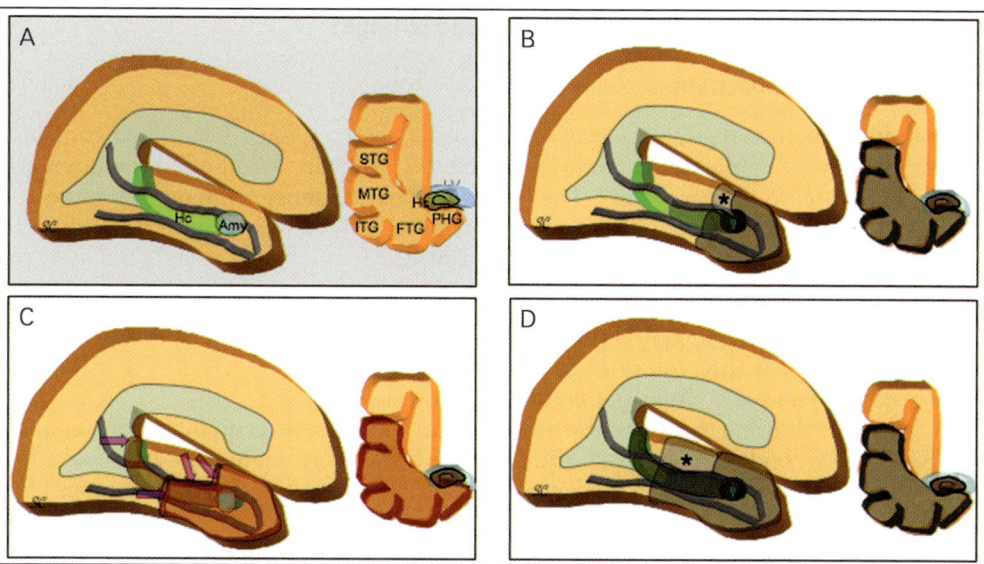

Figure 1. Schematic representations of an anterior temporal lobectomy.
A. Schematic representation of the right temporal lobe: hippocampus (green), amygdala (blue circle). STG: superior temporal gyrus; MTG: middle temporal gyrus; ITG: inferior temporal gyrus; FG: fusiform gyrus; PHG: parahippocampal gyrus; Hc: hippocampus; LV: temporal horn of the ventricle; Amy: amygdale. **B.** Technique described by Falconer and by Spencer. **C.** Temporal disconnection performed at the Grenoble University. **D.** Large temporal lobectomy performed at the Grenoble university. The posterior limit of the resection of the lateral cortex depends on SEEG findings, and includes the entire hippocampus. * extension of the resection on the right side.

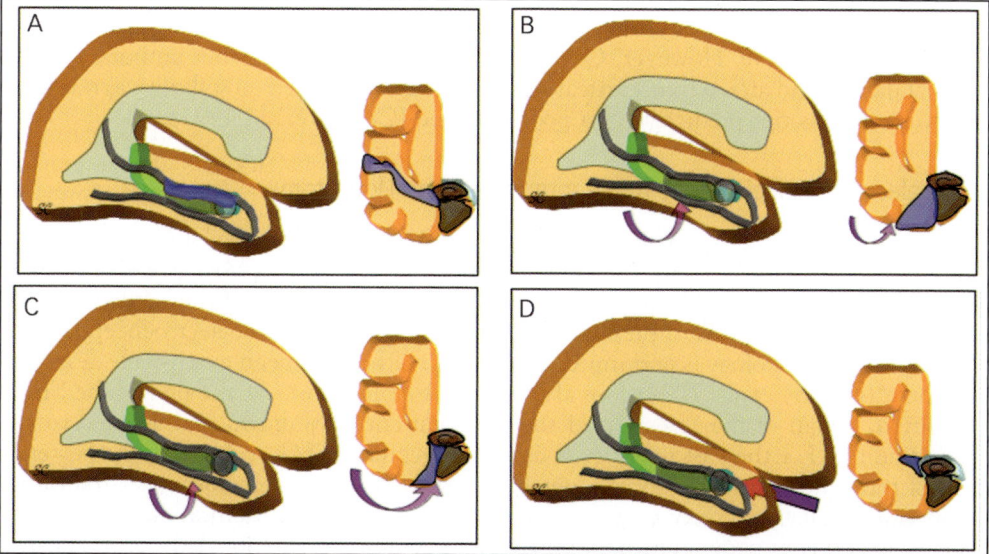

Figure 2. Schematic representations of selective amygdalo-hippocampectomy.
A. Transcortical technic described by Olivier. **B.** Infratemporal technique described by Hori. **C.** Transparahippocampal technic described by Park. **D.** Transylvian approach described by Yasargil.

Surgical techniques: advantages and disadvantages

Anterior temporal lobectomy

Several different techniques of subtotal temporal lobectomy have been described since the early reports of Penfield and Baldwin (Penfield & Baldwin, 1952) and Rasmussen and Jasper (Rasmussen & Jasper, 1958). The classic ATL is the most common procedure and was first described by Falconer (Falconer & Taylor, 1968). Here we will report the technique described by Spencer (Kim & Spencer, 2001).

During a standard temporal craniotomy and when anterior temporal exposure is maximal, a measurement from the temporal pole is taken of 3.5 cm to the first temporal gyrus. This vertical line serves as the posterior boundary of the neocortical resection. The neocortex is then gently removed, while preserving the superior temporal gyrus. The removal is extended to the fusiform gyrus and the inferior gyrus with the use of an ultrasonic aspirator (CUSA). The second step is to open the temporal horn, a key anatomical landmark. The choroid plexus is protected by a cottonoid and removal identifies the hippocampus. The temporal lobe is retracted laterally using a retractor. A microscope is then used and the resection of the floor of the temporal horn is performed, advancing medially. The tail of the hippocampus is identified at the level of the quadrigeminal plate. After this step, the superior limit of the amygdala resection is defined by a line going from the anterior tip of the temporal horn to the "knee" of the middle cerebral artery. Below this line, the amygdala is removed and microdissection allows one to remove the head of the hippocampus after having coagulated small perforating vessels supplying the hippocampus. This coagulation must be performed cautiously and far away from the parent vessel. Finally, the hippocampus is totally removed with the fimbria.

A tailored surgical approach was described by Walker (1967) and consisted of utilizing electrocorticography to adapt the length of the hippocampus to be removed. Alarcon et al. (1997) advocated the resection of the "leading regions" of spiking in order to achieve better seizure outcome. However, Cendes and collaborators, like other authors, pointed out that during, and after a transcortical selective resection, increased spiking was routinely observed and was not predictive of a poor outcome (Cendes et al., 1993).

Stereoelectroencephalography-based anterior temporal lobectomy

Our group in Grenoble currently performs the classic ATL as described above for the vast majority of cases. However, in some circumstances, particularly in MRI-negative cases or when discrepancies exist between surface EEG, clinical description of the seizure, neuropsychological data and MRI, a presurgical evaluation using the stereoelectroencephalography (SEEG) methodology is performed. This latter method has been extensively described elsewhere (Kahane et al., 2004) (see also chapter by Blumcke). At the end of the SEEG evaluation, a plan of the resection of the temporal cortex is drawn and adapted to the SEEG findings. For the vast majority of cases that require SEEG evaluation, the posterior limit of the temporal neocortex is adapted accordingly. In rare circumstances, the SEEG allows us to limit the resection of the temporal pole, preserving the non-atrophic hippocampus, which is of paramount importance to the dominant side in MRI-negative cases. The surgical technique used in this circumstance is driven by the SEEG findings which provide not only electrical information, but also a precise anatomical map of the region. Indeed, all the veins and arteries are identified during the surgical planning of SEEG, and functional mapping is also performed by electrical stimulation of the depth electrodes. We routinely perform a straight-line incision and then a circle-shaped craniotomy ("trephine"), 50 mm in diameter, centred by neuronavigation on the T1-T2 sulcus. Using the CUSA, the first temporal gyrus is then removed subpially (the posterior limit differs between the dominant and non-dominant side) and the posterior T2 and T3 cortex is subsequently cut vertically from the temporal basis up to the T1-T2 sulcus. We then enter the horn of the ventricle which is usually easily reached by neuronavigation, entering the white matter located at the depth of the T1-T2 sulcus. The hippocampus, the parahippocampus and the amygdala are removed *en bloc* by CUSA. The sylvian and choroidal fissure are never opened in order to prevent any injury to the vessels or the third nerve. The hippocampus is removed posteriorly up to the retrothalamic level. We then spray the cavity with "tissucol" fibrin glue which, in our experience, prevents the occurrence of an arachnoid cyst or subdural collection in the temporal fossa.

Advantages

This procedure is adapted to the patient and takes into account, besides the clinical history and MRI findings, the anatomo-clinical correlation of seizures. It is advocated when a large epileptogenic network is suspected and can lead to a very good outcome (80% Engel Class Ia).

Disadvantages

This technique requires invasive presurgical evaluation with depth electrodes and requires an experienced team with stereotactic tools.

Temporal anterior disconnection developed at Grenoble University

Rather than removing the anterior temporal lobe, we have recently described the possibility of disconnection (Chabardès *et al.*, 2008). This technique requires the same presurgical evaluation as described above and is indicated in non-lesional cases. The practical realisation of anterior temporal disconnection requires the same tools and same strategies as described for ATL but also requires the total preservation of all the vessels to avoid ischaemia-induced brain swelling. This technique has been developed as a proof of concept in order to validate the hypothesis that disconnecting the epileptogenic zone is sufficient to cure the patient.

Transcortical selective amygdalo-hippocampectomy approach (Niemeyer, 1958; Wheatley, 2008)

Originally described by Niemeyer in 1958, the transcortical sAHE approach consists of the removal of the amygdala and the first 3 cm of the hippocampus through the middle temporal gyrus (Niemeyer, 1958).

Neuronavigation is used in planning and at intraoperative stages of surgical dissection. For craniotomy, a standard curvilinear fronto-temporal flap based at the root of the zygoma is the incision most often used. The second most common type of incision is a linear skin incision made from the root of the zygoma superiorly. After incising the dura, the middle temporal gyrus (MTG) is identified. The posterior limit of incision on the MTG is based on neuronavigation and is usually 5 cm from the anterior temporal pole. Some centres also use the central sulcus as a landmark and limit posterior extent of neocortical incision to the pre-central sulcus on the dominant side. Entering the horn of the ventricle is achieved through the MTG with a sucker or the CUSA. The direction is parallel to the superior temporal gyrus (STG)/MTG sulcus through the white matter of the temporal stem. At this stage, a neuronavigation system is very helpful and one must be cautious not to go above the ventricular horn.

The CUSA is advanced into the lateral ventricular sulcus. The first landmarks identified are the choroid plexus and the choroidal fissure at the deep medial border of the ventricle. The subsequent landmark identified is the lateral ventricular sulcus, which is the demarcation between the hippocampus and the collateral eminence. The lateral ventricular sulcus is the point of entry into the parahippocampal gyrus. The parahippocampul gyrus is emptied first by use of the CUSA. Once this step is completed, the hippocampus can then be folded down into the space previously occupied by the parahippocampal gyrus. This allows a longitudinal view of the hippocampus throughout its length. At the medial border of the hippocampus, lateral to the choroid plexus and choroidal fissure, a white matter tract, the fimbria fornix system, is encountered. This is removed from the head of the hippocampus to the hippocampal posterior resection margin. The sucker or CUSA is then brought perpendicularly across the hippocampus down to the hippocampal sulcus. The same can be done at the anterior border of the hippocampal resection. The hippocampus is now only connected to the mesial structures by its adherence to the hippocampal sulcus which is divided. Resection of the parahippocampal gyrus and the body of the hippocampus is completed, sparing the hippocampal sulcus.

The amygdala, the uncus, and the head of the hippocampus can then be approached. Usually, 50 to 70% of the amygdala is removed only because the superior part of the amygdala is not well delineated and, once again, the navigation system can be of some help. Usually, perforant arteries are also individually identified, which are a good landmark to prevent removal of the amygdala. At this level, one must be cautious since injury to perforant arteries is a possible cause of capsular infarct. After this resection is complete, the head of the hippocampus, as well as the anterior entorhinal cortex, extending from the previously emptied parahippocampal gyrus, are resected. The uncus is easily identified as it dips over the tentorial edge and is resected. At the end of this procedure, performed subpially, the third nerve and the carotid nerve are seen through the arachnoid film. The optic tract located more superiorly is a good superior landmark.

Advantages

The transcortical approach provides a very clear view of the whole hippocampus which can be resected posteriorly. The relief of the amygdala can be easily detected. The choroidian fissure is not opened, which prevents any injury of the vessels within (posterior cerebral vessels). This technique is aimed at preserving cognitive functions and limiting neuropsychological deficit (mainly verbal memory loss).

Disadvantages

The middle temporal gyrus is breached, only sometimes damaging a small portion of neocortex. This elegant technique cannot be applied in patients with regional seizure onset, as the temporal pole is preserved. Memory decline is allegedly prevented using this technique but no robust evidence of this notion has been reported so far and contradictory results have been published.

Variant of the transcortical selective amygdalo-hippocampectomy (Olivier, 2000)

In this variant, the authors used neuronavigation and performed a transcortical approach throughout the superior bank of the second temporal gyrus, subsequently joining the superior temporal sulcus, descending across the white matter of the temporal stem and entering the temporal horn of the ventricle. This allows subpial removal of the amygdala, uncus, anterior hippocampus and entorhinal cortex.

Advantages/disadvantages

This technique was developed in order to prevent cognitive decline in patients with MTLE. It appears to be safe and technically less demanding than the other selective techniques. However, even if this technique proves to effectively prevent seizures, no definitive conclusion with respect to ATL can be drawn regarding the possibility of preventing cognitive decline.

Anterior (transsylvian) selective amygdalo-hippocampectomy (Yasargil, 1967)

The proximal approach through a pterional craniotomy was developed by Yasargil in 1967 for the microsurgical treatment of saccular aneurysms of the circle of Willis, fronto-orbital and temporobasal arteriovenous malformations, cavernomas, and extrinsic and intrinsic tumours (Yasargil, 1967). He first used this approach for sAHE in patients with intractable MTLE in 1973 and reported the first 100 cases of surgery in 1993 (Yasargil *et al.*, 1993). This is the first selective approach described and employed which aimed to spare the lateral neocortex.

Surgical technique

A pterional craniotomy and opening of the proximal, 3-5 cm (anterior) section of the sylvian fissure is carried out. A pial incision, 15-20 mm long, is then made lateral to the M_1 segment of the middle cerebral artery between the origins of the temporal polar and anterior temporal arteries. On completion of this dissection of the fissure, the amygdala is gradually removed in its lateral and basal portions towards the crural and ambient cisterns. Once this is achieved, the temporal horn is explored in an anteroinferomedial axis. The hippocampus and parahippocampus are approached between the choroidal fissure, along the anterior sector of the transverse fissure and collateral sulcus, medial to the fusiform gyrus. The anterior two thirds (2.5-3.0 cm long) of the hippocampus-parahippocampus is resected in an *en bloc* fashion or using the CUSA, facilitated by the anterior approach, although the posterior third of the hippocampus-parahippocampus is not resected.

Advantages

The proximal (anterior) transsylvian-transamygdalar approach to the mesial temporal structures permits the selective resection of two thirds of the amygdala and hippocampus-parahippocampus and preserves overlying T1, T2, T3, and T4 gyri, as well as the related subcortical connective fibre systems and other essential components of the temporal white matter. Volumetrically, approximately 70% of the amygdala is resected, including the lateral, anterior, basal, and cortical nuclei of the amygdala. However, the areas medial to the optic tract, such as the neighbouring amygdalostriatal zone, are not intentionally explored or removed. It has been advocated that preserving the posterior third of these structures also avoids injury to the vasculature of the lateral geniculate body, especially occlusion of the branches of the anterior choroidal artery (AChA) which might prevent severe visual field defects. Furthermore, this technique was developed to spare the lateral cortex which could prevent cognitive and verbal memory impairment especially when the dominant side is concerned.

Disadvantages

(1) This is a challenging surgical procedure, even for an experienced microsurgeon. The openings made in the sylvian fissure and transamygdala route are small. This technique is also based on the dissection of the vessels of the sylvian and choroidal fissures and anatomical variations are frequently encountered in the pattern and distribution of the temporal branches of the M_1 segment. This approach may lead to injury of the vessels and to vasospasm.

(2) The lateral parts of the parahippocampal gyrus may not be readily identified and may thus remain unresected. Also, the medial part of the fusiform gyrus may be inadvertently removed. sAHE reaches only the anterior portion of the hippocampus after a large removal of the amygdala and retraction back into the ventricle. This approach does not permit resection of the temporal pole which is frequently involved in MTLE (Chabardès et al., 2005).

(3) Although rare, damage to the visual system is possible. If the geniculate branches of the AChAs are damaged, an upper quadrantanopia is produced. Damage to the branches supplying optic radiation and continuing through the retrolenticular and sublenticular segments of the internal capsule may produce a homonymous hemianopia.

Transsylvian-transcisternal mesial en bloc resection (Vajkoczy, 1998)

Surgical technique

The standard pterional approach, with a frontolateral craniotomy and semicircular opening of the dura above the sylvian fissure down to the sphenoidal ridge and orbit, releasing CSF from the cisterns, is the same as that described by Yasargil. This technique requires the dissection of the medial aspect of the hippocampus through a large opening of the choroidal fissure, identification of the third nerve and coagulation of vessels from the choroidial fissure to the mesial temporal lobe.

After circumferential arachnoidal coagulation and cortical incision, the entire parahippocampal gyrus, including the uncus, the perirhinal, entorhinal, and posterior parahippocampal cortex, as well as the amygdala and anterior hippocampus, are resected *en bloc* to the midmesencephalic level. Control over the hippocampus resection is tailored by following the medial wall of the opened ventricle. The extent of the resection is limited laterally by the temporal horn and posteriorly by the "midmesencephalon." For lesions involving the dorsal aspect of the mesial temporal lobe, the resection is extended posteriorly by approximately 10 mm.

Advantages

This technique is the same as the sAHE described by Yasargil but with improved anatomical orientation and preservation of the lateral and temporo-basal cortex. Resection *en bloc* allows complete removal of the amygdala, the whole hippocampus and the parahippocampal gyrus.

Disadvantages

This technique requires manipulation of the vessels within the choroidal fissure and may create transient third nerve palsy as well as injury to the vessels and vasospasm in about 10% of cases.

Selective transinsular hippocampectomy, sparing the amygdala and neocortex (Levesque, 2008)

Surgical technique

A frontotemporal craniotomy is performed by neuronavigation. The sylvian fissure is exposed without drilling the pterion. Using a microscope, the preoperative entry points are identified and the sylvian cistern is exposed between the temporal and frontoparietal operculum. The inferoposterior insular sulcus is then exposed along an avascular region. Using microsurgical instruments, a 1-cm longitudinal keyhole incision is made along the inferior sulcus of the insula. The lateral horn of the ventricle is opened and the dorsal hippocampus is identified from the anterior tip of the ventricle to the trigone region.

The choroidal fissure remains unexposed and no attempt is made to identify the optic tract, located superiorly and mesially to it. Further dissection is carried out inferiorly, leading to the ambiens cistern. The posterior hippocampus is transected along a coronal plane at 3 cm from the pes to reach the initial posterior lateral dissection. The pia of the entorhinal-parahippocampal gyrus is incised and the entorhinal hippocampus is elevated to produce an *en bloc* specimen.

Advantages

This method avoids opening the choroidal fissure, preserving any injury of the vessels or any transient third nerve palsy. The major advantage of this selective hippocampectomy procedure is that the amygdala and neocortex are spared, allowing minimal cognitive and affective changes. Selective transinsular hippocampectomy is presumably safer than sAHE as it does not require drilling of the pterion and does not expose either the carotid artery, optic nerve or the origin of the anterior choroidal artery to the lateral ventricle. The authors have reported a significant improvement in verbal and memory scores compared with patients who received ATL.

Disadvantages

This technique requires the opening of the sylvian fissure with inherent risk of vessel injury and vasospasm. Selective transinsular hippocampectomy does not replace ATL in cases of regional temporal seizure onset associated with more widespread pathology. The incidence of hippocampal epilepsy without the involvement of the amygdala or temporal pole (Chabardès *et al.*, 2005) is very rare and limits the number of cases of patients who may benefit from this technique.

Subtemporal selective amygdalo-hippocampectomy (Hori *et al.*, 1993; 2007)

The technique of Hori *et al.* (2007) was reported in 26 patients and consisted of entering "the temporal horn at the lateral edge of the collateral eminence through the collateral sulcus after resecting the medial half of the fusiform gyrus. The entire hippocampal head is removed en bloc, including the entorhinal area, the amygdala and the innermost part of the uncus which are removed subpially to expose the anterior choroidal artery and the optic tract". Note that in this technique, the temporal stem is not removed, leaving the uncinate fascicle in place.

Advantages

The authors advocated no visual field defect (although only 10 cases were evaluated) and reported 2/10 cases with superior quadranopsia. They also advocated no verbal memory impairment. Entering the temporal horn through the fusiform gyrus implies less retraction of the temporo-basal cortex (see below) and may prevent injury of the vein of Labbé.

Disadvantages

Some retraction injury may occur to the anterior fusiform gyrus and the inferior temporal gyrus. The uncinate fasciculus and the temporal stem are not removed which leads to a necessity for long-term assessment of seizure outcome. In the present study, 14/26 (53%) patients were classified as Engel class I after a two-year follow-up period.

Subtemporal transparahippocampal amygdalo-hippocampectomy (Park et al., 1996)

The technique was applied in nine patients and consists of the removal of the hippocampus (anterior part), amygdala and parahippocampal gyrus, and can be summarized as follows. Following temporal craniotomy, a brain retractor is placed subtemporally at the level of the anterior uncus and CSF is drawn from the ambient cistern. Under the microscope, the oculomotor nerve is identified as an anatomical landmark for cortical incision on the uncus. The initial incision is usually located 10-15 mm posterior to the point at which the oculomotor nerve crosses the tentorial edge. The temporal horn is exposed by suction excision of the cortex and underlying white matter. The suction dissection is performed through the white matter, perpendicular to the inferior surface of the uncus to avoid the medial parahippocampal gyrus near the tentorial edge. Once the temporal horn is opened, the amygdala is identified from the head of the hippocampus. The choroidal fissure along the medial aspect of the hippocampus is visualized by gently elevating the body of the hippocampus. The connection between the amygdala and the hippocampus is divided by subpial aspiration and the parahippocampal gyrus overlying the inferolateral portion of the hippocampus is removed subpially. The head of the hippocampus is divided transversely in the direction of the tentorial edge. This allows complete separation of the hippocampus from the arachnoid membrane and its removal *en bloc*. Finally the amygdala facing the temporal horn is excised using the CUSA.

Advantages

This technique permits wide access to the hippocampus, amygdala, parahippocampal gyrus, and uncus, allowing the surgeon to remove the structures by direct visualisation. During the operation, the temporal stem, but also the fusiform gyrus, is spared, leading to less neocortical damage.

Disadvantages

As is the case for the technique of Hori et al., the temporal pole and the uncus fascicle are left in place, which may not be optimal for good long-term seizure outcome. Furthermore, access to the mesial structures requires retraction of the temporobasal cortex with possible injury to veins and temporobasal cortex

Gamma knife surgery (Regis et al., 1995)

Jean Regis at Marseille University was the first to apply gamma knife (GK) surgery to treat MTLE (Regis et al., 1995) using a 24-gy marginal dose. Long-term outcome in 15 patients after five years follow-up showed promising results (Bartolomei et al., 2008) with 60% of cases considered to be seizure-free (Engel class I). Seizure cessation occurred with a mean delay of 12 (± 3) months after GK radiosurgery, often preceded by a period of increasing aura or seizure occurrence (in 6/15 patients).

Advantages

This technique requires only one day of hospitalisation and does not require any rupture of the skin or cranium. In MRI-negative cases without HS, preliminary results indicated no memory decline when the dominant side was targeted.

Disadvantages

Following the procedure of GK surgery, a dramatic increase of auras can occur and should thus be anticipated. GK surgery is a sophisticated technique which requires an experienced and dedicated team.

Seizure outcome

Surgery for temporal lobe epilepsy is today considered a better option in terms of clinical effect and health economics. However, surgical techniques differ among teams and no data have so far been reported to favour sAHE over ATL. However, the choice of a more selective approach can make sense when "pure" mesiotemporal onset, involving the hippocampus, amygdala, parahippocampal gyrus or entorhinal cortex, has been identified. In MTLE cases, the temporal pole is part of the epileptogenic zone in about 50% of cases, which may be a cause for failure following selective surgical techniques.

Comparison between selective and non selective surgery

ATL (or cortico-amygdalo-hippocampectomy [CAH]) is now the classic gold standard procedure to treat intractable patients suffering from temporal lobe epilepsy. sAHE is the alternative method employed for surgical treatment of MTLE. Although few studies comparing the two techniques have so far been reported in the literature, a summary of the data regarding seizure outcome following ATL or sAHE is described below. Several studies have compared seizure outcome between selective and non-selective procedures, of which some are represented in *Table I*.

Regarding seizure control, both ATL and sAHE appear to score equally well. Tanriverdi et al. (2008) reported 100 cases surgically treated by sAHE (n = 50) or ATL (n = 50): 40% of the patients who underwent ATL and 58% of those who underwent sAHE were seizure-free (Engel Class Ia), whereas favourable (Engel Classes I and II) seizure outcomes

Table I. Seizure outcome: Comparison between sAHE and CAH
CAH: cortico-amygdalo-hippocampectomy; sAHE: selective amygdalo-hippocampectomy
(adapted from Olivier & Tanriverdi, 2009)

Reference	Number of patients		Follow-up (years)	Seizure outcome
	CAH	sAHE		
Renowden et al., 1995	50	17	2	Similar
Arruda et al., 1996	37	37	1	Similar
Mackenzie et al., 1997	72	28	1	Better in CAH
Clusmann et al., 2002	83	126	3	Similar in adults
Clusmann et al., 2004	35	27	4	Better in CAH in children
Paglioli et al., 2006	80	81	6	Similar
Bate et al., 2007	82	32	1	Better in CAH
Tanriverdi et al., 2008	50	50	5	Similar

were noted in 82% and 90% of patients who had undergone ATL and sAHE, respectively. They concluded that both ATL and sAHE could lead to similarly favourable seizure control in patients with MTLE. However, they did not mention the rationale for choosing ATL or sAHE; one can imagine that the best candidates were offered sAHE, which could have biased the outcome when comparing the two techniques. Surprisingly, they reported no difference between the two techniques regarding the impairment of verbal memory (Tanriverdi et al., 2009) (see below). In a longer study, reported by Paglioli (2006), of 161 patients with MTLE-HS with mean follow-up of 5.8 years, outcomes were not found to be significantly different between surgical techniques with regards to the Engel outcome class or subclass, except for Class IB. Five (6.3%) of the 80 patients who had undergone ATL still reported auras at the last follow-up visit (Engel Class IB), despite being free of complex partial seizures, whereas none of the 81 patients who had undergone sAHE experienced auras at the last follow-up visit.

The choice for the best surgical option is still debatable and no robust trials, with appropriate design for evidence-based medicine (i.e. class 1) which allow comparison between ATL and selective approaches, have been performed so far.

■ Memory outcome

It has been noted for many years that the temporal lobes are involved in the primary organisation of sensory inputs. The role of dominant (usually left) temporal lobe in language processing and memory is well established. Thus, a decline in verbal memory following dominant lobe surgery is anticipated. With the advancement in imaging and use of preoperative and intraoperative language mapping, the risks of memory impairment after temporal surgery have become much less, however, memory deficits still occur in temporal lobe surgery. This has been a research area of significant interest and surgical techniques have been adapted for many years in order to minimize the extension of neocortical resection in an attempt to prevent memory or cognitive decline. On the other hand, the best outcome of seizure control is obtained when the whole epileptogenic zone is removed, which sometimes encompasses mesial, but also antero-mesial, structures (Bartolomei et al., 2001). Significant decline in aspects of verbal memory, for example, poor recall of prose passages (Rausch & Ary, 1990) and difficulty with word list learning (Hermann et al., 1994) have been reported in the past. The few studies presented here indicate a possible advantage of sAHE over CAH in memory performance, especially on the dominant side. However, Lutz et al. (2004) found that left-sided surgery led to a decline in verbal memory, independent of the surgical approach.

A comparison of neuropsychological outcome following different surgical procedures undertaken for temporal lobe epilepsy is sumarized in *Table II*. Tanriverdi (2009) retrospectively evaluated data from 256 patients who underwent surgery for MTLE. Of these, 123 patients underwent CAH (63 right side and 60 left side), and 133 underwent sAHE (61 on the right side and 72 on the left side). A comprehensive neuropsychological test battery was assessed before and one year after surgery, and the results were compared between the surgical procedures. In this study, intellectual functions were assessed by WAIS-R full intelligence quotient (FIQ), verbal intelligence quotient (VIQ) and practical intelligence quotient (PIQ). Verbal learning and memory were evaluated by WMS-R (Wechsler Memory Scales) and RAVLT (Rey Auditory Verbal Learning Test). Non-verbal memory was tested with recall of simple geometric figures in immediate and delayed test mode.

General intelligence was shown to increase after epilepsy surgery. VIQ was particularly affected after sAHE. Significant deterioration was seen in verbal learning and recognition after left-sided sAHE. Non-verbal memory improvement was noted in left-sided surgery for temporal epilepsy, irrespective of the type of surgery. There was a slight decline in figural learning and memory in right-sided CAH. Poor memory outcome was shown to be associated with longer seizure duration prior to surgery and/or late surgery.

In the study by Paglioli and colleagues (Paglioli et al., 2006), surgical outcome data were prospectively collected for 2-11 years for 161 consecutive patients with MTLE-HS. Of these, 80 patients underwent ATL and 81 sAHE. Preoperatively, 58% of the patients had verbal memory scores 1 standard deviation (SD) below the normal mean. One third of the patients with preoperative scores in the normal range worsened after surgery, although this outcome was not related to the surgical technique. In contrast, one third of those whose preoperative scores were less than 2 SD experienced improvement after surgery. Of the 50 patients whose left side had been surgically treated, memory scores were improved in nine (18%) patients by more than 1 SD. Seven of these nine (78%) had undergone sAHE ($p = 0.05$). It was concluded that postoperative verbal memory scores may improve in patients who undergo selective resection of sclerotic hippocampus in the dominant temporal lobe if verbal memory is already documented preoperatively to be compromised. However, patients with near normal verbal memory may worsen after surgery if the site of surgery is the dominant temporal lobe, by either a selective or non-selective technique.

Table II. A comparison of neuropsychological outcome following different surgical procedures undertaken for temporal lobe epilepsy
sAHE: selective amygdalo-hippocamopectomy (reproduced from Tanriverdi with permission)

Reference	No of patients		FU duration (months)	Neuropsychology
Wieser & Yasargil, 1982	5	6	21	sAHE: less impairment
Goldstein & Polkey, 1992	25	21	15	No difference
Goldstein & Polkey, 1992	58	15	6	sAHE: less impairment
Goldstein & Polkey, 1993	19	23	< 6	sAHE: short-term beneficial effect on memory
Wolf et al., 1993	30	17	6	No difference
Renowden et al., 1995	50	17	24	sAHE: better for VIQ and non verbal memory
Helmstaedter et al., 1996	22	21	3	sAHE: better for immediate recall
Jones-Gotman et al., 1997	23	25	18	No difference in seizure-free patients
Helmstaedter et al., 1997	21	15	12	sAHE: better for non verbal memory
Pauli et al., 1999	16	26	NA	sAHE: better for verbal memory
Hadar et al., 2001	14	14	NA	sAHE: better for recall
Clusmann et al., 2002	83	126	38	sAHE: better for verbal memory
Lacruz et al., 2004	91	15	11	No difference
Clusmann et al., 2004	35	54	12	sAHE: less impairment in children
Hader et al., 2005	20	16	NA	No difference
Paglioli et al., 2006	45	41	36	sAHE: better for verbal memory
Morino et al., 2006	17	32	12	sAHE: better for memory function
Tanriverdi & Olivier, 2007	36	36	12	sAHE: less decline for verbal memory
Helmstaedter et al., 2008	35	62	12	sAHE: better for non verbal memory in right-sided resections
Shin et al., 2009	14	23	12	No difference

In 1997, Jones-Gotman et al. already reported that "learning and recall for words was impaired in groups with resection from the left temporal lobe, irrespective of whether mediobasal structures were spared or temporal neocortex was spared" (Jones-Gotman et al., 1997). They suggested that the presumed benefit of selective approach regarding memory impairment should be balanced with the necessity to offer seizure freedom to those patients who often require larger temporal resection.

Quality of life

The principal aim of surgery for temporal lobe epilepsy is the control of seizures in terms of frequency and intensity. Other aims include reduced complications and an improved sense of well being, reflected in patients' perception of quality of life (QOL). It has been shown that positive subjective changes in quality of life evolve gradually and may consolidate over two years in some cases. For example, in a five-year prospective study on QOL following temporal lobe epilepsy surgery by Cunha and Oliveira, enhancement of social function was evident 6 months after surgery and subsequently became more gradual (Cunha & Oliveira, 2010). A patient usually undergoes surgery a relatively long time after the onset of the first seizure including a period of pharmacotherapy and time spent in decision making regarding surgery. Adjustment disorders in the first few months after surgery are also reported (Wilson et al., 2005). For these reasons, assessment of the quality of life is advised after a two-year postoperative period.

Tanriverdi et al, published their findings of a prospective longitudinal study evaluating QOL, 12 years after epilepsy surgery. They found that gainful employment is the important factor in subjective perception of QOL by the patient after surgery. In turn, being seizure-free, mood, ability to drive, family and social functioning are factors which influence employment status. In a study described by Elsharkawy et al. (2009), 222 patients who underwent epilepsy surgery between 1991 and 2003 responded to a self-administered international epilepsy-specific questionnaire (the QOLIE-31). The QOL showed a steep, non-linear increase within the first years of seizure freedom and remained relatively stable thereafter. Cognitive function showed continuous improvement parallel to seizure freedom. Univariate analyses showed that seizure freedom, presence of auras, intake of anti-epileptic drugs (AEDs), severity of AED-related side effects, and driving a car were significantly correlated with all subscales of QOLIE-31. Furthermore, employment status, psychiatric problems, and the presence of a partner were significantly correlated with some subscales. So far, no relationship between quality of life and surgical technique has been reported.

To summarize, those who became seizure-free after surgery (Engel Class 1A, IB) have a better quality of life. However, in the study of Cunha & Oliveira (2010), patients, as a whole, had a significant improvement in their quality of life after surgery, even if they were not totally seizure-free. This raises the possibility that, even for patients for whom surgery is not expected to achieve total control of seizures, the benefits on quality of life should be taken into account for the decision to perform surgery.

Conclusion and future

Surgery is now a well established procedure to treat patients suffering from temporal lobe epilepsy. Different techniques have been described, from ATL, also referred as CAH, to more selective ones which aim to spare the lateral neocortex. More recently, gamma knife surgery has been advocated as a possible surgical option, especially in those patients with MRI-negative epilepsy. When a larger epileptogenic network is suspected, based on clinical, electrical and or imaging data, it may be mandatory to evaluate these patients with depth electrodes, using the SEEG methodology, and to perform a more generous temporal lobectomy, adapted to SEEG findings.

However, most patients with temporal epilepsy are treated by ATL or sAHE. Based on the literature, the choice of the technique is still debated as no clear advantages, in terms of seizure outcome or memory or quality of life, have been demonstrated so far, probably due to the fact that the so called "selective techniques" are not so selective. A consensus based on a number of published reports indicates the necessity to remove the amygdala, the whole hippocampus and the parahippocampal gyrus in MTLE, as well as the temporal pole when more regional onset is suspected.

References

- Alarcon G, Garcia Seoane JJ, Binnie CD, Martin Miguel MC, Juler J, Polkey CE, et al. Origin and propagation of interictal discharges in the acute electrocorticogram. Implication for pathophysiology and surgical treatment of temporal lobe epilepsy. *Brain* 1997; 120: 2259-82.
- Baily P, Gibbs F. The surgical tratment of psychomotor epilepsy. *JAMA* 1951; 145: 365-70.
- Bancaud J, Angelergues R, Bernouilli C, Bonis A, Bordas-Ferrer M, Bresson M, et al. Functional stereotaxic exploration (stereo-electroencephalography) in epilepsies. *Rev Neurol* 1969; 120: 448.
- Bancaud J, Angelergues R, Bernouilli C, Bonis A, Bordas-Ferrer M, Bresson M, et al. Functional stereotaxic exploration (SEEG) of epilepsy. *Electroencephalogr Clin Neurophysiol* 1970; 28: 85-6.
- Bartolomei F, Hayashi M, Tamura M, Rey M, Fischer C, Chauvel P, Regis J. Long-term efficacy of gamma knife radiosurgery in mesial temporal lobe epilepsy. *Neurology* 2008; 70: 1658-63.
- Bartolomei F, Wendling F, Bellanger JJ, Regis J, Chauvel P. Neural networks involving the medial temporal structures in temporal lobe epilepsy. *Clin Neurophysiol* 2001: 112: 1746-60.
- Cendes F, Dubeau F, Olivier A, Cukiert A, Andermann E, Quesney LF, Andermann F. Increased neocortical spiking and surgical outcome after selective amygdalo-hippocampectomy. *Epilepsy Res* 1993: 16: 195-206.
- Chabardès S, Kahane P, Minotti L, Tassi L, Grand S, Hoffmann D, Benabid AL. The temporopolar cortex plays a pivotal role in temporal lobe seizures. *Brain* 2005; 128: 1818-31.
- Chabardès S, Minotti L, Hamelin S, Hoffmann D, Seigneuret E, Carron R, et al. Temporal disconnection as an alternative treatment for intractable temporal lobe epilepsy: techniques, complications and results. *Neurochirurgie* 2008; 54: 297-302.
- Cunha I, Oliveira J. Quality of life after surgery for temporal lobe epilepsy: a 5-year follow-up. *Epilepsy Behav* 2010; 17: 506-10.
- Elsharkawy AE, May T, Thorbecke R, Ebner A. Predictors of quality of life after resective extratemporal epilepsy surgery in adults in long-term follow-up. *Seizure* 2009; 18: 498-503.
- Falconer MA. Surgery of temporal lobe epilepsy. *Proc R Soc Med* 1958; 51: 613-6.
- Falconer MA, Taylor DC. Surgical treatment of drug-resistant epilepsy due to mesial temporal sclerosis. Etiology and significance. *Arch Neurol* 1968; 19: 353-61.
- Feindel W, Leblanc R, de Almeida AN. Epilepsy surgery: historical highlights 1909-2009. *Epilepsia* 2009; 50 (Suppl 3): 131-51.
- Feindel W, Penfield W, Jasper H. Localization of epileptic discharge in temporal lobe automatism. *Trans Am Neurol Assoc* 1952; 56: 14-17.
- Gibbs A, Gibbs E, Lennox W: Cerebral dysrythmias of epilepsy. Measures for their control. *Arch Neurolo Psychiat* 1938; 39: 298-314.
- Hori T, Tabuchi S, Kurosaki M, Kondo S, Takenobu A, Watanabe T. Subtemporal amygdalohippocampectomy for treating medically intractable temporal lobe epilepsy. *Neurosurgery* 1993; 33: 50-6; 56-7 (discussion).

- Hori T, Yamane F, Ochiai T, Kondo S, Shimizu S, Ishii K, Miyata H. Selective subtemporal amygdalohippocampectomy for refractory temporal lobe epilepsy: operative and neuropsychological outcomes. *J Neurosurg* 2007; 106: 134-41.
- Jones-Gotman M, Zatorre RJ, Olivier A, Andermann F, Cendes F, Staunton H, et al. Learning and retention of words and designs following excision from medial or lateral temporal-lobe structures. *Neuropsychologia* 1997; 35: 963-73.
- Kaada B. Somato-motor, autonomic and electrocortigraphic responses to electrical stimulation of "rhinencephalic" and others structures in primates, cats and dogs: a study of responses from th elimbic, subcallosal, orbito-insular, piriform and temporal cortex, hippocampus-fornix and amygdala. *Acta Physiol Scand* 1951; 24: 1-262.
- Kahane P, Minotti L, Hoffmann D, Lachaux J, Ryvlin P. Invasive EEG in the definition of the seizures onset zone: depth electrodes. In: Rosenow FLH (ed.). *Presurgical Assessment of the Epilepsies with Clinical Neurophysiology and Functional Imaging*. Elsevier, 2004, pp. 109-133.
- Kim R, Spencer D. Surgery for mesial temporal sclerosis. In: Lüders H, Comair Y (eds.). *Epilepsy Surgery*. Philadelphia: Lippincott Williams and Wilkins, 2001, pp. 643-652.
- King JT, Jr., Sperling MR, Justice AC, O'Connor MJ. A cost-effectiveness analysis of anterior temporal lobectomy for intractable temporal lobe epilepsy. *J Neurosurg* 1997; 87: 20-8.
- Levesque MF. Selective hippocampectomy sparing amygdala and neocortex for temporal lobe epilepsy. In: *Neurosurgical Operative Atlas*. Thieme Publishers, 2008, pp. 11-5.
- Lutz MT, Clusmann H, Elger CE, Schramm J, Helmstaedter C. Neuropsychological outcome after selective amygdalohippocampectomy with transsylvian *versus* transcortical approach: a randomized prospective clinical trial of surgery for temporal lobe epilepsy. *Epilepsia* 2004; 45: 809-16.
- Niemeyer P. The transventricular amygdala-hippocampectomy in temporal lobe epilepsy. In: Baldwin M, Bailey P (eds.). *Temporal Lobe Epilepsy*. Springfield: Charles C Thomas, 1958, pp. 461-82.
- Olivier A. Transcortical selective amygdalohippocampectomy in temporal lobe epilepsy. *Can J Neurol Sci* 2000; 27 (Suppl 1): S68-76; S92-66 (discussion).
- Paglioli E, Palmini A, Portuguez M, Azambuja N, da Costa JC, da Silva Filho HF, et al. Seizure and memory outcome following temporal lobe surgery: selective compared with nonselective approaches for hippocampal sclerosis. *J Neurosurg* 2006; 104: 70-8.
- Park TS, Bourgeois BF, Silbergeld DL, Dodson WE. Subtemporal transparahippocampal amygdalohippocampectomy for surgical treatment of mesial temporal lobe epilepsy. Technical note. *J Neurosurg* 85: 1996: 1172-6.
- Penfield W, Baldwin M: Temporal lobe seizures and the technique of subtotal temporal lobectomy. *Ann Surg* 1952; 136: 625-34.
- Penfield W, Cone W. Elementary principles of the treatment of head injuries. *Can Med Assoc J* 48: 1943: 99-104.
- Penfield W, Paine K. Results of surgical therapy for focal epileptic seizures. *Can Med Assoc J* 1955; 73: 515-31.
- Rasmussen T, Jasper H: Temporal lobe epilepsy: indications for operations and surgical technique. In: Baldwin M, Bailey P (eds.). *Temporal Lobe Epilepsy*. Springfield: Charles C Thomas, 1958, pp. 440-60.
- Rausch & Ary, 1990: auteurs? titre? Revue? Volume? Pagination?
- Regis J, Peragui JC, Rey M, Samson Y, Levrier O, Porcheron D, et al. First selective amygdalohippocampal radiosurgery for "mesial temporal lobe epilepsy". *Stereotact Funct Neurosurg* 1995; 64 (Suppl 1): 193-201.
- Tanriverdi T, Dudley RW, Hasan A, Jishi AA, Hinai QA, Poulin N, et al. Memory outcome after temporal lobe epilepsy surgery: corticoamygdalohippocampectomy *versus* selective amygdalohippocampectomy. *J Neurosurg* 2009.

- Tanriverdi T, Olivier A, Poulin N, Andermann F, Dubeau F. Long-term seizure outcome after mesial temporal lobe epilepsy surgery: corticalamygdalohippocampectomy *versus* selective amygdalohippocampectomy. *J Neurosurg* 2008; 108: 517-24.
- Tanriverdi T, Poulin N, Olivier A. Life 12 years after temporal lobe epilepsy surgery: a long-term, prospective clinical study. *Seizure* 2008; 17: 339-49.
- Vajkoczy P, Krakow K, Stodieck S, Pohlmann-Eden B, Schmiedek P. Modified approach for the selective treatment of temporal lobe epilepsy: transsylvian-transcisternal mesial en bloc resection. *J Neurosurg* 1998; 88: 855-62.
- Walker AE. Temporal lobectomy. *J Neurosurg* 1967; 26: 642-9.
- Wheatley BM. Selective amygdalohippocampectomy: the trans-middle temporal gyrus approach. *Neurosurg Focus* 2008; 25: E4.
- Wieser HG, Yasargil MG. Selective amygdalohippocampectomy as a surgical treatment of mesiobasal limbic epilepsy. *Surg Neurol* 1982; 17: 445-57.
- Wilson SJ, Bladin PF, Saling MM, Pattison PE. Characterizing psychosocial outcome trajectories following seizure surgery. *Epilepsy Behav* 2005; 6: 570-80.
- Yasargil MG. Development of diagnosis and surgical therapy of cerebrovascular diseases. *Schweiz Med Wochenschr* 1967; 97: 1734-6.
- Yasargil MG, Wieser HG, Valavanis A, von Ammon K, Roth P. Surgery and results of selective amygdala-hippocampectomy in one hundred patients with nonlesional limbic epilepsy. *Neurosurg Clin N Am* 1993; 4: 243-61.

Predictors of seizure outcome following resection for mesial temporal lobe epilepsy

Alois Ebner

Epilepsy Clinic Mara, Epilepsy Center Bethel, Bielefeld, Germany

---

Virtually all patients or patient caregivers ask how likely it is that they will become seizure free, or at least free of disabling seizures (Engel class I), after planned epilepsy surgery. Thus, a clinician must be able to estimate the likelihood of improvement in a patient's seizure disorder following surgery with relatively high accuracy. Generally, the clinicians' answer to such questions is based on similar cases and postoperative follow-up. In many cases, especially those with extratemporal and extramesial-temporal epilepsies, comparisons are difficult to draw as very few cases are similar with regards to localization and extension of the epileptic focus (Ebner, 2000). The situation is a little different for those patients who suffer from focal epilepsy due to hippocampal sclerosis (HS) since this form of epilepsy is a relatively homogeneous condition and is also the most frequently surgically treated epileptic disease worldwide. Nevertheless, data regarding outcome differ between centres and reflect degrees of seizure freedom between 40% and 90%, depending on the follow-up time (Tanriverdi *et al.*, 2008; Dupont *et al.*, 2006). This review addresses the identification of possible predictors of seizure outcome based on history and/or results of presurgical work-up with a short review of the literature regarding predictors of outcome in mesial temporal lobe epilepsy (MTLE). Finally, the results of the Bethel Epilepsy Surgery Program are discussed.

■ Review of the literature

Tonini *et al.* (2004) published a meta-analysis of the literature to the year 2000 addressing the problem of predictors of epilepsy surgery outcome. Of the 47 articles included, the majority reported outcome of surgical interventions in temporal lobe epilepsies. They found that febrile seizures (odds ratio [OR]: 0.48; 95% confidence interval [CI]: 0.27-0.83), mesial temporal sclerosis (MTS) (OR: 0.47; 95% CI: 0.35-0.64), tumours (OR: 0.58; 95% CI: 0.42-0.80) abnormal MRI (OR: 0.44; 95% CI: 0.29-0.65), EEG/MRI concordance (OR: 0.52; 95% CI: 0.32-0.83), and extensive surgical resection (OR: 0.24; 95% CI: 0.16-0.36) were the strongest prognostic indicators of seizure remission. Predictors of unfavourable outcome were the presence of epileptiform discharges in postoperative EEG (OR: 2.41; 95% CI: 1.37-4.27) and the application of invasive techniques in presurgical evaluation (OR: 2.72; 95% CI: 1.60-4.60).

Table I shows the results of studies published between 2000 and 2008 which investigated predictors of outcome in patients surgically treated for temporal lobe epilepsy with HS. The following positive predictors were identified:
- seizure-free at two years follow-up (Foldvary *et al.*, 2000; Lee *et al.*, 2006);
- ipsilateral interictal spikes with regards to HS (Villanueva *et al.*, 2004);
- no switch of lateralization of ictal EEG activity (Lee *et al.*, 2006);
- history of febrile convulsion (Wieshmann *et al.*, 2008);
- hippocampal atrophy on MRI (Wieshmann *et al.*, 2008; Hardy *et al.*, 2003; Villanueva *et al.*, 2004; Jeong *et al.*, 2005);
- ipsilateral hypometabolism on FDG-PET (Dupont *et al.*, 2006);
- less than 20 seizures per month (Villanueva *et al.*, 2004);
- younger age at time of surgery (Jeong *et al.*, 2005), although seizures occurring within four weeks after surgery predicted a less favourable outcome (Tezer *et al.*, 2008).

Table I. Results of studies investigating predictors of outcome in patients surgically treated for temporal lobe epilepsy with hippocampal sclerosis between 2000 and 2008
IED: interictal epileptiform discharges; FC: febrile convulsion; HA: hippocampal atrophy; PO: postoperatively

	Seizure-free at 2 years	Ipsilateral IED	No switch of EEG seizure pattern	FC	HA	PET ipsilateral hypometabolism	<20 seizures per month	Seizure within 1 month PO	Age at surgery
Foldvary et al., 2000	+								
Wieshmann et al., 2008				+	+				
Lee et al., 2006	+		+						
Hardy et al., 2003					+				
Dupont et al., 2000						+			
Villanueva et al., 2004		+			+		+		
Tezer et al., 2008								−	
Jeong et al., 2005					+				+

Experiences of the Bethel Epilepsy Surgery Program

The majority of studies exploring predictors of outcome after surgical treatment show that the presence of a structural lesion on MRI indicates a favourable postoperative seizure outcome. This is especially the case when unilateral hippocampal atrophy, combined with increased signal in FLAIR-weighted coronal images, is present; a finding which is highly suggestive of HS. Despite the presence of unilateral HS on MRI, outcome is variable, indicating that HS alone is not solely predictive of postoperative seizure outcome.

We hypothesized, therefore, that as well as a patient's history, the results of tests usually applied in non-invasive preoperative work-up also carry some prognostic information. Our results regarding history, seizure semiology, interictal and ictal surface EEG, and psychiatric findings are presented.

History

Surgical outcome was much more favourable in patients with MTLE and a history of complex febrile convulsions (CFCs) compared to patients who had no history of febrile convulsions. CFCs were only reported when it was clear from medical records or parents' reports that the febrile seizures lasted more than 15 minutes, showed focal ictal/post-ictal signs, or appeared as status epilepticus.

Of 84 patients who underwent epilepsy surgery with more than two years follow-up, 60 (71%) became free of disabling seizures (Engel class I). Postoperatively, 91% of patients with a history of CFCs became free of disabling seizures (Engel class I), while only 64% of patients without a history of febrile seizures became free of disabling seizures (Engel class I) postoperatively (Janszky et al., 2003). Only the history of CFC was associated with surgical outcome; (OR: 5.9, 95% CI: 1.26-27.7; $p = 0.023$).

In another study (Janszky et al., 2005), we found that epilepsy duration is the most important predictor for long-term surgical outcome: 90% of patients with an epilepsy duration of 10 years or less were free of disabling seizures (Engel class I) five years after surgery, whereas those with an epilepsy duration of 30 years or longer only had a 33% chance of being free of disabling seizures. The study included 171 patients (100 females and 71 males, aged 16-59 years) who had undergone presurgical evaluation, including video-EEG, MRI-defined HS, and temporal lobectomy.

The results of this study additionally showed that predictors of long-term surgical outcome of TLE with HS are different from those variables which predict short-term outcome. Secondarily generalised seizures (SGTCS) and ictal dystonia were associated with a worse outcome over two years. Both of these variables together with older age and longer epilepsy duration were also related to a worse outcome over three years. Ictal limb dystonia, older age and longer epilepsy duration were associated with long-term surgical failure, evaluated five years postoperatively. In order to determine the independent predictors of outcome, we calculated multivariate analyses. The presence of SGTCS and ictal dystonia independently predicted the poor two-year outcome, longer epilepsy duration and ictal dystonia predicted the poor three-year outcome and longer epilepsy duration ($p = 0.003$) predicted the poor five-year outcome.

Semiology

In the study by Gyimesi et al. (2007), we investigated the pathophysiology of patients' ability to react during the conscious (aura) phase of complex partial seizures (CPS) originating from the temporal lobe. Video recordings of CPS experienced by 130 adult patients who had undergone epilepsy surgery for intractable medial temporal lobe epilepsy were reviewed. All patients were instructed to push an alarm button when they felt an aura. We defined pre-ictal reactivity as the ability to push the alarm button before the complex partial (unconscious) phase of seizures. Seventy-seven patients (59%) pushed the alarm button before seizures. Patients with pre-ictal reactivity were significantly younger, more often had lateralized EEG seizure patterns, and had better postoperative outcome: 83% of patients with ability to react before a seizure became free of disabling seizures (Engel class I), while only 59% of patients without ability to react before a seizure became free of disabling seizures (Engel class I), postoperatively. It was concluded that the ability to react before a CPS is associated with a circumscribed region involved at seizure onset and spread, as well as being free of disabling seizures (Engel class I), postoperatively.

EEG

Interictal epileptiform discharges (IEDs) are widely known to be a good prognostic sign when lateralized to the temporal area harbouring HS. This was also found in our study exploring the predictive value of surface EEG findings in patients with MTLE (Schulz et al., 2000). However, the new finding described here is the prognostic value of a so-called lateralization "switch". This phenomenon is defined as an EEG seizure pattern which starts over one temporal area and switches to the other side with a different frequency after some time, thereby showing contralateral progression. Postoperatively, 82.8% of patients with regionalized EEG seizures without contralateral propagation, but only 45.5% of patients with contralateral propagation ($p = 0.007$), became free of disabling seizures (Engel class I); 84.6% of patients with 100% IED lateralized to one temporal lobe, but only 52.2% with less than 100% ($p = 0.015$). The highest predictive value was reached when interictal and ictal findings were combined following surgery with a minimum follow-up of one year; 88.9% of patients with 100% IED lateralized to one temporal lobe with combined regionalized ictal EEG, 73.7% of patients with either variable, and only 33.3% of patients with <100% IED lateralized to the same temporal lobe with combined contralateral ictal EEG propagation ($p = 0.007$) were free of disabling seizures (Engel class I). It was concluded that the switch of lateralization or bitemporal asynchrony in ictal scalp EEG and bitemporal IED are most probably an index of bitemporal epileptogenicity in MTS and are associated with a worse outcome. Very similar results were reported in the same year by Lee et al. (2000), who used depth electrodes in a cohort of patients with HS. They found that 47% of patients with a switch of lateralization, referred to as a "distinct secondary electrographic seizure" (DSES) were not seizure-free (compared to 45.5% in our study), whereas 84% without DSES became seizure-free (compared to 82.8% in our study). It would therefore seem appropriate to analyze the ictal scalp EEG (as well as ictal depth electrode recordings) with regards to the presence or absence of distinct contralateral seizure activity, since this information may be used to predict a favourable or less favourable outcome.

Psychiatric findings

Psychiatric evaluations are routinely carried out in all patients selected for epilepsy surgery in our program. Of 100 patients suffering from MTLE with HS who underwent surgery between 1991 and 1996, there was a clear correlation between the presence of psychiatric symptoms and postoperative seizure outcome. Of 72 patients with a psychiatric diagnosis, only 43% were free of disabling seizures (Engel class I) two years after the operation, whereas of the 28 patients without any psychiatric problems 89% were free of disabling seizures (Engel class I). In a second group of 91 patients who underwent surgery after 1996, the following data was determined:
- of 24 patients who did not have a psychiatric diagnosis, 75% became free of disabling seizures (Engel class I) two years after the operation;
- of 13 patients with a psychiatric diagnosis on axis 1 and 24 patients with a psychiatric diagnosis on axis 2, 69% and 58% became free of disabling seizures (Engel class I), respectively;
- of 30 patients with psychiatric diagnoses on both axis, *i.e.* showed psychiatric syndromes and personality disorders, only 52% were free of disabling seizures (Engel class I) (Koch-Stoecker, 2002).

In conclusion, the data would seem to indicate that increased psychopathology is associated with poorer postoperative seizure outcome.

Conclusion

Several factors, as outlined in the review of the literature over the last 20 years, have been identified which have some predictive value with regards to postoperative seizure outcome after epilepsy surgery in the temporal lobes, mainly in patients with HS. However, as Hardy *et al.* (2003) point out, many factors which have been previously described to predict favourable outcome in the overall group of patients receiving temporal lobe resections for intractable epilepsy are, in fact, predictors of MTS and lose their predictive value when the subgroup of patients with confirmed MTS is examined.

In our own studies involving patients with HS, as demonstrated by MRI, we have found this finding, as an independent variable, and other information taken from the history or results of non-invasive preoperative work-up, to be useful in enabling us to obtain additional prognostic information which can be used to counsel patients confronted with the decision to undergo epilepsy surgery.

A history of CFCs, the ability to react before the onset of a complex partial seizure, the duration of MTLE of less than 10 years, ipsilateral interictal and ictal EEG findings, and the absence of a psychiatric diagnosis are all predictors of a favourable outcome when MRI shows unilateral HS.

References

- Dupont S, Tanguy ML, Clemenceau S, Adam C, Hazemann P, Baulac M. Long-term prognosis and psychosocial outcomes after surgery for MTLE. *Epilepsia* 2006; 47: 2115-24.
- Ebner A. Preoperative evaluation in epilepsy surgery: some principal considerations In: Lüders H (ed.). Epilepsy Surgery, vol. 2. London: Lippincott-Raven, 2000, pp. 177-83.

- Foldvary N, Nashold B, Mascha E, Thompson EA, Lee N, McNamara JO, et al. Seizure outcome after temporal lobectomy for temporal lobe epilepsy: a Kaplan-Meier survival analysis. *Neurology* 2000; 54: 630-4.
- Gyimesi C, Fogarasi A, Kovács N, Toth V, Magalova V, Schulz R, et al. Patients' ability to react before complex partial seizures. *Epilepsy Behav* 2007; 10: 183-6.
- Hardy SG, Miller JW, Holmes MD, Born DE, Ojemann GA, Dodrill CB, Hallam DK. Factors predicting outcome of surgery for intractable epilepsy with pathologically verified mesial temporal sclerosis. *Epilepsia* 2003; 44: 565-8.
- Janszky J, Schulz R, and Ebner A Clinical features and surgical outcome of medial temporal lobe epilepsy with a history of complex febrile convulsions. *Epilepsy Res* 2003; 55: 1-8.
- Janszky J, Pannek HW, Janszky I, Schulz R, Behne F, Hoppe M, Ebner A. Failed surgery for temporal lobe epilepsy: predictors of long-term seizure-free course. *Epilepsy Res* 2005; 64: 35-44.
- Jeong SW, Lee SK, Hong KS, Kim KK, Chung CK, Kim H. Prognostic factors for the surgery for mesial temporal lobe epilepsy: longitudinal analysis. *Epilepsia* 2005; 46: 1273-9.
- Koch-Stoecker S. Psychische Störungen im Kontext epilepsiechirurgischer Eingriffe bei Temporallappenepilepsien. [Thesis] Bethel, Bielefeld, 2002.
- Lee KH, Park YD, King DW, Meador KJ, Loring DW, Murro AM, Smith JW. Prognostic implication of contralateral secondary electrographic seizures in temporal lobe epilepsy. *Epilepsia* 2000; 41: 1444-9.
- Lee SA, Yim SB, Lim YM, Kang JK, Lee JK. Factors predicting seizure outcome of anterior temporal lobectomy for patients with mesial temporal sclerosis. *Seizure* 2006; 15: 397-404.
- Schulz R, Lüders HO, Hoppe M, Tuxhorn I, May T, Ebner A. Interictal EEG and ictal scalp EEG propagation are highly predictive of surgical outcome in mesial temporal lobe epilepsy. *Epilepsia* 2000; 41: 564-70.
- Tanriverdi T, Olivier A, Poulin N, Andermann F, Dubeau F. Long-term seizure outcome after mesial temporal lobe epilepsy surgery: corticalamygdalohippocampectomy *versus* selective amygdalohippocampectomy. *J Neurosurg* 2008; 108: 517-24.
- Tezer FI, Akalan N, Oguz KK, Karabulut E, Dericioglu N, Ciger A. Predictive factors for postoperative outcome in temporal lobe epilepsy according to two different classifications. *Seizure* 2008; 17: 549-60.
- Tonini C, Beghi E, Berg AT, Bogliun G, Giordano L, Newton RW, et al. Predictors of epilepsy surgery outcome: a meta-analysis. *Epilepsy Res* 2004; 62: 75-87.
- Villanueva V, Peral E, Albisua J, de Felipe J, Serratosa JM. Prognostic factors in temporal lobe epilepsy surgery. *Neurologia* 2004; 19: 92-8.
- Wieshmann UC, Larkin D, Varma T, Eldridge P. Predictors of outcome after temporal lobectomy for refractory temporal lobe epilepsy. *Acta Neurol Scand* 2008; 118: 306-12.

The role of automated seizure detection and prediction

Christoph Kurth

Epilepsiezentrum Kork, Kehl-Kork, Germany

Epilepsy is characterized by recurrent, spontaneous and suddenly occurring seizures which cannot be anticipated by most patients (Schulze-Bonhage et al., 2006). Unforeseen disturbance of consciousness, mood, memory, sensation, personality and/or movement are the most disabling clinical features. For a quarter of all epileptic patients worldwide (around 50-60 million), epilepsy cannot be controlled sufficiently by antiepileptic drugs or epilepsy surgery (Annegers, 1996). Improvement of diagnostic procedures and the development of alternative therapeutic strategies based on seizure detection or prediction may reduce morbidity and mortality as well as greatly improve the quality of life for these patients.

The aim of the first seizure detection systems which emerged in the 1970s and 1980s was the improvement of long-term video-EEG monitoring by off-line detection of epileptic seizures using recorded EEG data. The time for reviewing the EEG would be reduced significantly by an effective seizure detection algorithm with high sensitivity. The rate of false positives in this context is a less critical aspect because even with a high rate of false alarms, the amount of data would be reduced significantly. Due to increasing computational power, on-line processing of EEGs has become possible within the last 10 years. The development of new mathematical methods for signal and information processing such as expert systems, artificial neural networks or the theory of non-linear systems (chaos theory) has led to improvements in detection algorithms. Today, implementation of seizure detection algorithms in on-line warning systems or closed-loop therapeutic devices is under extensive discussion.

Nevertheless, seizure detection algorithms suffer from an important drawback since they are based on the detection of ongoing seizure activity on the EEG. If seizure detection algorithms are to be used to trigger therapeutic interventions, a significant subclinical time interval between the beginning of the seizure on the EEG and the beginning of the clinical symptoms is necessary to apply the intervention. Due to the limited nature of these subclinical seizure periods (in temporal lobe epilepsy up to around 10 seconds), one is restricted to rapidly acting interventions such as (deep) brain stimulation (Morrell, 2006) or local application of drugs (Stein et al., 2000). Therefore a method to *predict* the occurrence of a seizure could further open therapeutic possibilities, making the time period for intervention significantly longer. In addition to deep brain stimulation and local drug administration, systemic application of drugs or more experimental approaches, such as focal cooling of brain areas (Hill et al., 2000), may be possible. Most studies in the field of seizure prediction published in the 1990s showed very promising results. Unfortunately these findings, based on the theory of non-linear systems, could not be reproduced in recent evaluations (Mormann et al., 2007).

■ Seizure detection

Seizure detection can be defined as the detection of an ongoing epileptic seizure. The aim of early seizure detection is the identification of seizure patterns on the EEG prior to the onset of clinical symptoms. While off-line detection is used retrospectively to reduce a large amount of EEG data, on-line detection requires a fast algorithm for "just in time" EEG analysis and can also be applied to intervention systems.

Seizure detection is possible because of the uniformity of patients' seizure patterns. The typical ictal EEG pattern in temporal lobe epilepsy, detected from surface electrodes in the temporal region, is rhythmic sustained theta activity which evolves in time and space. Often starting with a flattening of the EEG followed by low amplitude fast theta activity, signal amplitude may increase during the seizure and frequency decreases, while seizure activity spreads to other brain regions. Seizure onset, based on surface EEG, may be very focal, although a widespread onset detected from all electrodes of a hemisphere is also possible. In some patients, delta-rhythms or repetitive spike-waves may be seen. Often clinical symptoms start before the seizure pattern occurs and EEG patterns are significantly disturbed by artefacts (Wieser, 1983). Thus, in many cases, seizure detection based on recordings from surface electrodes would only be appropriate for monitoring situations. Due to the variability of seizure pattern, it is very difficult to develop a generic algorithm which would work well for all patients, without adapting to individual seizure characteristics of the EEG.

Typical seizure activity recorded from invasive electrodes can be characterized as a flattening of the EEG followed by a low amplitude fast activity in the beta band which shows an increase in amplitude and often a decrease in frequency during the seizure. Seizure spread to other regions may also be seen on surface electrodes, depending on the implantation scheme. Repetitive spiking or spike-waves may also be seen. Very often, seizure activity from invasive electrodes starts several seconds before rhythmic patterns from the surface electrodes and clinical symptoms can be seen (Wieser, 1983). Thus, for early seizure detection in most patients with temporal lobe epilepsy, an invasive recording is necessary.

Since the 1970s, various algorithms for automated seizure detection have been proposed. Most of them are based on a statistical approach which evaluates the characteristics and ongoing changes in seizure activity compared to the normal background EEG. Therefore, a delay of up to several seconds between seizure onset on the EEG and the detection of a significant change in the recording cannot, in principle, be avoided. Early algorithms rely on the detection of an increase in signal amplitude (Prior et al., 1973), EEG flattening (Harding, 1993) or sustained rhythmic activity (Gotman, 1982, Webber et al., 1996). Spectral analysis by short time Fourier transformation (STFT) was used for pre-processing to reduce the amount of information to be analysed (i.e. Gabor, 1998, Srinivasan et al., 2005, Polat & Günes, 2007). The calculated spectrum tells us which frequencies and how much of these frequencies exist in a defined time window of the EEG recording, but due to the fact that the EEG changes in time (non-stationary signal), and time information is lost during STFT, it is not possible to provide exact information as to when an incident happened during the time window evaluated. Thus, it is not possible to know which frequencies exist at what time intervals; using a narrow window frequency, resolution is poor and using a wide window frequency, time resolution is poor. To overcome this significant drawback, wavelet transformation (WT) was applied to the EEG analysis as an alternative to STFT (i.e. Subasi et al., 2005; 2007). WT is a multi-resolution analysis which examines a signal at different frequencies with different resolutions. It is more suitable for signal components with short duration of higher frequency and longer duration of lower frequency. Davey et al. (1989), Dingle et al. (1993), Tzallas et al. (2006), and Argoud et al. (2006) reported extensive use of spatial context information. Some authors calculated non-linear parameters such as entropies (Kannathal et al., 2005) or Lyapunov exponents (Güler et al., 2005) for pre-processing the EEG data. Features extracted from the EEG were used as an input for a large number of different classification methods; expert systems rely on a knowledge base with a large number of facts and rules which are applied, along the lines of "if™ then™" statements, to decide whether or not the characteristics of an EEG sample are consistent with a seizure pattern (Davey et al., 1989). Artificial neural networks (ANN) can be defined as information processing, highly parallel organized systems simulated on computers. They consist of a large number of simple computational elements, densely connected by modifiable links. An internal representation of a set of patterns can be developed by a training process which can be understood as a non-linear statistical analysis of the data. ANNs are able to generalise features from the training set and classify new patterns after the training period even if the signal-to-noise ratio is unsatisfactory (Rummelhart et al., 1986). In contrast to heuristic methods or expert systems, it is not necessary to provide explicit rules or parameters. Since many problems associated with seizure detection are similar to those of spike detection, techniques for spike detection, for example with self-organising neural networks (Kohonen Feature Map) (Kurth et al., 2000), can also be applied to seizure detection without the need for pre-processing of the data (Kurth & Steinhoff, 1997). Other approaches based on ANN have been used, for example by Gabor (1998), Srinivasan et al. (2005), Tzallas et al. (2007) and Schad et al. (2008). Nearest neighbourhood classifiers are based upon calculation of the similarity between high-dimensional feature vectors and reference vectors (Qu & Gotman, 1997) and require training with a template seizure. In contrast, systems based on probability analysis and Bayes' theorem (Grewal & Gotman, 2005) only require a single initial training with representative seizure and non-seizure EEG data from several patients in order to generate a test statistic. Decision trees were used by Polat and Günes (2007). Adaptive neuro-fuzzy inference systems apply fuzzy logic technology which is based on computing with "degrees of truth" rather than the usual Boolean "true or false" (1 or 0) (Kannathal et al., 2005). Fuzzy logic systems and feed-forward neural networks are essentially equivalent (Hong-Xing & Chen, 2000).

For patients evaluated with invasive electrodes, sensitivity of the different methods ranged between about 60% and 100% (rate of false positives: 0.1 to 1 per hour) and for patients evaluated with surface electrodes, sensitivity was between about 70% and close to 100% (rate of false positives: 0.02 to more than 5 per hour) depending on the algorithms and the EEG data used. The pre-processing of EEG data using Lyapunov exponents or entropies (Güler et al., 2005, Kannathal et al., 2005) performed satisfactorily when compared with the results of non-linear signal analysis in the field of seizure prediction.

Detection of ictal tachycardia, which is frequent in temporal lobe epilepsy (Leutmezer et al., 2003), could also be used in some patients for the identification of epileptic seizures. Because the increase of heart rate may occur at least a minute before clinical symptoms, this method may be appropriate for early seizure detection in some cases.

Evaluation of body or limb movements by accelerometry can be useful for the detection of seizures with motor activity (myoclonic, clonic, tonic and other types of movement patterns) (Nijsen et al., 2005). This method may be used as either a warning system or for the reduction of data during video-EEG monitoring.

In summary, some detection methods are already sensitive enough to be used in warning and intervention systems. The rate of false positives may be acceptable for clinical use of EEG monitoring, but remains relatively high for intervention systems.

■ Seizure prediction

"Seizure prediction" means anticipation of a seizure before it starts and is based on the hypothesis that gradual changes in the dynamics of the EEG precede a seizure which can be detected by mathematical methods. Clinical observations which support this hypothesis include: preictal changes in cerebral blood flow, oxygen availability, blood oxygen-level-dependent signal on fMRI, spike rate on EEG or heart rate (Mormann et al., 2007). However, establishing an exact definition which may be useful for seizure prediction is far from trivial (Lehnertz et al., 2007). The feasibility of prediction algorithms for therapeutic purposes depends on two time intervals. The "seizure occurrence period" (SOP) can be defined as the period during which the seizure is predicted to occur, and corresponds to the interval between the minimum and maximum time between prediction and occurrence of a seizure in a patient (Winterhalter et al., 2002). The SOP may vary significantly between different patients and may last several hours in some patients. The "seizure prediction horizon" (SPH) is the shortest possible time window for therapeutic interventions following detection of seizure precursors. SPH must be sufficiently long for successful clinical application of the planned intervention, in case of a warning. Since the exact time of seizure onset is unknown, interventions should have an effect which lasts for at least the duration of the SOP. During seizure detection for intervention purposes, the short intervention horizon between detection of a subclinical seizure pattern and the occurrence of clinical symptoms is challenging, the main problem in seizure prediction being the long prediction horizons. Any prediction algorithm produces a certain number of false alarms. A high rate of false positives together with a long SPH is a very unfavourable combination. For a broad acceptance of prediction algorithms, the rate of false positives should be lower than 50% (Schelter et al., 2007).

In the following example, a typical patient with temporal lobe epilepsy has one seizure a week. Sensitivity of a hypothetical prediction algorithm which triggers a warning system should be 90% and the rate of false positives should be two in 24 hours (0.08 per hour), which would appear to be a relatively good result. Given an SOP of half an hour, 94% of the warnings are false positives and the patient waits for a seizure which does not occur for an hour on a seizure-free day. With an SOP of three hours, the patient will spend six hours a day waiting for a seizure because of a false alarm. If the rate of false positives is just a little worse with three warnings in 24 hours (0,12/hour), 96% of the alarms are false positives and the time the patient waits without a seizure occurring rises to nine hours a day. Unfortunately, optimisation of the algorithm parameters to reduce the rate of false positives will not solve this problem, because tuning an algorithm to reduce false positives usually results in a decline of sensitivity (Winterhalder et al., 2003). The negative effects of false positive results depend on the intervention system chosen. In the case of a warning system, the patient will prepare him or herself for an upcoming seizure for the duration of the SOP. Thus, acceptance of a system with a high rate of false positives and long SOPs will be low, due to the psychological stress and alarms which may no longer be taken seriously. Interventions such as drug administration or brain stimulation may cause side-effects which contribute to significant impairment of brain function. Frequent application of interventions may lead to a loss of efficacy.

For the first seizure prediction algorithm evaluations in the 1970s and 1980s, preictal changes in the EEG were found only a few seconds before seizure onset in many patients and therefore discussion of SOP and SPH were not necessary. In these early studies, linear analysis techniques, such as pattern recognition, analysis of spectral data and auto-regressive modelling, were used to predict seizures by searching for hidden information on the EEG (Lehnertz et al., 2007).

In the 1990s and early 2000s, the extensive exploration of mathematical methods based on the theory of non-linear dynamics was justified by the fact that brain activity is dominated by complicated non-linear neuronal interactions. A large number of studies using parameters, such as decrease of spatio-temporal complexity, Lyapunov coefficient, dynamical similarity, phase synchronization, accumulated signal energy or correlation dimensions (Iasemidis et al., 1990; Lehnertz & Elger 1998; Martinerie et al., 1998; Le van Quyen et al., 2000; 2001; Mormann et al., 2000; Litt et al., 2001; Navarro et al., 2002) were published, many of which produced very encouraging results. Since 2003, several studies have tried to replicate these optimistic results based on extensive databases with a significantly poorer outcome (Mormann et al., 2007). The similarity index was re-evaluated by Winterhalder et al. (2003), the correlation dimension by Aschenbrenner-Scheibe et al. (2003), the accumulated energy by Maiwald et al. (2004) and the Lyapunov coefficient by Lai et al. (2004). According to Mormann et al. (2007) and Lehnertz et al. (2007), the earlier optimistic results appeared to be due to the application of highly optimised algorithms, for the detection of unknown preictal patterns on the EEG, for small and selected data sets (seizure type, signal-to-noise ratio, artefacts, duration of recording, state of vigilance, etc.). Moreover, all of these methods were limited to univariate measures, evaluating the signal of only one electrode. Therefore, it was impossible to investigate interactions between different brain regions (Lehnertz et al., 2007). Neuronal synchronization and spread of seizure activity could not be taken into consideration. In order to examine the interdependencies between the EEG signal of different channels, bi- or multivariate measures, such as non-linear interdependence (Arnhold et al., 1999), phase synchronisation (Bialonski & Lehnertz, 2006) or artificial neural networks, based on leaky integrate-and-fire neurons (Schad et al., 2008), were used.

In 2005, Mormann et al. published a study which evaluated several linear and non-linear uni- and bivariate measures. They used a technique called "seizure time surrogates" (Andrzejak et al., 2003) to prove that a prediction method performed better than chance; surrogate seizure onset times were generated by randomly exchanging inter-seizure intervals. A method for seizure prediction is better than chance only if the algorithm for a number of different surrogate data performs significantly worse than for the original data. By applying this technique to univariate linear and non-linear measures, including measures which have been extensively discussed in former papers, such as Lyapnov coefficient, correlation dimension and accumulated energy, none performed better than a random predictor. Significant results were only documented for multivariate measures of synchronization.

To date, prospective studies have been seldom reported (Mormann et al., 2007), and for some, superiority was not proven over a random predictor as described above (Iasemidis et al., 2003, D'Alessandro et al., 2005). In the study of Chaowalitwongse et al. (2005), methodological problems, due to the use of optimized analysis parameters, were discussed.

In summary, to date, no algorithm for seizure prediction, applicable to practical clinical use in a seizure intervention system, has been developed, and it is furthermore not yet possible to draw a convincing conclusion from the literature (Mormann et al., 2007). So far, algorithms exhibit insufficient sensitivity and a rate of false positives which is much too high for patients to accept. Moreover, only slow and limited progress has been made in this field over the last few years. Hughes (2008) reviewed 68 reports from 33 centres working in this field; only 14 (21%) included sufficient information regarding the time between seizure prediction and occurrence of seizures and 11 (16%) reported negative, non-specific or inconsistent findings.

■ Future perspectives

An important problem in the evaluation of seizure prediction and detection algorithms is the tendency towards in-sample optimisation with analysis parameters being adapted to limited EEG samples of one patient. Careful statistical validation with a prospective evaluation of longer periods of unselected, continuous EEGs of several patients, including periods of rest, sleep and activity, is necessary, as demonstrated by the dependence of the performance of two seizure prediction methods (Schelter et al., 2006). Furthermore, it is yet to be proved that a prediction algorithm performs better than chance using techniques such as time series surrogates. Sensitivity and rate of false positive warnings should be determined in the context of the SPH and SOP (Winterhalder et al., 2003). If seizure detection algorithms are evaluated, delay times between the beginning of the seizure and detection should be reported. For non-generic prediction algorithms, EEG samples of long duration, which include several seizures, are required in order to adapt the parameters of the method to the individual patient and further adapt EEGs with seizures to evaluate the method. In temporal lobe epilepsy, spontaneous seizure frequency is often limited to just a few seizures a month and recording of ten or more seizures under EEG monitoring conditions will become difficult in many cases. Moreover, little is known about the effect of antiepileptic drugs on preictal EEG dynamics (Lehnertz & Elger, 1997) and seizure provocation by fast tapering of medication during video-EEG recording. A continuous high seizure frequency may also cause non-deliberate bias effects. If patients are sent home with implanted recording systems, they would have to report upon their seizures themselves. Problems such as a selection and response bias or unawareness of a seizure in the context of self-reports have been discussed by Litt and Krieger (2007) and Blum et al. (1996).

A large number of studies in the past were based on the hypothesis that preictal changes in EEG may be adequately modelled by methods derived from the theory of non-linear dynamics, but there is still very little known about the mechanisms of ictogenesis and consecutive preictal changes in the EEG (Hughes, 2008). Astonishingly, some more recent studies have found relevant preictal changes in a larger distance from the ictal onset zone (*e.g.* Mormann *et al.*, 2003). There may also be significant differences in the preictal dynamics of the EEG depending on the localization of the seizure onset zone and the underlying pathology (Mormann *et al.*, 2007). Several studies have found that high frequency oscillations (Schiff *et al.*, 2000, Worrell *et al.*, 2004) or phase demodulation (Kalitzin *et al.*, 2005) on the EEG may play a role in the initiation of seizures.

One ambitious aim of on-line early seizure detection, as well as seizure prediction, is the development of a closed-loop treatment device which would be able to interrupt an upcoming seizure before it becomes clinically relevant by, for example, electrical brain stimulation or local application of antiepileptic drugs. Continuously recorded EEG from implanted electrodes would be evaluated on-line. In the event of an upcoming seizure being detected, an intervention would be automatically triggered to stop the pathological activity. EEG processing would continue until a new seizure is recognised and another trigger would be sent to the intervention system, and so on. Currently, the performance of seizure prediction algorithms is too limited for such an application. Early seizure detection may be applicable to fast-acting interventions, however, whether an upcoming seizure can be aborted after detection or whether the brain, as Mormann *et al.* (2007) suggests, "has already passed a *point of no return* and is in a state that will inevitably progress into a clinical seizure manifestation", still remains an open question. For electrical stimulation systems, it is also an open question as to whether closed-loop stimulation on demand, with its high technical impact, is superior to open-loop stimulation schemes with fixed stimulation protocols, such as those used for vagal nerve stimulation. Efficacy and tolerability, as well as wearing-off phenomena after longer use of both kinds of stimulation settings, will have to be evaluated very carefully. Moreover, it is unknown whether the electrode used for recording EEG in a closed-loop system is the necessary and sufficient electrode for stimulation. The use of stimulation electrodes, different from the recording electrode, may be more appropriate, however, no acute side effects of the stimulation should be apparent to the patient.

The question as to whether only clinical events should be included in the evaluation of detection or prediction algorithms, as reported in most studies thus far (Mormann *et al.*, 2007), is only relevant for off-line analyses of EEG data. In applying on-line seizure detection to the EEG recordings in patients with temporal lobe epilepsy, each detected event should be handled as an upcoming seizure of clinical relevance because all seizures in these patients start subclinically. For seizure prediction algorithms, it is not known whether clinical events differ from subclinical activity with regards to preictal EEG changes.

In summary, although an effective algorithm for seizure detection or prediction may be developed in the future, a large number of questions and problems presently remain unanswered.

References

- Andrzejak RG, Mormann F, Kreuz T, Rieke C, Kraskov A, Elger CE *et al.* Testing the null hypothesis of the non-existence of the pre-seizure state. *Phys Rev E* 2003; 67: 010901.
- Annegers JF. The epidemiology in epilepsy. In: Wyllie E (ed). *The Treatment of Epilepsy: Principle and Practice*. Baltimore: Williams & Wilkins, 1996, pp. 165-72.
- Argoud FIM, Azevedo de FM, Neto JM, Grillo E. SADE [3]: an effective system for automated detection of epileptiform events in long-term EEG based on context information. *Med Biol Eng Comput* 2006; 44: 459-70.

- Arnhold J, Grassberger P, Lehnertz K, Elger CE. A robust method for detecting interdependencies: application to intracranial recorded EEG. *Physica D* 1999; 134: 419-30.
- Aschenbrenner-Scheibe R, Maiwald T, Winterhalder M, Voss HU, Timmer J, Schulze-Bonhage A. How well can epileptic seizures be predicted? An evaluation of a nonlinear method. *Brain* 2003; 126: 2616-26.
- Bialonski s, Lehnertz K. Identifying phase synchronization clusters in spatially extended dynamical systems. *Phys Rev E* 2006; 74: 051909.
- Blum DE, Eskola J, Bortz JJ, Fisher RS. Patient awareness of seizures. *Neurology* 1996; 47: 260-4.
- Chaowalitwongse W, Iasemidis LD, Pardalos PM, Carney PR, Shiau DS, Sackellares JC. Performance of a seizure warning algorithm based on the dynamics of intracranial EEG. *Epilepsy Res* 2005; 64: 93-113.
- D'Alessandro M, Vachtsevanos G, Esteller R, Echauz J, Cranstoun S, Worell G, et al. A multifeature and multi-channel univariate selection process for seizure prediction. *Clin Neurophysiol* 2005; 116: 506-16.
- Davey BLK, Fright WR, Caroll GJ, Jones RD. Expert system approach to detetion of epileptiform activity in the EEG. *Med Biol Eng Comput* 1989; 27: 365-70.
- Dingle AA, Jones RD, Caroll GJ, Fright WR. A multistage system to detect epileptiform activity in the EEG. *IEEE Trans Biomed Eng* 1993; 40: 1260-8.
- Gabor AJ. Seizure detection using a self-organizing neural network: validation and comparison with other detection strategies. *Electroencephalogr Clin Neurophysiol* 1998; 1007: 27-32.
- Gotman J. Automatic recognition of epileptic seizures in the EEG. *Eelectroencephalogr Clin Neurophysiol* 1982; 54: 530-40.
- Grewal S, Gotman J. An automatic warning system for epileptic seizures recorded on intracerebral EEGs. *Clin Neurophysiol* 2005; 116: 2460-72.
- Güler NF, Übeyli ED, Güler I. Recurrent neural networks employing Lyapunov exponents for EEG signals classification. *Expert Syst Appl* 2005; 29: 506-14.
- Harding GW. An automated seizure monitoring system for patients with indwelling recording electrodes. *Electroencephalogr Clin Neurophysiol* 1993; 86: 428-37.
- Hill MW, Wong M, Amarakone A, Rothmann SM. Rapid cooling aborts seizure-like activity in rodent hippocampal-entorhinal slices. *Epilepsia* 2000; 41: 1241-8.
- Hong-Xing L, Chen CLP. The equivalence between fuzzy logic systems and feed forward neuralnetworks. *IEEE Trans Neural Net* 2000; 11: 356-65.
- Hughes JR. Progress in predicting seizure episodes with nonlinear methods. *Epilepsy Behav* 2008; 12: 128-35.
- Iasemidis LD, Sackellares JC, Zaveri HP, Williams WJ. Phase space topography and the Lyapunov exponent of electrocorticograms in partial seizures. *Brain Topogr* 1990; 2: 187-201.
- Iasemidis LD, Shiau DS, Chaowalitwongse W, Sackellares JC, Pardalos PM, Principe JC, et al. Adaptive epileptic seizure prediction system. *IEEE Trans Biomed Eng* 2003; 50: 616-27.
- Kalitzin S, Velis D, Suffczynski P, Parra J, Lopes da Silva F. Electrical brain stimulation paradigm for estimating the seizure onset site and the time to ictal transition in temporal lobe epilepsy. *Clin Neurophysiol* 2005; 116: 718-28.
- Kannathal N, Choo ML, Acharya UR, Sadasivan PK. Entropies for detection of epilepsy in EEG. *Comput Meth Prog Biomed* 2005; 80: 187-94.
- Kurth C, Steinhoff BJ. Automated seizure detection in continuous EEG recordings by a Kohonen Feature Map. *Epilepsia* 1997; 38: 154.
- Kurth C, Gillam F, Steinhoff BJ. EEG spike detection with a Kohonen Feature Map. *Ann Biomed Eng* 2000; 28: 1362-9.
- Lai YC, Harrison MA, Frei MG, Osorio I. Controlled test for predictive power of Lyapunov eponents: their inability to predict epileptic seizures. *Chaos* 2004; 14: 630-42.

- Le van Quyen M, Martinerie J, Baulac M, Varala F. Anticipating epileptic seizures in real time by a nonlinear analysis of similarity between EEG recordings. *Neuroreport* 1999; 10: 2149-2155.
- Le van Quyen M, Martinerie J, Navarro V, Boon P, D'Have M, Adam C, et al. Anticipation of epileptic seizures from standard EEG-recordings. *Lancet* 2001; 357: 183-8.
- Lehnertz K, Elger CE. Neuronal complexity loss in temporal lobe epilepsy: effects of carbamazepine on the dynamics of the epileptogenic focus. *Electroencephalogr Clin Neurophysiol* 1997; 103: 376-80.
- Lehnertz K, Elger CE. Can epileptic seizures be predicted? Evidence from nonlinear time series analysis of the brain electrical activity. *Phys Rev Lett* 1998; 80: 5019-23.
- Lehnertz K, Mormann, F, Osterhage H, Müller A, Prusseit J, Chernihovskyi A, et al. State-of-the-art of seizure predicition. *J Clin Neurophysiol* 2007; 24: 147-53.
- Leutmezer, et al. Electrocardiographic changes at the onset of epileptic seizures. *Epilepsia* 2003; 44: 348-54.
- Litt B, Esteller R, Echauz J, D'Alessandro M, Shor R, Henry T, et al. Epileptic seizures may begin hours in advance of clinical onset: a report of five patients. *Neuron* 2001; 30: 51-64.
- Litt B, Krieger A. Of seizure prediction, statistics and dogs. *Neurology* 2007; 68: 250-1.
- Martinerie J, Adam C, Le van Quyen M, Baulac M, Clemenceau S, Renault B, et al. Epileptic seizures can be anticipated by non-linear analysis. *Nat Med* 1998; 4: 1173-6.
- Maiwald T, Winterhalder M, Aschenbrenner-Scheibe R, VossHU, Schulze-Bonhage A, Timmer J. Comparison of three nonlinear seizure prediction methods by means of the seizure prediction characteristic. *Physica D* 2004; 194: 357-68.
- Mormann F, Lehnertz K, David P, Elger CE. Mean phase coherenceas a measure for phase synchronization and its application to the EEG of epilepsy patients. *Physica D* 2000; 144: 358-69.
- Mormann F, Kreuz T, Rieke C, Andrzejak RG, Kraskov A, David P, et al. On the predictability of epileptic seizures. *Clin Neurophysiol* 2005; 116: 569-87.
- Mormann F, Andrzejak RG, Elger CE, Lehnertz K. Seizure prediction: the long and winding road. *Brain* 2007; 130: 314-333.
- Morrel M. Brain stimulation for epilepsy: can scheduled or responsive neurostimulation stop seizures? *Curr Opin Neurol* 2006; 19: 164-8.
- Navarro V, Martinerie J, Le van Quyen M, Clemenceau S, Adam C, Baulac M, et al. Seizure anticipation in human neocortical partial epilepsy. *Brain* 2002; 125: 640-55.
- Nijsen T, Arends J, Griep P, Cluitmans P. The potential value of 3-D accelerometry for detection of motor seizures in severe epilepsy. *Epilepsy Behav* 2005; 7: 74-84.
- Polat K, Günes S. Classification of epileptiform EEG using a hybrid system based on decision tree classifier and fast Fourier transform. *Appl Math Comput* 2007; 187: 1017-26.
- Prior PF, Virden RSM, Maynard DE. An EEG device for monitoring seizure discharges. *Epilepsia* 1973; 14: 367-72.
- Qu H and Gotman J. A patient-specific algorithm for the detection of seizure onset in long-term EEG monitoring: possible use as a warning device. *IEEE Trans Biomed Eng* 1997; 44: 115-22.
- Rumelhart DE, Hinton GE and Williams RJ. Learning internal representation by error propagation. In: Rumelhard DE, McCalland JL (eds). *Parallel Distributed Processing*, vol. 1, Cambridge, MA: MIT Press, 1986.
- Schad A, Schindler K, Schelter B, Maiwald T, Brandt A, Timmer J, et al. Application of a multivariate seizure detection and prediction method to non-invasive and intracranial long-term EEG recordings. *Clin Neurophysiol* 2008; 119: 197-211.
- Schulze-Bonhage A, Kurth C, Carious A, Steinhoff BJ, Mayer T. Seizure anticipation by patients with focal or generalized epilepsy: A multicentre assessment of premonitory symptoms. *Epi Res* 2006; 70: 83-8.

- Schelter B, Winterhalder M, Maiwald T, Brandt A, Schad A, Timmer J, et al. Do false predictions of seizures depend on the state of vigilance? A report from two seizure-prediction methods and proposed remedies. *Epilepsia* 2006; 47: 2058-70.
- Schelter B, Winterhalder M, Feldwisch H, Wohlmuth J, Nawrath J, Brandt A, et al. Seizure predicition: The impact of long prediction horizons. *Epilepsy Res* 2007; 73: 213-7.
- Schiff SJ, Colella D, Jacyna GM, Hughes E, Creekmore JW, Marshall A, et al. Brain chirps: spectrographic signatures of epileptic seizures. *Clin Neurophysiol* 2000; 111: 953-8.
- Srinivasan V, Eswaran C, Siraam AN. Artificial neural network based epileptic detection using time-domain and frequency-domain features. *J Med Sys* 2005; 29: 647-60.
- Stein AG, Eder HG, Blum DE, Drachev A, Fisher RS. An automated drug delivery system for focal epilepsy. *Epilepsy Res* 2000; 39: 103-14.
- Subasi A, Alkan A, Koklukaya E, Kiymik MK. Wavelat neural network classificationof EEG signals by using AR model with MLE preprocessing. *Neural Networks* 2005; 18: 985-97.
- Subasi A. EEG signal classification using wavelet feature extraction and a mixture of expert model. *Exp Syst Appl* 2007; 32: 1084-93.
- Tzallas AT, Karvelis PS, Katsis CD, Fotiadis DI, Giannopoulos S, Konitsiotis S. A method for classification of transient events in EEG recordings: application to epilepsy diagnosis. *Meth Inf Med* 2006; 45: 610-21.
- Tzallas AT, Tsipouras MG, Fotiadis DI. Automatic Seizure detection based on time-frequency analysis and artificial neural networks. *Comput Intell Neurosci* 2007; 13: 1-13.
- Webber WRS, Lesser RP, Richardson RT, Wilson K. An approach to seizure detection using an artificial neural network (ANN). *Eelectroencephalogr Clin Neurophysiol* 1996; 98: 250-72.
- Wieser HG. *Electroclinical features of the psychomotor seizure*. Stuttgart, New York: Gustav Fischer Verlag, 1983.
- Winterhalder M, Maiwald T, Voss HU, Aschenbrenner-Scheibe R, Timmer J, Schulze-Bonhage A. The seizure prediction characteristic: a general framework to assess and compare seizure prediction methods. *Epilepsy Behav* 2003; 4: 318-25.
- Worrell G, Parish L, Cranstoun S, Jonas R, Baltuch G, Litt B. High frequency oscillations and seizure generation in neocortical epilepsy. *Brain* 2004; 127: 1496-506.

Behavioural approaches: a critical review

Bernhard J. Steinhoff

Epilepsiezentrum Kork, Kehl-Kork, Germany

One of the major burdens for patients with epilepsy is the uncertainty of, and circumstances relating to, the next epileptic seizure. Most probably, the high proportion of patients with additional psychiatric disorders, such as depression and anxiety, would be markedly lower if patients were able to have confidence in reliable predictors of probable seizures. A patient who believes in the ability to predict seizures worries less about his/her disease (Jacoby, 1992) and has higher quality of life scores (Au *et al.*, 2002).

Some epileptic syndromes are characterised by typical seizure-related provocative situations and circumstances such that patients may actively reduce the probability of seizure relapses by avoidance of such situations. Moreover, individual and mostly anecdotal experiences of anticonvulsive behavioural mechanisms are tempting approaches for patients with active epilepsies both to overcome the insecurity mentioned above and to actively participate in an anticonvulsive treatment beyond the pure prophylactic antiepileptic drug treatment.

This review summarizes the most relevant literature addressing this topic which plays a major role in many discussions with patients and relatives, especially in cases of intractable epilepsy syndromes.

■ Avoidance of precipitants

According to Aird (1988), the control of seizure-provocative factors is the clue to gaining seizure freedom in 14% of intractable epilepsy syndromes. More than 40 different seizure-inducing factors including emotional stress, changing states of vigilance, sleep deprivation, disturbed water and acid-base status, sensory stimuli, and intake or discontinuation of drugs have been reported in the literature. According to patients, emotional reactions play a dominant role as a seizure-precipitating factor, an observation which is not concurred by doctors (Aird, 1983).

For idiopathic generalised epilepsy syndromes, the probability of achieving seizure freedom, without chronic intake of antiepileptic drugs, by simply improving life hygiene is considerably higher than in patients with focal epilepsies (Wolf & Okujava, 1999). However, significant improvements in the setting of neurobehavioural treatment, including the improvement of knowledge about the disease with coherent consequences for individual lifestyle, were also reported in patients with temporal lobe epilepsies (Andrews et al., 2002).

■ Sleep and sleep deprivation

One of the most important and most thoroughly investigated seizure-provoking factors is sleep deprivation, particularly for idiopathic generalised epilepsy syndromes but also, to a lesser extent, focal epilepsies (Frucht et al., 2000; Mendez & Radtke, 2001). Following stress, sleep deprivation was the second most frequently quoted seizure precipitating factor in the questionnaire study of Frucht and co-workers (2000). For some patients, especially with idiopathic generalised epilepsies, the avoidance of severe sleep deprivation is a crucial factor to achieve seizure freedom. On the other hand, for patients with juvenile myoclonic epilepsy (JME), who experience epilepsy onset frequently in adolescence, it may be more helpful to consider effective antiepileptic drug therapy than to risk social deprivation by introducing rigid modifications of a life-style which usually includes some sleep deprivation and alcohol experience at that time of life. Finally, the knowledge that sleep deprivation and, in many societies, alcohol are important risk factors may help to avoid high risk situations following potentially hazardous activities the day before, such as swimming or driving. The highest seizure risk is observed within 48 hours after relevant sleep deprivation (Kotagal, 2001). In this respect, the problem of uncertainty, with regards to when the next seizure occurs, is partially reduced in such cases. This aspect should be addressed during the recovery of patients. Since sleep and fatigue are other important potential trigger factors for seizures (Frucht et al., 2000), patients should still consider maintaining a regular sleep-wake cycle in most instances.

■ Alcohol

Alcohol intake may be another relevant precipitating factor particularly for adolescents sensitive to sleep deprivation. In spite of some controversial discussions (Hauser et al., 1988), it again appears that patients with idiopathic generalised epilepsies, and especially JME, are particularly sensitive to alcohol as a seizure-provocative factor. Alcohol was quoted as a clinically relevant risk factor by 51% of patients with JME (Pedersen & Petersen, 1998). Acceptable alcohol limits have been proposed for patients with epilepsy (Krämer, 2000), however, it is most probably essential to discuss this topic carefully and on an individual basis in order to achieve the best possible balance between behavioural avoidance of unnecessary risks and exaggerated caution and overprotection.

■ Photosensitivity

It is assumed that approximately 5% of all epilepsy patients are sensitive to external photic stimuli (Takahashi et al., 2001) which may be presented, among other potential hazardous circumstances, via television, video-games, flickering neon tubes or in discotheques (Takahashi et al., 2001). It should be pointed out that, in the context of this textbook, photosensitivity in patients with mesial temporal lobe epilepsy is extremely rare (Fiore et al., 2003). Most patients with photoparoxysmal responses suffer from idiopathic generalised or progressive myoclonic epilepsy syndromes. The best known example of a paroxysmal photosensitive effect is the so-called "pokemon monster incident" when several hundred Japanese children developed photoconvulsive responses whilst watching a sequence of a popular TV cartoon consisting of deep red low luminance 12 Hz flicker stimuli (Takahashi & Tsukahara, 1998). When photosensitivity is demonstrated, patients may considerably reduce their risk by avoiding typical hazardous situations, such as: the use of additional light sources while watching TV, avoidance of being too close to the light source by using remote controls, using monocular view in high risk situations and the use of appropriate polarising sun glasses or optical filters which erase deep red light and lower the light intensity (Anyanwu, 1999; Wilkins et al., 1999; Jain et al., 2001; Takahashi et al., 2001).

■ Counteractive measures

Uncertainty and the lack of control are common themes in daily life for epilepsy patients and are partly responsible for psychosocial problems (Hermann et al., 1990; Gehlert, 1994; Amir et al., 1999). The use of better methods to cope leads to less anxiety and depression (Rosenbaum & Palmon, 1984).

Suitable candidates for counteractive mechanisms should usually have some sort of reliable warning such as premonitory symptoms. These are defined as events which are semiologically different from the seizures themselves and characterized by either longer intervals between the event and the seizure (Lee & No, 2005; Schulze-Bonhage et al., 2006) or auras which represent simple partial seizures and usually occur seconds to minutes prior to the more intense seizure phase patients wish to avoid (Lee & No, 2005). Several counteractive measures have been advocated in order to actively suppress or prevent seizures. Self-control strategies of any kind are especially attractive among patients who are not seizure-free on antiepileptic drug treatment. It is not surprising that the number of patients actively using self-control techniques is considerably higher among patients with intractable rather than medically well controlled epilepsies (Cull et al., 1996; Rajna et al. 1997; Spector et al., 2000).

The most important approaches comprise psychological treatment, namely behavioural therapy and biofeedback techniques. Among the various psychological, motor, sensory or combined approaches, other advocated methods include: the arrest of incipient seizures, the control of specific provocative factors in reflex epilepsies, and the control of non-specific factors which increase seizure susceptibility, as well as other miscellaneous methods (Antebi & Bird, 1993; Bourgeois, 1996). Most authors agree that cognitive behavioural therapy and psychological support are appropriate to reduce depression, manage stress, reduce negative emotions, increase self-efficacy, and strengthen the social network (Davis et al., 1984; Ried et al., 2001).

Whether or not psychological treatment also has a convincing antiepileptic effect is a controversial matter and methodologically difficult to assess. Whereas some mostly uncontrolled open and often questionnaire-based studies report such an effect (Gillham, 1990; Schmid-Schönbein, 1998; Spector et al., 2000; Andrews et al., 2002; Lee & No, 2005), other studies could not reproduce convincing antiepileptic efficacy beyond the unquestionable positive impact on the management of the disease (Tan & Bruni, 1986; Au et al., 2003). The efficacy rates reported vary widely and range from 13% to about 80% (Schmid-Schönbein, 1998; Spector et al., 2000; Andres et al., 2002).

EEG biofeedback

EEG biofeedback is based on the principles of operant conditioning. Patients are educated in training sessions to influence their own EEG. Target changes include the enhancement of the so-called "sensorimotor rhythm" (SMR), namely midline activity in the fast alpha and slow beta range with suppression of slow activity, as well as the reduction of slow cortical potentials (SCPs) (Sheth et al., 2005; Sterman, 2000; Lubar et al., 1981; Rockstroh et al., 1993).

Most studies addressing these techniques are open and not controlled, and based on case studies. Using the SMR approach, these case studies have reported impressive clinical improvement rates of up to 82% (Lubar et al., 1981), whereas in an open study using the SCP approach, which mainly aims to reduce contingent negative variation (CNV), a one-year responder rate of more than 50% and a third of seizure-free patients were described (Rockstroh et al., 1993). Patients with simple partial seizures responded better than those with complex partial or secondary generalised seizures (Kotchoubey et al., 2001). Controlled studies are few and difficult to perform. A statistically significant therapeutic effect was reported in a group of patients undergoing self-control of respiratory parameters compared to a group of patients with optimised drug therapy and psychological counselling (Kotchoubey, et al., 2001). Since the galvanic skin response (GSR), which measures the electrical resistance of the skin of the hand, inversely corresponds with the amplitude of the CNV, GSR biofeedback training has also been applied to epilepsy. In a study of 18 patients (10 with verum therapy, eight with sham control biofeedback), 60% of the patients undergoing the therapy had statistically significant seizure reduction of more than 50%, relative to patients with sham control biofeedback (Nagai et al., 2004).

Critical data assessment

A critical review of the published material concerning psychological treatments of epilepsy including EEG biofeedback stated that, in view of methodological deficiencies and the limited number of individual studies, there is no current evidence to support the use of these treatments (Ramaratnam et al., 2005).

Conclusion

Behavioural approaches in epilepsy address the avoidance of seizure-provoking factors and the goal of self-control prior to or during seizures by voluntary counteractions. For epilepsy syndromes in which provoking factors such as various external stimuli are clearly identified, the avoidance of such factors may be crucial. This is mainly the case in idiopathic generalised and progressive myoclonic epilepsy syndromes which are usually more sensitive to sleep deprivation, alcohol withdrawal or photic stimulation than focal epilepsies. However, it is necessary to demonstrate unequivocally, in each case, whether or not such external stimuli provoke seizures. Although the avoidance of seizure-provoking factors may be very helpful, patients and relatives should certainly also avoid behaviour which is too cautious or overprotective, since this may lead to social burdens and even anxiety disorders. In such cases, a well-tolerated and effective antiepileptic drug treatment would most probably better contribute to achieving a satisfying quality of life.

The concept of behavioural control of seizures is attractive, since the major trauma for patients with epilepsy is the lack of control concerning the time of occurrence and the intensity of seizures. In cases where self-control is effective, it is mandatory that the seizure itself does not preclude voluntary actions; only patients with premonitory symptoms, long-lasting auras or other simple partial seizures at onset may be suitable candidates.

References

- Aird RB. The importance of seizure-inducing factors in the control of refractory forms of epilepsy. *Epilepsia* 1983; 24: 567-83.
- Aird RB. The importance of seizure-inducing in youth. *Brain Dev* 1988; 10: 73-6.
- Amir M, Roziner I, Knoll A, Neufeld MY. Self-efficacy and social support as mediators in the relation between disease severity and quality of life in patients with epilepsy. *Epilepsia* 1999; 40: 216-24.
- Au A, et al. Predicting the quality of life in Hong Kong Chinese adults with epilepsy. *Epilepsy Behav* 2002; 3: 350-7.
- Au A, Chen F, Li K, Leung P, Li P, Chan J. Cognitive-behavioral group treatment program for adults with epilepsy in Hong Kong. *Epilepsy Behav* 2003; 4: 441-6.
- Antebi D, Bird J. The facilitation and evocation of seizures. A questionnaire study of awareness and control. *Br J Psychiatry* 1993; 162: 759-64.
- Andrews DJ, Reiter JM, Schonfeld W, Kastl A, Denning P. A neurobehavioral treatment for unilateral complex partial seizure disorders: A comparison of right- and left-hemisphere patients. *Seizure* 2002; 9: 189-7.
- Anyanwu E. Evaluation of the laboratory and environmental factors that induce seizures in photosensitive epilepsy. *Acta Neurol Belg* 1999; 99: 126-32.
- Bourgeois BFD. Behavioral and social therapy. In: Wallace S (ed). *Epilepsy in Children*. London: Chapam Hall, 1996, pp. 557-9.
- Cull CA, Fowler M, Brown SW. Perceived self-control of seizures in young people with epilepsy. *Seizure* 1996; 5: 131-8.
- Davis GR, Armstrong HE Jr, Donovan DM, Temkin NR. Cognitive-behavioral treatment of depressed affect among epileptics: preliminary findings. *J Clin Psychol* 1984; 40: 930-5.
- Fiore LA, Valente K, Gronich G, Ono CR, Buchpiguel CA. Mesial temporal lobe epilepsy with focal photoparoxysmal response. *Epileptic Disord* 2003; 5: 39-43.
- Frucht MM, Quigg M, Schwaner C, Fountain NB. Distribution of seizure precipitants among epilepsy syndromes. *Epilepsia* 2000; 41: 1534-9.
- Gehlert S. Perceptions of control in adults with epilepsy. *Epilepsia* 1994; 35: 81-8.
- Gillham RA. Refractory epilepsy: an evaluation of psychological methods in outpatient management. *Epilepsia* 1990; 31: 427-32.
- Hauser WA, Ng STKC, Brust JCM. Alcohol, seizures and epilepsy. *Epilepsia* 1988; 29: 66-78.
- Hermann BP, Whitman S, Wyler AR, Anton MT, Vanderzwagg R. Psychosocial predictors of psychopathology in epilepsy. *Br J Psychiatry* 1990: 156: 98-105.
- Jain S, Woodruff G, Bissessar EA. Cross polarized spectacles in photo-sensitive epilepsy. *J Pediatr Ophthalmol Strabism* 2001; 38: 331-4.
- Jacoby A. Epilepsy and the quality of everyday life. Findings from a study of people with well-controlled epilepsy. *Soc Sci Med* 1992; 34: 657-64.
- Kotagal P. The relationship between sleep and epilepsy. *Semin Pediatr Neurol* 2001; 8: 241-50.

- Kotchubey B, et al. Modification of slow cortical potentials in patients with refractory epilepsy: a controlled outcome study. *Epilepsia* 2001; 42: 406-16.
- Krämer, G. Epilepsie: Antworten auf die häufigsten Fragen. 2nd ed. Stuttgart: Trias, 2001.
- Lee SA, No YJ. Perceived self-control of seizures in patients with uncontrolled partial epilepsy. *Seizure* 2005; 14: 100-5.
- Lubar JF, et al. EEG operant conditioning in intractable epilepsies. *Arch Neurol* 1981; 38: 700-4.
- Nagai Y, Goldstein LH, Fenwick PB, Trimble MR. Clinical efficacy of galvanic skin response biofeedback training in reducing seizures in adult epilepsy: a preliminary randomized controlled study. *Epilepsy Behav* 2004; 5: 216-23.
- Mendez M, Radtke RA. Interactions between sleep and epilepsy. *J Clin Neurophysiol* 2001; 18: 106-27.
- Pedersen SB, Petersen KA. Juvenile myoclonic epilepsy: Clinical and EEG features. *Acta Neurol Scand* 1998; 97: 160-3.
- Rajna P, et al. Hungarian multicentre epidemiologic study of the warning and initial symptoms (prodrome, aura) of epileptic seizures. *Seizure* 1997; 6: 361-8
- Ramaratnam, S, Baker, GA, Goldstein, LH. Psychological treatment for epilepsy. *Cochrane Database Syst Rev* 2005; 19: CD0030309.
- Ried S, Specht U, Thorbecke R, Goecke K, Wohlfarth R. MOSES: an educational program for patients with epilepsy and their relatives. *Epilepsia* 2001; 42 (Suppl 3): 76-80.
- Rockstroh B, et al. Cortical self-regulation in patients with epilepsies. *Epilepsy Res* 1993; 14: 63-72.
- Rosenbaum M, Palmon N. Helplessness and resourcefulness in coping with epilepsy. *J Consult Clin Psychol* 1984: 52: 244-53.
- Schmid-Schönbein C. Improvement of seizure control by psychological methods in patients with intractable epilepsies. *Seizure* 1998; 7: 261-70.
- Schulze-Bonhage, A, Kurth C, Carius A, Steinhoff BJ, Mayer T. Seizure anticipation by patients with focal and generalized epilepsy: a multicentre assessment of premonitory symptoms. *Epilepsy Res* 2006; 70; 83-8.
- Sheth RD, Stafstrom CE, Hsu D. Nonpharmacological treatment options for epilepsy. *Semin Pediatr Neurol* 2005; 12: 106-13.
- Spector S, Cull C, Goldstein LH. Seizure precipitants and perceived self-control of seizures in adults with poorly-controlled epilepsy. *Epilepsy Res* 2000; 38: 207-16
- Sterman MB. Basic concepts and clinical findings in the treatment of seizure disorders with EEG operant conditioning. *Clin Electroencephalogr* 2000; 31: 45-55.
- Tan SY, Bruni J. Cognitive-behavior therapy with adult patients with epilepsy: a controlled outcome study. *Epilepsia* 1986; 27: 225-33.
- Takahashi T, Tsukahara Y. Pocket monster incident and low luminance visual stimuli: special reference to deep red stimulation. *Acta Paediatr Jpn* 1998; 40: 631-7.
- Takahashi Y, et al. Optical filters inhibiting television-induced photosensitive seizures. *Neurology* 2001; 57: 1767-73.
- Wilkins AJ, et al. Treatment of photosensitive epilepsy using coloured glasses. *Seizure* 1999; 8: 444-9.
- Wolf P, Okujava N. Possibilities of non-pharmacological conservative treatment of epilepsy. *Seizure* 1999; 8: 45-52.

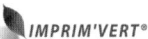